Milady's Skin Care Reference Guide

Mark Lees, Ph. D.

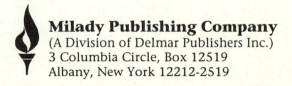
Milady Publishing Company
(A Division of Delmar Publishers Inc.)
3 Columbia Circle, Box 12519
Albany, New York 12212-2519

NOTICE TO THE READER

Credits:

Publisher: Catherine Frangie
Developmental Editor: Joseph Miranda
Senior Project Editor: Laura V. Miller
Art/Design Supervisor: Susan V. Mathews
Production Manager: John Mickelbank
Freelance Project Editor: Pamela Fuller

Copyright © 1994
Milady Publishing Company
(A Division of Delmar Publishers Inc).

For information address:
Milady Publishing Company
(A Division of Delmar Publishers Inc.)
3 Columbia Circle, Box 12519
Albany, NY 12212-2519

Printed in the United States of America
Published simultaneously in Canada
by Nelson Canada
a division of The Thomson Corporation

1 2 3 4 5 6 7 8 9 10 XXX 00 99 98 97 96 95 94

Library of Congress Cataloging-in-Publication Data

Lees, Mark.
      Milady's skin care reference guide / Mark Lees.
          p.   cm.
      Includes index.
      ISBN 1-56253-071-2
      1. Skin—Care and hygiene.
   RL87.L36   1994
   616.5—dc20

                                                                      93-28236
                                                                           CIP

DEDICATION

This book is dedicated to my parents, Richard and Virginia Lees.
Thank you for your lifelong encouragement.

Contents

Acknowledgments

Very special thanks to the following people and organizations for contributing in many ways to this book. The author very much appreciates their efforts.

Editors and staff of Milady Publishing Company: Cathy Frangie, Amy Clinton, Pamela Fuller, Joe Miranda.

Reviewers: Nancy A. Gooding; Charles Mizzelle ; Louise Williams.

Erica Miller, Correlations, Inc., Dallas, Texas.

Rube Pardo, M.D., Ph.D., Dept. of Dermatology, University of Miami.

Samuel J. LaMonte, M.D., Facial Plastic Surgeon, Pensacola, Florida.

Kirk Smith, M.D., Plastic Surgeon, Pensacola, Florida.

David Wanetik, Skin Culture Institute, New York, New York.

Howard Murad, M.D., Murad Skin Research Laboratories, Los Angeles, California.

Rebecca James, Cosmetic Chemistry Instructor, UCLA.

Francosmetics/Rene Guinot, Inc., Beverly Hills, California.

Johnson & Johnson

My wonderful staff, family, and friends for putting up with me while I was writing this book.

Timothy Berger, M.D., Dermatologist, San Francisco, California.

Michael Bond, M.D., Dermatologist, Memphis, Tennessee.

Melvin Elson, M.D., Dermatologist, Nashville, Tennessee.

George Fisher, M.D., Dermatologist, Pensacola, Florida.

Figures 12-2, 12-3, 12-5, 12-6, 12-8 are reprinted from *Acne Morphogenesis and Treatment* by Gerd Plewig, M.D. and Albert M. Kligman, M.D., Ph.D.; permission of publishers, Springer-Verlafg, New York, U.S.A., Heidelberg, Berlin, Germany.

About the Author

Dr. Mark Lees is recognized throughout the world as a leader in the field of professional skin care and esthetics. He holds a M.S. in Health and a Ph.D. in Health Sciences. He has lectured for professional, consumer, and medical groups throughout the United States and has made appearances in both Europe and Australia.

He holds numerous awards and titles including:

> The CIDESCO International diploma—the highest earned professional skin-care title in the world.

> Paramedical Educator of the Year from the Advanced esthetics Training Institute of St. Louis.

> The "AMY" Award for Esthetician of the year from *American Salon* magazine.

> The Academy of Legends Award from *Dermascope* magazine.

> The Rocco Bellino Award for Outstanding Education from the Chicago Cosmetologists' Association.

Dr. Lees is former Vice-President of the American Association of Esthetics (CIDESCO—U.S.A. Section); former National Chairman of EstheticsAmerica, the esthetics division of the National Cosmetology Association; and is Director of Board Certification for Aestheticians International Association.

He has been quoted and interviewed by *Glamour* magazine, NBC News, *The Miami Herald*, *The Washington Post*, and many other publications. He has authored a chapter on esthetics and cosmetology in *Esthetic Dentistry*.

He is president of Mark Lees Skin Care, Inc., and his products are available in fine salons and dermatology clinics throughout the United States and Canada. He also owns and directs his own clinic in Pensacola, Florida.

Letter to the Reader

When I was originally approached about writing this book, I thought about how much I would have appreciated a book that told me everything I needed to know about the real day-to-day practice of skin care, a book that answered questions about advanced treatment, unusual conditions, and communicating with referring physicians.

While I have always felt that I received an outstanding education in esthetics, there was so much that I never saw or worked with until I was out in the **real world**!

This book is that book. I have tried to reconstruct every subject and condition that I have seen in my last 14 years as a practicing esthetician. All practitioners make mistakes—I did too! I hope that by using this book the reader will be able to avoid making some of these mistakes and will learn about more advanced subjects that an esthetician sees every day.

I also hope that schools will incorporate this book into their curriculums, helping to better prepare future estheticians for the world they will operate in.

This profession is very rewarding, and in the near future many bridges will be built between the esthetics and medical communities. I hope that this book will help improve this relationship.

The best of luck to you in this fabulous profession and always remember, when you think you're through learning, you're through!

Mark Lees, Ph.D.

CIDESCO Diplomate

Pensacola, Florida

1

Advanced Anatomy and Physiology of the Skin

In this chapter you will learn about the anatomy and functions of cells. You will also recognize different types of tissues and their functions. You will learn, in detail, about the different layers of the skin and functions of various reactions that take place in the different layers of skin. Skin penetration will be studied, as well as some techniques for better penetrating, moisturizing, and conditioning treatments for the skin.

Before we can fully understand how to treat cosmetic disorders of the skin, we must first fully understand the functions and activies of the body, more specifically, the **cell**. The cell is almost a self-contained factory of life. Cells are the building blocks of the human body. Within each cell, many chemical and physical processes constantly take place. To simplify, let's think of the cell as a very, very small living body. This is, of course, an oversimplification, but it will help us understand the many miraculous functions that happen inside each cell of the human body.

The Structure of the Cell

Much like the skin that covers our bodies, the cell is protected by an outer shell known as the **cell membrane** (Figure 1-1). The cell membrane gives the cell structure and shape and contains the many internal parts of the cell. The cell membrane is made of a network of lipids (fatty matter) and protein. The cell membrane possesses a function known as **selective permeability**. Selective permeability means that the cell membrane can let substances into the cell, such as food, water, and oxygen. It can also let substances out of the cell, such as waste and carbon dioxide. The cell is furnished food, water, and oxygen by the blood. Blood is also the vehicle that carries waste materials and carbon dioxide away from the cell membrane and eventually out of the body. Blood itself is made up of cells.

FIGURE 1–1 Structure of the cell

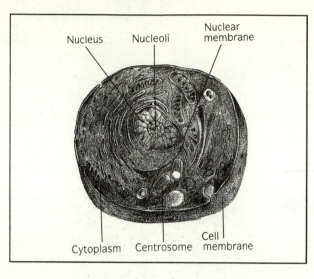

Inside the cell is a fluid called **cytoplasm**. Cytoplasm is made of water and other substances. It has a gel-like consistency. Cytoplasm allows other structures to move around inside the cell. If you think of the cell as a human body, the cytoplasm would play the part of the blood, allowing transportation within the cell.

Organelles

Organelles are small structures within the cell that each have their own function. You can think of organelles as being miniature body organs in the cell. For many years, scientists did not know about the existence of organelles. But as science progressed, these super-small structures were discovered.

Inside the cell cytoplasm, there is a structure that is formed like a maze, sort of like a house of mirrors at a carnival. This maze is called the **endoplasmic reticulum**. This network of material forms little canals within the cytoplasm that allow substances and other organelles to move around. Think of the endoplasmic reticulum as blood vessels within the body.

The **mitochondria** are the "lungs" and the "digestive system" of the cell. The mitochondria can be thought of as the cell's nutritionist. They convert oxygen and nutrients so that they can be used as energy by the cell. The mitochondria are also responsible for converting oxygen to carbon dioxide, which is an essential part of the oxygen usage system within the body. The mitochondria have "departments" that also control the amount of water and other substances that are allowed into the cytoplasm at particular times. As a "digestive factory" they help to break down simple sugars, fats, and parts of proteins called

amino acids. These are broken into smaller units that can more easily be used by the cell for energy. The **Golgi apparatus** is a storage mechanism, helping to store proteins for later conversion to manufacture other necessary chemicals when the cell needs them. Think of the Golgi apparatus as a tiny "silo," storing fuels for a future date.

Ribosomes are very small organelles that help build protein structures that the cell needs. They are the protein "construction division" of the cell.

Lysosomes are the "demolition crew" of the cell. They manufacture enzymes that help to break apart large molecules entering the cell so that they can be more easily converted to other necessary chemicals and substances. Lysosomes also are the "self-destruct" mechanism for the cell. When a cell dies, the lysosome releases enzymes that help to destroy the cell membrane.

Vacuoles are often one of the biggest organelles. They are the "storage vats" for waste and excess food supplies.

A Day in the Life of a Cell

Let's go through an oversimplified yet representative "day in the life of a cell." The blood cells deliver foods for the cell that have already been substantially broken down by the digestive system, absorbed through the intestinal wall, and absorbed by the blood. The blood also delivers fresh oxygen from the lungs. First the cell membrane acts as a "guard," allowing certain substances into the cytoplasm. Once inside, they may be guided to their destination by the canals of the endoplasmic reticulum. The lysosomes start breaking down the large protein molecules. The ribosomes are building or "rebuilding" the proteins that the cell needs at the time. The mitochondria serve as a "power plant" making usable energy for the cell from the variety of proteins, sugars, oxygen, and fats that have arrived. Excess food product and waste from production are stored in the vacuoles. The Golgi apparatus stores proteins to use later for manufacturing enzymes and hormones. After production is over, waste materials and carbon dioxide are released by the cell membranes to the blood. The blood takes the waste away to the lungs, where the carbon dioxide is breathed out, and to the kidneys, which filter out the other waste.

The Nucleus

We have discussed some of the respiratory, digestive, and synthesis functions of the cell. But what controls these many functions? Where is the "brain" of the cell? Centered in the cytoplasm is a large structure called the **nucleus**. The nucleus of the cell is made largely of protein and is also responsible for building certain proteins. It contains fibers called **chromatin**. Chromatin is largely responsible for cell division, which will be discussed later. The chromatin is made of a mixture of protein and special chemicals called **nucleic acids**. The most important of these acids is deoxyribonucleic acid, better known as DNA. DNA is a long, spiral-shaped molecule, which looks like a twisted ladder. The DNA has the power to duplicate itself, and within it are the "directions" for running the cell operations. Therefore, it may pass on instructions to new cells as it duplicates, insuring that each type of cell will know the "blueprint" for life.

Cells divide and reproduce by a process known as mitotic division, or **mitosis**. Hereditary traits for the cell are found in small structures in the DNA called **genes**. When the cell divides, the chromatin fibers line up and are seen as **chromosomes**. The entire "blueprint" is duplicated in the DNA, and the cell splits into two separate cells, both containing the exact same DNA, and genes (Figure 1-2). By this process cells are constantly reproducing themselves, carrying out the same functions.

Cell Specialization

Many types of cells are found within the human body. Groups of cells that perform the same function are called **tissues**. There are many different types of tissue.

Muscular tissue is of three types, which include visceral muscle, skeletal muscle, and cardiac muscle.

Visceral muscle is responsible for involuntary muscle actions. Involuntary muscle actions are movements that happen subconciousnessly. Movement of the lungs expanding and contracting, muscles of the intestines, and muscles of the digestive system are involuntary muscles. In other words, these muscle structures operate on "automatic pilot." Involuntary muscles are also known as smooth muscle tissue.

Skeletal muscles are responsible for the movement of the bones and the body's physical motion. Because these muscle cells have stripes or **striations**, they are also known as striated

FIGURE 1–2 Indirect division of the human cell

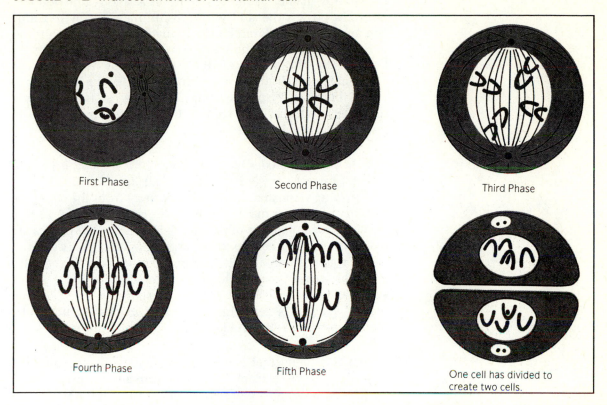

First Phase

Second Phase

Third Phase

Fourth Phase

Fifth Phase

One cell has divided to create two cells.

muscles. Skeletal muscles are responsible for voluntary movement and therefore are known as voluntary muscles. These muscles are controlled by the conscious brain, which means the brain directly controls their movement. Walking across a room to pick up an object is a motion in which the brain has complete control and is an example of a voluntary muscle action.

Cardiac muscle tissue used to be considered an involuntary smooth muscle, but it has since been established that this tissue is also striated, so it is classified in a separate category. Cardiac muscle is both striated and involuntary.

Connective tissue are groups of cells that specialize in providing support and cushioning for the body. **Cartilage** and **ligaments** are examples of connective tissue. They help to connect bones to each other, and bones to muscle. The ear and nose are made of **cartilage**.

Skeletal tissue makes up the bones in the body.

Nerve tissue are cells that control the brain and the nerves. Nerve cells transmit messages to all parts of the body. There are many types of nerve cells in the skin, which will be discussed later in this chapter. Think of the nerves as a long line of dominoes that possess the ability to transmit messages by touching one another. This "domino effect" enables the nerves to transport commands from the brain and information to the brain. Let's pretend that you accidentally touch a hot stove. The heat and pain nerve cells in the skin transmit the feeling up the body to the brain in a split second. The brain, in turn, sends a response in another split second, telling your arm muscles to immediately remove your hand from the hot stove.

Liquid tissue includes blood and lymph. The blood is responsible for carrying oxygen and food to all the cells in the body, and carrying waste and carbon dioxide away from the cells. The majority of blood is made of a substance called **plasma**. Plasma makes up the liquid part of the blood. Floating in the plasma are red blood cells, or **red corpuscles**, whose function is to complete oxygen-carbon dioxide transport to and from all the cells. The other main type of blood cells are white blood cells, or **white corpuscles**, which are largely responsible for defending the body against bacterial invasion. Much more about the white blood cells will be discussed in the chapter on immunity.

Lymph is a liquid that bathes all the tissues of the body and helps to filter wastes from the bloodstream and the body. Filters in the lymph system are present in many areas of the body such as the armpits, groin, and neck. These filters are called **lymph nodes**. When you are sick, sometimes you will have swollen areas in your neck or other areas. This is because the lymph is filtering debris and dead bacteria from the body, attempting to rid the body of these wastes. The lymph nodes swell when they are filtering lots of debris.

Adipose tissue is fat tissue. Fat, although it has a bad reputation, contributes to many functions within the body. It helps cushion all the other types of tissue. Imagine sitting on a sofa that had no cushions. It would be very hard and would break more easily if it was dropped or damaged. Fat helps the body in the same way, helping to soften injuries and protect the organs. Fat also is needed to produce hormones and other chemicals necessary for life.

Endothelial tissue lines the walls of the intestines, lungs, and other internal organs.

Epithelial tissue lines the outer body surfaces. The skin is an example of epithelial tissue.

Physiology of the Skin

The skin is comprised of three major layers (Figure 1-3). The **subcutaneous layer** the most internal layer of the skin. It contains large layers of fat to provide cushion for the internal organs, as previously discussed. Winding through the subcutaneous layer are blood vessels and lymph vessels, again insulated by fat tissue. The subcutaneous layer also contains nerve endings called **lamellated corpuscles,** which are responsive to pressure.

FIGURE 1–3 Histology of the skin, hair, and glands

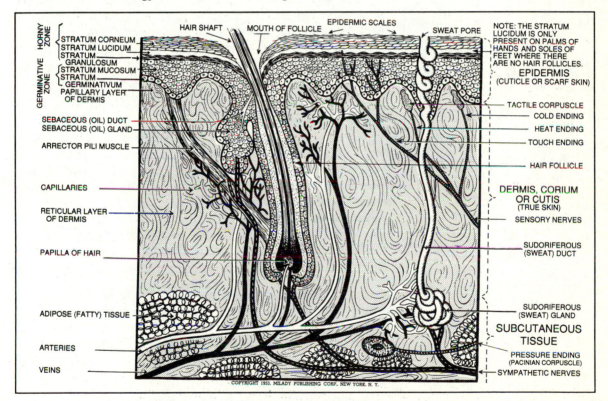

The **dermis** is the next layer toward the skin surface. The dermis is often called the "live" layer of the skin. The upper part of the dermis is called the **papillary layer**, containing the **dermal papillae**. Think of the dermal papillae as a "handlike" structure that attaches itself to the **epidermis**, the outermost of the three layers. The dermal papillae look like fingers "holding" the two layers together. Inside the papillae are many small blood vessels called capillaries, spiraling through the papillae. Also found in the papillary layer are some nerves sensitive to firm touch, called **Meissner's corpuscles**. These nerves sense deep touch. As an experiment, gently touch your hand. Next, exert more pressure on your hand. Doesn't it have a completely different feeling? This is because deeper nerves are stimulated when the skin is touched or pushed in a firmer manner.

The lower, more internal area of the dermis is called the **reticular layer**. The reticular layer contains a multitude of structures and activity. **Collagen** and **elastin fibrils** intertwine throughout the reticular layer. Both of these fibers are made of protein and are examples of connective tissue. They give the skin firmness and elasticity. Collagen is not flexible and gives skin its firmness and inability to stretch very much. Elastin is the fibrous structure that gives skin elasticity and the ability to "bounce back." Fat globules are also in this layer, as well as numerous blood vessels (arteries and veins), lymph vessels, and nerve endings that are sensitive to pain, heat, cold, and pressure. The base or bottom part of the hair follicle is also found in the reticular layer, as well as the **sudoriferous glands** or sweat glands, and the **sebaceous (oil) glands**.

The sebaceous glands secrete an oily mixture of fats and lipids. There are a number of different substances within sebaceous secretions. These include **triglycerides**, **sphingolipids**, **glycolipids**, **phospholipids**, **cholesterol**, **ceramides**, as well as **fatty acids** and **waxes**. These secretions work together as **sebum** to help form a moisture barrier on the skin's surface to help keep in moisture, hinder the growth of bacteria, and provide "mortar" for the cells. In other words, they help the cells stick together as a protective barrier for the inner skin and body.

The sudoriferous glands produce sweat. There are two kinds of sweat glands: the **apocrine** glands and the **eccrine** glands. The apocrine glands are present in the groin area and the armpits. They produce a thicker form of sweat and are basically responsible for producing the substance that, when in contact with bacteria, produces body odor.

The eccrine glands are abundant on the face and other parts of the body. They are present in extremely large numbers in the palms of the hands and the soles of the feet.

Sweat is a mixture of water, salt, urea, uric acid, ammonia, broken down proteins (amino acids), simple sugars, and vitamins. Sweat is the function of the body that controls temperature. As sweat evaporates, it helps to cool the surface of the skin. Some wastes are excreted by sweat, but body temperature regulation is its major function. When looking through a microscope, eccrine glands take the form of a spiral tube, much like the inside of a refrigerator. Apocrine glands are branched, appearing more like blood vessels off a major artery.

The epidermis, which is the major part of the skin that the esthetician treats, is made up of five basic layers.

The basal layer is the innermost layer of the epidermis. Within it are **melanocytes,** the cells that are "pigment factories" for the skin. Different color skin types have the same number of melanocytes, but people of certain races and ethnic backgrounds simply carry genes that make the melanocytes produce more **melanin** or pigment. Sunlight, injuries to the skin, and hormones can also stimulate melanin production. This is what causes an individual to become tan after a day at the beach. The primary function of melanin is to shield and protect the skin from damaging sun rays or injury. It is the body putting up a "parasol" to deflect ultraviolet rays. So, essentially a "healthy-looking" tan is actually the body defending itself from something unhealthy. The melanocytes "inject" melanin into the cells at the basal layer, and as they drift upward toward the surface, the cells are eventually shed from the surface. This is what causes the "loss" of a tan.

The basal cells are constantly dividing through mitosis, constantly pushing upwards to the outside of the skin. As they divide and move toward the surface, the intercellular structures discussed earlier begin to change. They produce a protein called **keratin**, which is the "magic" that helps protect the skin against invasion. As the cells change they also produce a variety of fats, or lipids, which help hold the keratinized cells together, much the way mortar holds a brick wall together.

Protein keratin synthesis begins in the basal layer, where fibrils of keratin begin to form out of the cytoplasm in the cell. As the cells move up from the basal layer, they start to form the next cellular layer, or **stratum**. The spiny layer, or **stratum spinosum**, is so called because the cells appear to have little spines or thorns on the outside of the cell membranes. In this layer the cells change shape from cubelike to multi-sided.

The next layer is the **stratum granulosum**, or granular layer. The granular looking cells are filled with a substance called **keratohyalin**, which helps to form keratin from the microtubule structures first formed in the basal cell layer. Keratohyalin is produced by the endoplasmic reticulum, as previously discussed. The nuclei of the dying cells are breaking down, and the cell is dying. In the granular stage new lipids are formed, which will again help to serve as a medium or "mortar" for the outer cell layer.

The next layer of the skin is the **stratum lucidum,** or clear layer, so called because it appears lucid or clear upon microscopic examination. It is filled with a substance called **eleidin,** which is produced from keratohyalin, and will eventually form keratin.

The outermost layer of the epidermis is called the **stratum corneum,** or "horny" layer, so called because the cells are piled up on top of one another in layers and have a horny appearance on the microscopic surface. Cells in this layer are referred to as **corneocytes**. In the "mortar" of the "bricks" in this layer are small structures called **lamellar bodies**. Lamellar bodies are thought to be produced during the stage of keratinization in the granular layer of the skin. Their function is to produce more lipids, which will serve to permit certain substances in and out of the corneum. In other words they will permit certain substances into the "mortar" of the cell layer and will allow certain gases and toxins produced by the skin to escape through the same pathway. The fats formed by the lamellar bodies serve almost the same purpose as the cell membrane discussed earlier. They possess the characteristic of selective permeability.

Let's take a minute to review the process of keratinization. The epidermis is divided into five layers:

1. The basal layer, which is a live layer, where the cells are dividing and constantly pushing upward. The melanocytes are also present in this layer. As cells drift upwards through the five layers they die. In the process of dying, they form keratin, a resilient protein that will eventually serve to protect the skin from invasion.

2. The spiny layer, where the shapes of the cells have changed.

3. The granular layer, where keratin continues to form, and where fats that will makeup the "mortar" begin to form.

4. The clear layer, where the process of keratinization continues.

5. Ultimately the cells reach the top of the skin in the horny layer or stratum corneum, where they become the "bricks" in the outer, protective layer of skin. The cells are filled with keratin protein. The lamellar bodies are small "fat factories" and help to produce mortar to seal between the cellular "bricks," but have the unique ability to allow certain substances in and out of the skin.

Skin Penetration

Not long ago, scientists and physicians believed that the skin was a barrier to almost everything. Suddenly, about a decade ago, it was discovered that a number of substances could indeed penetrate the skin. Drugs were developed that were absorbed **transdermally**, which means that these drugs penetrate the epidermis and the dermis, and then are absorbed into the bloodstream. This discovery opened new pathways for many treatments, including treatment of heart irregularities and motion sickness.

One of the first signs that the skin is more penetrable than first thought was the incident in which the antibacterial hexachlorophene was found to penetrate the skin readily, and hence was taken off the over-the-counter market and is now only available by prescription.

A variety of tests have been developed to measure skin penetration of substances, using techniques involving dyes and substances that have been "labeled" with radioactive compounds. These radioactive substances can be measured in the tissue or the blood to determine the amount and level of penetration.

Routes of Penetration

The investigation of skin penetration is still largely theoretical. Although we know that many substances can penetrate the skin to varying degrees, we know that many cannot. The issue of drug claims versus cosmetic claims influences the following few paragraphs. Please be careful with the claims you make for cosmetics. For more information on this issue, please read the chapter on claims for cosmetics.

It is generally accepted that there are four means of penetrating the skin (Figure 1-4). Certain substances can penetrate the skin through the following routes:

1. The hair follicle, which is essentially a hollow tube that begins with its opening at the epidermis and ends with its root in the dermis. It is theoretically possible that small enough substances could go into the hair follicle and end up a lot closer to the blood vessels, since the hair follicle extends into the dermis. The inner walls of the follicle are lined with epidermal cells. The layers of the epidermis basically dip into the follicle. The problem here is that the space is relatively limited, since the hair follicles occupy a relatively small proportion of the entire epidermis.

FIGURE 1–4 Various routes of skin penetration: through the sebaceous glands, the follicle wall, and intercellular and transcellular routes. *Courtesy Francosmetics, Inc.-René Guinot.*

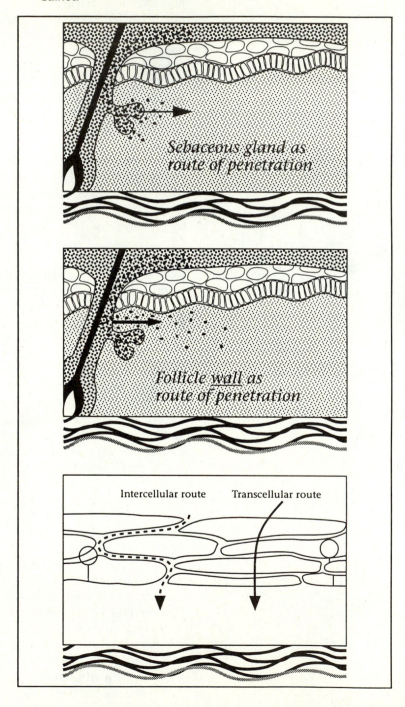

2. The sebaceous glands may also provide a pathway for certain substances. Many of these glands empty directly into the hair follicle; however, some of the apocrine glands may be not associated with a hair follicle.

3. The sudoriferous duct, which is relatively small compared to the size of a follicle (pore) opening.

4. The intercellular ("mortar") fluids are probably the best vehicle for penetration of the epidermis. Its surface area is large. But how do we penetrate the stacks of keratinized corneocytes, which are impermeable to many substances? The fatty fluid holding the cells together is actually permeable by certain substances.

Remember that earlier in the chapter we discussed how cells migrate from the basal layer to the corneum. In this process they die and form keratin, but also manufacture new lipids, along with the lamellar bodies that secrete more lipids into the intercellular cement.

These lipids in the intercellar cement will accept similar substances. In other words, theoretically, if we can make substances that are similar to the lipids in the intercellular cement, these substances may be readily accepted by the intercellular cement.

Other factors that affect skin penetration include the specific area where penetration is attempted. The order of permeability of various areas of the body are, in descending order: the genitals, head, trunk, and finally the arms and legs. So the face is generally more accepting of skin penetration than the back, and so forth. The forehead seems to be the most penetrable area of the skin on the face.

The size of the corneocytes may play an important role in penetration potential. The forehead's corneocytes are smaller than other areas on the face. The thickness of the stratum corneum may also be a factor. Another issue is the condition of the skin being treated. Torn or injured tissue, or skin that has a rash or abrasion, may be more easily penetrated. This is simply explained. The corneocytes are not as thick in such areas.

The size of the molecule being penetrated has a big effect on its permeability. Large proteins like collagen are not permeable. They are simply too big to go between the cells. However, smaller molecules with more affinity for lipids like sodium PCA (a humectant), retinoids, squalane, and fat-soluble vitamins such as vitamins A, D, and E seem to have good permeability. Some large molecules such as collagen do not need to penetrate the skin to be useful cosmetically. Collagen is a substantive, which means that it adheres readily to the surface of the corneum, helping to bind water and reduce water loss from within the epidermis. Cleansers, sunscreens, and makeup foundations are other examples of substances that should not be penetrated. They totally lose their cosmetic effectiveness at lower levels, assuming they could be penetrated at all. Keratolytics like salicylic acid need to stay on the surface because they work solely on the corneum; we do not want to dissolve other layers. However, for medicinal purposes, we would obviously want to penetrate the full epidermis in many cases. Cosmetically, moisturizers will work better and hold moisture for longer periods of time if they are able to penetrate deeper into the corneum.

Other Factors that Influence Penetration

The thickness of the stratum corneum will obviously have an effect on skin permeability. If there is a large buildup of dead cells on the surface, penetration is hindered. When applying a moisturizer, for example, an excessively thick corneum will not absorb the moisturizer as well. The buildup of cells is usually dry and brittle, due to the large amount of keratin present within each cell, and will "grab" the moisture from the moisturizer. Therefore, the lower corneum is less likely to benefit from the moisture treatment.

Excessive oily skin will have a layer of excess sebum on the surface, further slowing penetration. Doctors often apply a strong solvent such as acetone before applying chemical peel solutions. This is to cut the excess sebum on the surface, so that the chemical peeling solution can better adhere to and affect the desired area.

Temperature of the skin also influences its acceptance of preparations. Warm skin is generally more accepting. Heat causes activity within molecules, kind of "stirring up" the molecules in the intercellular cement and the cell activity itself. On the other hand, certain substances such as hydrocortisone are known to absorb better when cold compresses are applied to the area.

Salon Application Techniques for Good Absorption of Topical Preparations

Because some routes of penetration are more effective than others, some techniques can be used in the salon to get products to penetrate better. Moisturizing and conditioning treatments will be more effective if they can get deeper into the corneum.

Preparing the Skin for Treatment

Cleansing the skin helps rid the surface of dirt, dust, pollutants, makeup, and excess secretions such as sweat and sebum. Some dead keratinocytes (corneal cells) are removed during basic cleansing.

Using toners, fresheners and astringents helps to remove more excess sebum on the surface. Using these products both in the salon and at home will help to better prepare the surface for penetration of appropriate cosmetic treatment preparations.

The amount of alcohol, propylene glycol, and other solvents will have a direct effect on the amount of sebum removed. The oilier the skin is, the more solvent should be present in the toner. This process can work against us as well. For example, if you use a strong astringent on dry, dehydrated, thin, sensitive skin, and then apply a treatment that is too strong, it can irritate the skin instead of helping it. Be careful to choose the appropriate cleanser and toner for the skin type you are treating.

Removing cellular buildup—for skin types with excess corneum the use of mechanical, enzyme, or cosmetic peeling or other exfoliating treatments will help to remove excess corneocytes. Removing these dead cells will help improve the appearance of the skin in four ways.

1. Removing these dead keratinized cells will immediately improve the skin's surface appearance, making it look smoother and clearer. Removing the cells that surround wrinkles will make wrinkles look less apparent. If you think of a wrinkle as a ditch, a mound of dead cells on either side of the ditch will make the ditch look deeper, Removing the mounds will reduce the space between the bottom of the wrinkle and the skin surface, making it look less obvious.

2. Makeup will apply more evenly to a more even surface. Clients report that makeup applies much easier for up to two weeks after a good exfoliation.

3. Removal of the cells stimulates the skin, helping it look healthier, with improved surface circulation and glow.

4. Removing the cells increases physical penetration of moisture treatments or other preparations applied after the exfoliation.

Types of Exfoliation

Mechanical exfoliation means that the cells are mechanically removed by physically removing them from the skin. They are actually being "bumped" from the surface of the skin. Good examples of mechanical exfoliation are the use of a brushing machine or granulated scrub. "Peel-off" masks and drying preparations that are rubbed off are also good examples of mechanical exfoliatiion.

Enzyme treatment uses **proteolytic,** or protein dissolving, enzymes that actually dissolve the excess corneocyte buildup. Enzyme "peeling" is a common salon treatment that will be discussed in more detail in Chapter 18.

Chemical solvents and light chemical peeling are used to reduce excess corneocytes on the surface. Glycolic acid, resorcinol, salicylic acid, and lactic acid are chemicals used in this type of procedure, which will be discussed in more detail in Chapter 18.

Increasing Physical Absorption of Moisture Treatments

Besides improving the surface permeability by the skin preparation techniques we have just discussed, using various techniques or tools to increase absorption can make penetration of treatment preparations more likely.

Massage stimulates the skin both physically and thermostatically, meaning that the heat generated by friction with the skin actually warms the surface, as well as warming the preparation you are using . A good but gentle massage with the appropriate moisturizer will increase its penetration and effectiveness.

Selecting the right cream—Use the knowledge you obtain in this book to help select the right preparation. Manufacturers now develop preparations that are more readily accepted by the lipids in the intercellular cement. Creams that are very heavy or greasy may be less permeable due to the large size of the molecules in their base formulations.

Use of heat and cold will increase cream penetration. Infrared lamps and infrared "skin irons" release heat, which aids absorption. Heat masks and paraffin treatments produce similar results. Warning! Do not use direct heat on sensitive skin; red, irritated skin; or skin with enlarged or distended capillaries!

Cold penetration with cold "globes" may be more appropriate for sensitive skin. Globes are glass or plastic balls that contain cryogenic (extremely cold) liquids. You can cut irritation from globes by placing a large piece of gauze over the face after applying the treatment and before using the cold therapy.

High frequency treatment releases heat deeper into the skin layers, helping to stimulate the skin and increase product absorption.

Iontophoresis or **ionization** uses electrical current to polarize preparations into the skin (Figure 1-5). Ions are repelled into the skin by use of galvanic current. See Gerson, *Milady's Standard Textbook for Professional Estheticians* for further instructions on machine usage.

Use of masks over creams restricts evaporation of the creams, therefore increasing penetration.

Warning—some types of treatments should not be used with these penetration techniques and certain individuals are not good candidates for some of these techniques. Use common sense and follow manufacturers' instructions for all treatments, preparations, and devices.

FIGURE 1–5 Ionization

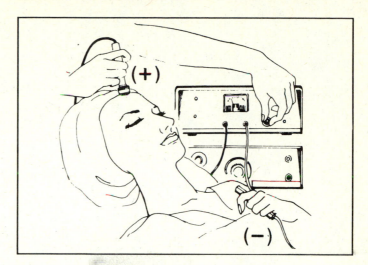

TOPICS FOR DISCUSSION

1. What is the function of the cell membrane?
2. What is selective permeability?
3. Why is the nucleus of the cell so important?
4. What is the difference between involuntary and voluntary muscles?
5. Discuss the three major layers of skin and the structures contained in each.
6. Discuss in detail methods for helping creams penetrate the skin better in the salon.

CHAPTER

2

The Immune System

The body's immune system is a very complex system. It is the body's defense mechanism against disease and other invaders. This chapter will describe how the immune system functions and some of the many reactions that take place in the body's fight against disease. You will learn the many immune functions of the skin and why the skin is one of the most important parts of the immune system.

The **immune system** is the body's mechanism for fighting disease. The immune system involves a complex series of specialized cells, the blood, the nervous system, organs, hormones, and many complex chemical reactions. When a person possesses the necessary substances and characteristics to avoid getting a disease, that person is said to be **immune** to that disease.

Let's suppose that your body is invaded by a pathogenic organism. A **pathogenic organism** is a type of bacteria, virus, or other one-celled organism that causes disease. This kind of bacteria is, of course, foreign material to the body. An antigen is a foreign substance that the body recognizes as foreign, and therefore attempts to defend against. The body will produce a special kind of protein called an **antibody** that helps to neutralize foreign organisms entering the body. When you have already had chicken pox, you cannot get chicken pox again. This is because your body produced antibodies the first time you had the illness. When your body builds antibodies to diseases when you are sick, the process is called **acquired immunity**. In other words, you acquired immunity to a future illness of the same type that you did not have before you were ill.

Natural immunity is immunity to certain diseases that you have had since you were born. You obtain the antibodies for natural immunity from your mother's blood and your parents' genes before you are born. In Chapter 1, we mentioned white blood cells. White blood cells are largely responsible for fighting disease in the immune system. White blood cells are produced by the bone marrow, but also by the spleen, liver, and lymph nodes.

There are 8,000 white blood cells per milliliter of blood. When the body has an infection, there may be up to 50,000 white blood cells per milliliter of blood. When the body has an infection, there may be up to 50,000 white blood cells per milliliter!

Components of the Immune System

There are two kinds of white blood cells. **Polymorphonuclear leucocytes** are referred to as **polymorphs**. Polymorphs are divided into three types: eosinophils, basophils, and neutrophils. Polymorphs attack bacteria and other pathogenic organisms in a process called **phagocytosis.** They surround foreign bodies and destroy them. They also help in disposing of **necrotic** (dead) tissue. Pus is defeated, dead polymorphs. You can understand this better if you think about a pimple. When acne bacteria take over a pore, polymorphs rush to the rescue. Some are killed by the bacteria and some die during the struggle. Their bodies are the main component of pus in the pustule.

A very large variety of white blood cell is called a **macrophage**. Macrophage means "large phagocyte." It acts as a guard, constantly patrolling the body looking for foreign invaders (Figure 2-1). Its cell membrane will surround and "swallow" bacteria. It is large enough to swallow and destroy even a hundred bacteria at a time. Macrophages can identify foreign bodies and determine that they are invaders, and not part of the body's cells. In other words, they can tell the difference between the body's own cells and foreign invading organisms.

FIGURE 2–1 A macrophage guarding the epidermis

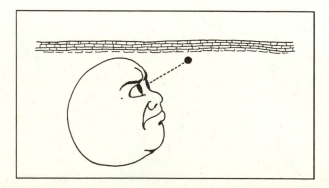

The other type of white blood cell is called the **lympho-cyte**. Lymphocytes are produced by the lymph nodes, the spleen, and the thymus gland. The thymus gland is located under the breastbone in the chest. It secretes hormones and helps to trigger synthesis of more lymph tissue.

There are two types of lymphocytes. They are called B-lymphocytes and T-lymphocytes, also known as **B-cells** and **T-cells**. T-cells are of three types. T-helper cells help alert the immune system. Think of T-helper cells as messengers. When a macrophage identifies a foreign organism, the T-helper cell runs to the lymph nodes, where another type of T-cell, the T-killer cell, is waiting. T-killer cells are activated and rush to the invasion site of the foreign organism. The T-killer cells work to kill the organisms. After the battle is won, another type of T-cell called T-suppressor cells stop the T-killer cells from fighting and signal them that the battle is over.

The T-helper cell also plays another role in the immune system. It signals the B-cells, which are in the lymph nodes. The B-cells make antibodies that are, as we discussed previously, proteins that help to prevent further infection or reoccurrence. Antibodies are also called **immunoglobu-lins**, called Igs by scientists. Igs float through the bloodstream and help protect against invasion by organisms they recognize.

Let's put all this information in perspective. Think of the body as a community. The immune system is the "fire department" (Figure 2-2). The macrophage is the fire patrol unit, constantly looking for "fires" (foreign organisms). If it spots a "fire," it holds it and checks it out, making sure it is not a "false alarm". Once the macrophage has established that the organism is real, it signals the T-helper cells, who rush to the "fire station" to alert the T-killer cells, who are waiting to "slide down the pole!" The T-killer cells rush to the scene, fiercely battling the "blaze" of foreign organisms, killing all the organisms. Watching the battle is the T-suppressor cell—sort of a lookout. When the "fire is out," the T-suppressor cells blow the whistle to let the T-killer cells know that the fire is under control. The T-helper cells have also alerted the B-cells in the lymph nodes. The B-cells start producing "fireproofing materials" (antibodies, Igs). The Igs serve as safety officers to make sure that this type of "fire" never starts again.

FIGURE 2–2 The Immune Fire Department

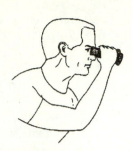

1. The macrophage spots a "fire" and signals the T-helper cells.

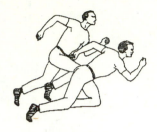

2. The T-helper cells run to the "fire department."

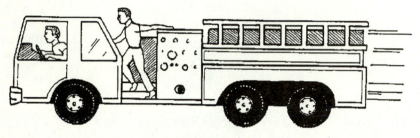

3. The T-killer cells rush to the scene of the "fire ."

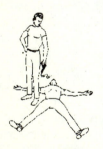

4. The T-killer cells kill invading organisms.

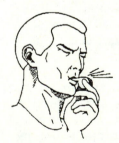

5. T-suppressor "blows whistle" to let T-killer cells know that everything is under control.

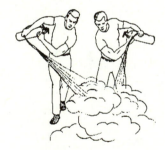

6. B-cells maufacture antibodies ("fireproofing"), helping to prevent another invasion.

How the Immune System Communicates with Itself

In Chapter 1 we discussed how DNA replicates itself in cell division and how each cell is a self-contained life system connected to other cells, specialized into the different tissues .

The information contained in the DNA of each cell allows the cell to duplicate an exact copy of itself, passing on the instructions from one cell generation to the next. This is a unique code in each individual person.

Just as the DNA is coded, so is the surface of the cell membrane. Each cell membrane has on its surface special codes called **receptors**. Receptors inform T-cells of what type of cell it is and that it is an "official" cell of the body and not an antigen (foreign body). The receptors on the cell membranes are made of special proteins. These proteins specifically fit similar protein structures on the surface of immune system cells, such as macrophages. It works like a lock and key (Figure 2-3). As long as the macrophage's "key" fits a cell's "lock," the macrophage recognizes the cell as part of the body's tissue. When the key does not fit, the macrophage starts the process of investigating the unidentified body.

The T-cells communicate with each other by releasing a hormone-type substance called **interleuken**. Interleuken is present in the cytoplasm of T-cells and is released as an alarm system when the T-cell is alerted to a foreign body. It is sort of like a skunk spraying when it is disturbed! The other T-cells receive a similar alarming message from the interleuken.

FIGURE 2–3 Lock and key of the membrane

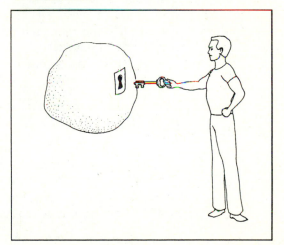

About Cancer

Cancer is one of the most intriguing and destructive diseases. Cancer starts in one cell. The cell becomes deformed and then duplicates through mitosis, but the process of mitosis does not stop. The abnormal cell keeps dividing, creating more and more cancerous cells.

With the thousands of cell duplications happening constantly in our bodies, some cells become **mutated**, or changed, from time to time. They become deformed and are recognized as deformed by the immune system. The immune system will kill these cells. So it is theoretically possible that cancerous cells develop periodically, but that these cells are usually killed by the immune system. However, when the immune system does not function properly, or when the cancerous cells divide too fast to be killed by the immune system, cancer as we know it develops.

Cancer cells can also "disguise" themselves. The T-cells are trained to react to receptors on the cell membrane that help them distinguish body cells from foreign bodies. In a cancerous cell, the cell membrane is actually the same as the membrane of a normal body cell. The T-cells cannot tell that the cell is cancerous. The T-cell treats the cell as a normal cell, ignores it, and does not attack. Cancerous cells that have abnormalities in their cell membrane may be recognized as unusual, but normal cell membranes will indicate no problem to the immune system. Cancer is abnormal cells duplicating out of control. This is how cancer can spread so quickly. Spreading of cancer is called **metastasis;** the cancer is said to be metastasizing.

T-cells, as we have already discussed, are produced by the thymus gland in the chest. The thymus gland is very productive early in life and then significantly reduces production. T-cells, unlike other body cells, live for about 60 years, then start to die. This may explain why older people are more likely to get cancer and illnesses of any kind.

Onco- means "tumor," and *-ology* means "the study of." **Oncology** is the study of cancer. Physicians who specialize in the treatment of cancer are called **oncologists**.

Let's review for a moment some things we learned in Chapter 1. In the nucleus of cells in our body lies the DNA. DNA contains instructions for running the cell. In the DNA are the genes, which determine our hereditary traits.

Among the genes are the oncogenes. Oncogenes play an important part in cell duplication. They help trigger the replication process. Everything is fine unless they get out of control. Scientists believe that oncogenes out of control may initiate the beginning of that one cancerous cell.

Cancer Causes

What specifically causes oncogenes to go out of control is not known. However, some substances are **carcinogenic**. *Carcinogenic* means "cancer-causing." Substances that are carcinogenic are called **carcinogens**. There are many well-known carcinogens. Let's start with the one discussed the most—smoking!

Smoke insults the body like almost no other substance. Smoke is, of course, foreign to the body. So the body tries to get rid of it like any other foreign substance. The chemicals within smoke kill cells. The cells have to work hard to repair the tissue damaged by the chemicals. This hurried process to repair the cells in the tissues, along with possible aggravation of the oncogenes by the chemicals, may cause abnormal cell replication and therefore cancerous cells. Because the body is stressed by the repair process, the immune system is overworked during this rebuilding process. The "tired" immune system is less likely to react well to invaders. So one effect of smoking is that it decreases immune functions in the body.

Many other substances can contribute to "slowing" of the immune system. Excessive alcohol, illegal drug use, stress, improper diet, too much fat, lack of exercise, and many other factors can contribute to malfunctions of the immune system. Let's think about these factors individually.

Alcohol in excessive amounts can cause a tremendous stress on all body systems. It is in fact a poison in significant quantities. Continual, repetitive damage is done day after day to the body of an alcoholic. Alcoholics also tend not to eat correctly, not to get enough sleep, and to cause themselves stress by creating problems for those around them.

Illegal drug use also damages the body. The effects are similar to that of alcohol. High stress levels, poor diet, and irritation to the tissues are all effects of drug use. Drug users also risk the danger of overdose, which often kills.

Stress insults every function of the body. Scientists and physicians are learning more and more about stress and its influence on disease. It is generally accepted that stress can be a factor in almost every disease. When the body is under stress, the immune system is overworked. **Immunosuppression** refers to the slowing of the immune system by any of the factors mentioned in this section.

Improper diet robs the body of its fuel—the fuel it needs to carry out all the chemical reactions that take place in every single cell in the body. Imagine how you would feel if you were not able to eat for several days. The cells cannot function properly without proper nutrition. And the immune system is made of cells!

Too much fat in the diet causes a buildup of cholesterol and triglycerides in the blood vessels. This **plaque** obstructs blood flow. How do cells receive their food and oxygen? From the blood! If the "road" is blocked, the supplies can not get through. And the cells of the immune system are on the delivery route.

Regular aerobic exercise such as walking, biking, aerobics, or swimming improve the oxygen transport system of the body. This means that the body gets more oxygen. Exercising regularly also can lower blood pressure, reduce cholesterol and triglycerides, and reduce stress. All of these factors we have just discussed involve one thing—common sense! Treat your body with respect and it will treat you with respect.

Free Radicals

Anyone who reads health magazines has heard of free radicals. **Free radicals** are oxygen atoms that are unstable, because they have lost an electron in their outer orbit (see Chapter 7). They are attracted to fats or lipids, which have extra electrons available to stabilize these oxygen atoms. The cell membrane is made up of lipids. These oxygen atoms attach themselves to the cell membrane. When enough free radicals attach themselves to the cell membrane, they reduce its permeability. Proteins, fats, carbohydrates, and oxygen cannot get into the cell. Wastes, toxins, and carbon dioxide cannot get out of the cell. Needless to say, the cell will eventually die.

DNA damage from free radicals can occur and is possibly a factor in skin cancer. It has also been suggested that hyperpigmentation is linked to free radicals. One of the biggest causes of free radicals is sun exposure.

While free radical oxygen atoms are a byproduct of many normal chemical reactions within the body, free radicals are also formed readily from smoking, alcohol, stress, and pollution. While free radicals can affect all the body cells, and are probably significantly responsible for the aging of the entire body, free radicals have a strong effect on the skin. We will discuss treating and preventing free radical formation in Chapter 9.

How Medicine Helps the Immune System

Vaccines

Vaccines are an artificial way of tricking the immune system into making antibodies, or Igs. Vaccines introduce very small amounts of antigen (foreign organisms) into the body. Not enough of the organism is introduced to cause the body to become ill, but enough that it triggers the B-cells to make immunoglobulins to protect against whatever organism is being used in the vaccination process.

Sometimes the vaccination process will produce minor symptoms of the illness. You have probably heard of people getting slightly ill after receiving a flu vaccine. In cases where small amounts of the organisms are enough to trigger disease, doctors sometime use dead viruses or irradiated organisms in vaccines. Irradiated organisms used in vaccines have been treated with some form of radiation before being used. They are still alive, but the radiation treatment renders the organisms unable to reproduce. These are sometimes called **modified live vaccines**.

Vaccines are available against a large variety of diseases, including polio, smallpox, measles, mumps, certain types of influenza (flu), and many other diseases.

Antibiotics

Antibiotics are drugs that are made from extracts obtained from living organisms. Penicillin is probably the best known form of antibiotic. It is derived from a type of mold. Antibiotics do not produce long-term, or active, immunity. They simply kill the bacteria.

Science has yet to develop much effective treatment for viruses. Viruses are different than bacteria in that they do not have the same characteristics as one-celled organisms. Viruses are particles instead of cells. They do not have the same structure as a cell. They invade the body by "injecting" themselves into healthy cells. They reproduce in great numbers inside the body cell, eventually killing the cell. When the cell dies, the many viruses are released to invade other cells.

The immune system is our best protection against viruses. Scientists have developed immune system stimulants and synthetic immunoglobulins that may help the body's own immune system fight viruses. However, no drugs to kill viruses are yet available that are as effective as antibiotics are against bacterial infections.

Sometimes antibiotics kill the wrong bacteria as well as the ones they were intended to kill. It is not unusual for someone taking antibiotics to have gastrointestinal disturbances while they are taking antibiotics. This is because the antibiotics also kill "good guy" bacteria while they are attacking the pathogenic organisms. Many bacteria present in our bodies help with necessary chemical reactions that happen within the body constantly. When these bacteria are killed by an antibiotic, normal body functioning may be affected.

The Immunity Role of the Skin

The fact that the skin is the outer shield of the body makes it an immune barrier. Keratin in the corneocytes helps to protect the body against invasion by foreign bodies and organisms. The fact that the skin will resist being punctured by a needle illustrates this point. If you press your finger against the point of a needle, the skin will not be pierced unless pressure is applied to the needle.

Microorganisms are found all over the surface of the skin at all times. These organisms generally do not penetrate the skin because of the layers of corneocytes preventing absorption. The **acid mantle**, or the layer of lipids and sweat secretions on top of the skin, help to kill many bacteria. What if we tear the skin or puncture it with that needle? When we puncture the skin, we break the barrier of the corneocytes and expose the broken skin and blood to the many microorganisms that are on the needle, as well as those on the surface of the skin.

Diseases that cause breaks in the skin surface, such as eczema, acne, and dermatitis, make the skin more susceptible to invasion by microorganisms. Dermatitis is often accompanied by a secondary infection such as a fungus or bacteria.

The second possibility for passing the barrier of the corneum is through the routes of skin penetration we discussed earlier. It is physically possible for a microorganism to penetrate the skin through the intercellular fluids or cement that we discussed in Chapter 1. But this organism would have to penetrate the corneum, its layers of keratinized cells, the acid mantle, and the intercellular cement.

Let's suppose that a microorganism gets through the outer layer. The microorganism is first noticed by the **Langerhans cell**. Langerhans cells are "guard" cells that constantly patrol the epidermis. Langerhans cells look like spiders, since one end has many tentacle-like structures called **dendrites**. On the other end of the Langerhans cell is a pseudopod. **Pseudopod** means "false foot." The Langerhans cell is able to extend this oval shaped foot to help it move.

When the Langerhans cell is stimulated by a foreign body, it breaks off a sample piece of the antigen. The Langerhans cell then presents the sample piece to the macrophage, which is present in the epidermis just under the Langerhans cell. The macrophage then identifies the antigen, and if it is indeed a pathogenic organism, it signals the T-cells to the rescue.

The Langerhans cells are particularly sensitive to sun exposure. A moderate amount of sun exposure will knock them out of commission for a few days. Repeated sun exposure may knock them out of commission long enough for skin cancer cells to get a good start. With the Langerhans cells "on sick leave" from the sun exposure, the skin is left vulnerable to other microorganisms. This lack of immune protection may also have a domino effect on other parts of the immune system within other parts of the body.

The keratinocytes in the epidermis also help to secrete a number of important immune substances. The keratinocytes secrete a protein substance called apolipoprotein-E, apo-E for short. Apo-E helps transport cholesterol, which makes up a part of the intercellular cement. Keratinocytes also help to neutralize potential carcinogens and produce two different forms of interleukin, the hormone-like substance that helps immune cells communicate. The keratinocytes also produce another substance called granulocyte macrophage colony stimulating factor (GM-CSF), which helps promote replication of the macrophages in the granular layer of the epidermis. Last but not least, the keratinocytes produce a substance very similar to that produced by the thymus gland. These hormones help cause T-cells to mature.

Also present in the epidermis are the Granstein cells, which are believed to play a part in suppressing immune function. It is theorized that the Granstein cells act similarly to T-suppressor cells in discontinuing actions of the immune system.

Scientists are now experimenting with a new yeast cell membrane derivative that may cause collagen production. The extract causes stimulation of the macrophage, which seems to reach down into the dermis with its pseudopod and stimulate the fibroblast, the dermal cell that activates collagen and elastin production. It may be theoretically possible to stimulate collagen and elastin production in this manner. This accomplishment might have significance in both the cosmetic and medical worlds, as stimulated production of collagen and elastin could help a number of problems ranging from wrinkles to improved wound healing.

Autoimmune Diseases

Autoimmunity is a condition where the immune system cannot distinguish the difference between antigens and its own body cells. The immune system essentially starts attacking the body cells. A good example of an autoimmune response is what happens sometimes after an organ transplant. We have all heard about a kidney transplant patient who "rejected" the new kidney. The immune system sees the new kidney as a foreign body and works to attack and reject the new kidney.

Autoimmune diseases also cause rejection, but the person's own body cells are being rejected.

Probably the most frequent condition that estheticians see involving autoimmunity is **lupus erythematosus**, usually called lupus. Lupus patients have developed antibodies to their own cells.

The body is constantly cleaning itself of dead body cells. In lupus, the lymphocytes also produce antibodies to these dead cells. While the lymphatic and blood systems are still trying to rid the body of these dead cells, the antibodies produced by the malfunctioning immune system bind themselves to the dead cells, creating "traffic jams" in the blood vessels. Damage to the blood vessels results.

Lupus mostly affects the skin, the joints, the nervous system, and the kidneys. The skin is marked by a butterfly-shaped rash on the cheeks. Sun exposure can cause sudden attacks of the disease.

Lupus is managed by medical specialists called rheumatologists or immunologists. They control the symptoms of lupus with steroids and other symptom-relieving drugs. These drugs may cause additional medical as well as esthetic problems. If you have a lupus patient in your skin-care practice, consult with the physician before beginning esthetic treatment. Let the doctor know what treatment you are planning to use and what topical preparations you will use. Most lupus patients can greatly benefit from esthetic treatment.

TOPICS FOR DISCUSSION

1. What is the function of the immune system?
2. What is the difference between acquired and natural immunity?
3. Describe the process of the immune system functioning on a foreign body.
4. What are some factors that suppress the immune system?
5. Discuss the skin's immune function.
6. What is an autoimmune disease? What is one of the most prevalent autoimmune diseases the esthetician sees?

3

AIDS

AIDS (Acquired Immune Deficiency Syndrome) is a devastating disease that will affect millions of people in the near future. In this chapter you will learn how the AIDS virus affects the immune system and the body. We will discuss how AIDS is transmitted and what can be done to prevent further spread of AIDS. We will discuss AIDS symptoms in the body, including many symptoms that may appear in the skin. Management of the AIDS patient will be reviewed so that you will be knowledgeable about the medical treatment of AIDS and AIDS-related conditions.

In the late 1970s doctors at a major California medical center noticed that they were treating an abnormally large number of young men with a relatively rare pneumonia called **pneumocystis carinii pneumonia**. All of the young men they were treating had one thing in common. They were all homosexuals. They also noticed that the patients had recurrent unusual infections of many types. The patients also had become very weak and had lost weight rapidly.

This was the beginning of the epidemic of the disease we now know as AIDS. The letters AIDS stand for Acquired Immune Deficiency Syndrome. It was obvious to these doctors that the immune systems of these patients was malfunctioning badly. Doctors in other major metropolitan areas started noticing the same disease affecting three major groups of individuals: intravenous drug users, male homosexuals, and persons who had received blood transfusions. It was evident that all of these groups had been affected by some sort of organism that was passed from individual to individual by the transmission of bodily fluids. Soon after the epidemic started, scientists isolated a virus they called HTLV-III. These letters stood for human t-lymphotropic virus (Type III). The letters for the virus have since been changed to HIV for **human immunodeficiency virus.**

As we learned in Chapter 2, viruses work by "injecting" themselves into healthy cells. Once they are inside the healthy cells, they reproduce in great numbers, eventually killing the cell. The cell ruptures, releasing millions of new viruses. Each of these new viruses can "inject" other cells, repeating the process and duplicating even more viruses. The HIV virus attacks T-cells, the main defense cells of the immune system discussed in Chapter 2. This virus eventually can completely destroy the immune system. Without a properly functioning immune system, the body's cells are left abandoned with no army of immune cells to protect them against invasion by microorganisms.

The reason that AIDS patients become ill with such rare diseases as pneumocystis carinii pneumonia is because the immune system can no longer fight off infections. AIDS patients are plagued by a variety of rare illnesses. These rare illnesses are called **opportunistic infections** because they are sicknesses that the immune system normally has no trouble fighting off. With an impaired immune system, however, these diseases are able to get a good foothold in the body and cause infection.

How People Get Infected with AIDS

The HIV virus has been linked to a similar virus in African green monkeys. The monkeys carry this similar virus but are not always affected by it. When viruses or other organisms duplicate many times, the DNA in the organism sometimes changes slightly. This change is called a **mutation**. Many scientists believe that the AIDS virus mutated in a human after the human was bitten by a monkey in Africa. The virus was then probably spread sexually. There are many, many cases of AIDS in Africa, mostly in heterosexuals. Because HIV attacks white blood cells, it can spread very rapidly in the body. Blood, as you know, flows through the body. There are some blood cells in every body fluid. Body fluids are blood, semen, urine, vaginal secretions, spinal fluid, tears, saliva, and amniotic fluids in pregnant women. Semen and blood appear to be the only real sources of infections. No infection from tears or saliva has ever been documented.

Intravenous drug users are infected by the AIDS virus by using dirty hypodermic needles that contain small amounts of blood from another person. When they inject their illegal drugs, they also inject the other person's HIV-infected blood.

Many patients who received blood transfusions before blood was being checked for HIV contamination became infected. Organ donors infected with HIV donated organs that were also contaminated, causing AIDS in some people. However, now that there are tests to screen blood and tissue donations, infection through receiving blood transfusions or organ transplants is highly unlikely.

The number one risk source for HIV infection is sexual intercourse. Sexual intercourse involves direct transmission of body fluids from one individual to another. The vagina, the penis, and the rectum all have many small blood vessels that can break during intercourse, causing direct exposure. When HIV-infected blood enters the body, infection can occur. Once the virus enters the body, it can spread very quickly. However, symptoms caused by the breakdown of the immune system may not be noticed for months or years.

Anyone who has been infected by the HIV virus can transmit the virus to others through sexual contact, whether or not that person has symptoms. During the early stages of the disease, it is virtually impossible to tell if an individual is infected by looking at that individual.

Testing for the AIDS Virus

When the body is infected with HIV, the B-cells produce antibodies to the virus. These antibodies can be identified by blood tests that are able to isolate the antibody.

The first test done for the HIV antibody is called the ELISA test. This test is a screening test for the HIV antibody. If the test is positive, this indicates that the patient has antibodies to the virus. Confirmation of a positive Elisa test is completed by a second blood test called a western blot test. If the second test is also positive, the patient definitely has HIV antibodies. Doctors refer to these patients as HIV-positive. Persons who do not have the virus or antibodies are called HIV-negative. HIV-positive individuals, as we said before, may not show symptoms of AIDS for months or years. Medical scientists believe, however, that all HIV-positive individuals will eventually develop AIDS symptoms.

Sometimes a person with HIV infection will not test positive for the virus immediately. Let's suppose an individual was exposed through sexual contact but did not test positive when he was tested for HIV two months later. However, several months later he tested positive for the virus. This delayed reaction occurs because the B-cells had not yet produced antibodies to the virus. The B-cells eventually produced antibodies, and they were identified during the later test. The period of time between exposure to the HIV virus and the time antibodies are made is called a window phase. Individuals will not test positive if there are no antibodies, because the test identifies the antibodies, not the virus. For high-risk individuals, several tests should be performed at intervals over a period of a year to eighteen months. During that time the individual must abstain from sexual contact to prevent the possibility of another window phase occuring.

The Symptoms of HIV Infection

Many small infections can occur in an HIV-positive person before strong symptoms develop. Strange skin rashes and lesions, repeated infections such as frequent flu-like symptoms, chronic tiredness, and other symptoms may be symptoms of HIV infection. Of course many other diseases can have these same symptoms. Because a person has symptoms like these does not necessarily mean the person is infected with HIV. However, the beginning of immune system breakdown may result in multiple minor infections.

ARC stands for AIDS-Related Complex. Persons with ARC have had some symptoms of illness and a positive HIV antibody test. ARC may result in unexplained weight loss, frequent flu-like symptoms, chronic tiredness, diarrhea, vomiting, and night sweats.

In order to call HIV infection AIDS, a person must both be HIV-positive and show signs of advanced immune system breakdown, identified by the presence of a definite opportunistic disease. We will discuss these diseases shortly. Doctors often refer to patients with these symptoms as having "full-blown" AIDS.

Common AIDS Symptoms

Pneumocystis carinii pneumonia affects AIDS patients. This form of pneumonia produces high fever, a horrible hacking cough due to fluid in the lungs, and almost always results in hospitalization.

Other forms of lung infection are also prevalent in AIDS patients. Fungal and yeast infections of the lungs are common, as well as fungal and yeast infections of the esophagus. Other forms of bacterial infection may also occur in the lungs. Some of these infections may occur simultaneously.

Swollen lymph nodes are also common in HIV-infected individuals. The immune system is trying to fight off infection, but is losing the battle. Swollen lymph nodes may indicate the presence of a large number of dead T-cells killed by HIV.

Dementia is an infection of the brain or cerebrospinal tissues. This may result in personality disorders or mental illnesses. Various forms of cancer are much more likely to occur in AIDS patients. Again, the immune system no longer can protect the body. **Chronic wasting syndrome** refers to rapid, unexplained weight loss. Any sort of recurrent infection may be a symptom. A simple infection may be treated with antibiotics, but reoccurs in a short period of time. These are only a very few general symptomatic diseases of AIDS. Again, it must be stressed that all of these diseases may occur in healthy, HIV-negative persons. But, they are most likely to occur when the immune system is not functioning well, as is the case with HIV infection. These diseases are sometimes called AIDS-indicator diseases. Doctors know that if an HIV-infected person has these diseases, AIDS is often indicated.

Treatment of AIDS and HIV Infection

At the time of this writing there is no cure for AIDS. It may be decades before we have a cure. There are very few true cures for viral infections. AIDS is caused by a viral infection, as are the common cold, types of influenza (the flu), and many other illnesses.

Scientists are investigating the possibility of developing a vaccine. A vaccine may be available before a cure is found. Developing a vaccine may involve injecting small particles of proteins from the HIV virus, which may cause development of antibodies to HIV without causing HIV infection.

For persons who already have AIDS, doctors can treat individual symptoms as they appear, but treatment is not always successful because of the depressed immune system of the AIDS patient. Medicine may help fight infection, but medicine has to count on the immune functions of the body taking over at some point. Prevention of repeat infections is also hard to count on with an impaired immune system.

Various antibiotics are used to treat the various diseases associated with AIDS. Radiation therapy and chemotherapy are used to fight cancers associated with AIDS. Again, however, when the body's immune system is not functioning well, the body cannot support the help it receives from drug therapy.

Full-blown AIDS may last for months or even years before an AIDS patient's immune system eventually cannot fight any more disease and the patient dies. Patients may also die from symptoms associated with various diseases. AIDS patients do not die of AIDS. They die of diseases caused by a disfunctional immune system.

For HIV-positive patients, doctors will closely monitor immune functions in the body. Once a patient is diagnosed as HIV-positive, doctors encourage patients to get regular tests to keep a close check on T-cell levels. By monitoring this number, doctors can help by administering drugs to help fight off infections. They can also provide treatment that helps slow the progression of the AIDS virus. One such drug is called *zidovudine*. Its trade name is Retrovir®, but is best known by the public as AZT.

Zidovudine causes problems for some HIV positive patients. In some cases it causes diarrhea, frequent tiredness, and sometimes anemia. **Anemia** is a condition in which the body does not have enough hemoglobin, the protein in red blood cells that transports oxygen throughout the body. An anemic person can become very weak.

Another problem with AZT is that it is sometimes ineffective against new strains of the virus. A **strain** is a variety of the virus. Unfortunately, the AIDS virus has already mutated at least once since the discovery of HIV. Doctors may need to develop other drugs to fight new strains of HIV. This obviously not only slows the possibility for a cure, it also provides more time for the virus to spread in already-infected persons, and in the meantime many more people will become infected.

Another form of disease prevention for HIV-infected persons is administration of a drug called pentamidine. Pentamidine is administered to HIV-positive patients via inhalation therapy. The patients breathe in an aerosol mist of the drug, which helps to protect the lungs from developing pneumocystis carinii pneumonia, the lung infection that frequently infects and kills AIDS patients. Treatments with pentamidine help to prevent infection.

Prevention of AIDS

The best treatment we have for AIDS right now is prevention. Prevention means taking steps to stop people from getting a disease. In this case, it means stopping people from becoming infected with the HIV virus. The best way to prevent the spread of the virus is through education. This is where the esthetician can play a very important part. If you are knowledgeable about AIDS you can help your clients understand the syndrome as well as answer questions about preventing the spread of AIDS. It is, therefore, very important that all estheticians, and in fact all health and personal care professionals, be aware of prevention techniques.

Prevention Techniques

There are basically only two ways to get HIV infection or AIDS through contact with infected individuals. Both ways involve the exchange of blood, blood products, or body fluids contaminated with the HIV virus between individuals.

Because sexual contact is the number one cause of the spread of AIDS, "safe sex" practices must be implemented. Any exchange of blood, semen, or vaginal fluids during sexual contact may cause HIV infection if one person is infected. Precautions must be carefully carried out to prevent exchange of these fluids. The absolute safest prevention technique is abstinence. **Abstinence** means that the persons do not engage in sexual intercourse at all. If sexual partners choose to have sexual intercourse, using a condom (rubber) is important. A latex condom is the only type that is safe to use. Some condoms are made of skin taken from lambs. Skin, as we discussed in Chapter 1, can be permeable. It is possible that a condom made of lambskin will leak semen and cause infection. Condoms must be worn throughout sexual relations, from start to finish.

Avoiding of body penetration is also helpful in preventing AIDS. When the penis enters any body orifice, such as the vagina, rectum, or mouth, the disease transmission possibility is greatly increased.

Monogamy means that two persons who engage in sex are faithful to one another and never have sex with any person except for their spouse or partner. Persons who have been in monogamous relationships for a period of ten or more years, or persons who are in a monogamous relationship where both persons have tested negative for HIV and have received medical counseling regarding proper HIV testing need not worry about HIV infection, as long as there are no other risk factors. Other risk factors include use of intravenous drugs.

The use of intravenous drugs (illegal drugs that are injected by a hypodermic needle into the body) is terrible for the health of any individual. Besides the many health risks that illegal drug use causes, HIV infection is also very possible. People who are addicted to intravenous drugs are often careless about health and hygiene. They use other addicts' needles or share needles that are dirty and contaminated with HIV or many other diseases. Direct injection of HIV-infected blood almost certainly leads to HIV infection.

Dispelling Myths About AIDS

When people do not fully understand something that is life-threatening like AIDS, they tend to be afraid. Because they are afraid, rumors often get started about how the disease spreads. Let's stop some of those rumors. These are the facts about AIDS.

1. The only way to get AIDS is to exchange blood or body fluids contaminated with blood from a HIV-infected person.

2. You cannot get AIDS from casual contact. Sitting next to someone who is infected cannot transmit HIV.

3. You cannot get AIDS by drinking after someone or sharing eating utensils.

4. You cannot get AIDS by hugging, touching, social kissing (on the cheek), or by eating food prepared by someone who is infected.

5. You cannot get AIDS from mosquito or insect bites.

6. No cases of AIDS have ever been associated with French kissing.

7. AIDS is not a gay disease. Anyone can become infected if they engage in unsafe sex or share needles with an infected person.

AIDS and the Esthetician

There have been a few incidences where a health-care worker became infected with HIV due to needle-stick injuries. This means that the health-care worker was accidentally stuck with a used, dirty needle. from a HIV-infected patient.

This, of course, can cause infection in the same way as intravenous drug users. It is very important that all health-care workers and personal-care workers take precautions to avoid such accidents.

We, of course, do not work with body fluids as health-care workers do. However, certain procedures performed by estheticians may sometimes result in very small amounts of blood surfacing on the skin. Extraction, waxing, tweezing, and electrolysis are examples of such procedures. Clients may express concern about your salon's techniques for sterilizing equipment to prevent HIV infection. Because we work in a field that sometimes involves contact with small amounts of body fluids and blood, we must take special precautions when handling clients. We must make sure to follow strict sanitation guidelines and make sure that all our utensils and equipment are thoroughly disinfected at all times. We will discuss techniques to prevent transmission of AIDS and many other diseases in the next chapter.

Skin Symptoms Associated with AIDS

Many symptoms of AIDS affect the skin. Because the skin is on the outside of the body, visible symptoms may be the first detectable sign of AIDS, ARC, or HIV infection. Because many of these symptoms are visible to the naked eye and are on the outside of the body, physicians rely on many of these symptoms to detect an infected person. The good thing about this is that skin symptoms may be identified early in infection and allow the physician to administer treatment before life-threatening conditions arise.

Again, it is important to remember that these symptoms may all be present in normal, healthy, HIV-negative individuals. The esthetician should never mention the AIDS relationship of these symptoms to the client. The esthetician should only refer these problems to a doctor, as you should for any medical condition.

The symptoms, which affect many people anyway, tend to be much more severe and chronic in HIV-positive persons. The treatments for these symptoms administered by physicians are often more intensive to treat skin problems associated with AIDS patients. Many of these symptoms may also affect mucous membranes, such as the inside of the mouth, rectum, vagina, and eye.

Herpes

Herpes is a virus that comes in many different forms. Most people think of genital herpes when they hear the word *herpes*. But, as we said before, there are many different herpes viruses, not all transmitted by sexual contact (Figure 3-1).

Cold sores, for example, result from one form of the herpes virus. Genital herpes is another form. In AIDS patients herpes flareups tend to be much more severe and happen more often. Physicians may give these patients antiviral medications to help the depressed immune system heal the lesions associated with a herpes infection.

Another form of herpes is called herpes zoster, better known as shingles. Shingles is actually an adult manifestation of chicken pox. It can be very painful. Shingles in HIV-positive patients is often much worse and widespread than in normal healthy individuals (Figure 3-2).

Warts

Warts are often recurrent and more widespread in HIV-positive patients. They may occur in unusual places such as the beard area, mouth, and tongue. Plantar warts on the feet or hands may also be present. The physician may find that these warts are

FIGURE 3–1   Herpes Type II in an HIV-positive patient. *Courtesy Rube J. Pardo, M.D., Ph.D.*

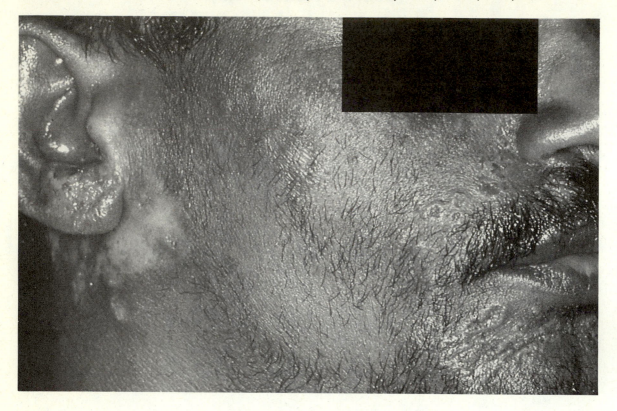

resistant to normal treatment. Venereal warts on the genitals, anus, and vagina are also often seen.

Molluscum contagiosum is often seen in normal children. It often looks like a large group of warts and is often seen on the face.

Infections

Impetigo is a bacterial infection, again often seen in small, normal children. In AIDS patients, again, the lesions can be much worse. Impetigo is characterized by multiple lesions, often in the mouth and chin area. They have a crusty top, but ooze transparent fluid. Impetigo is extremely contagious. Refer the patient to a physician immediately.

Mycosis infections are fungal infections. Many fungal infections can affect both the skin and the internal organs of the AIDS patient. Skin infections from fungi may be indicative of internal fungal infections in AIDS patients. Fungal infections may show many different forms of symptomatic lesions.

Folliculitis is an irritation of the hair follicle and is caused by a bacterial infection. The follicles appear inflamed, are in groups or patches, and often may appear as patches of very tiny pustules.

FIGURE 3–2 Shingles on the neck and face of an HIV-positive patient. *Courtesy Rube J. Pardo, M.D., Ph.D.*

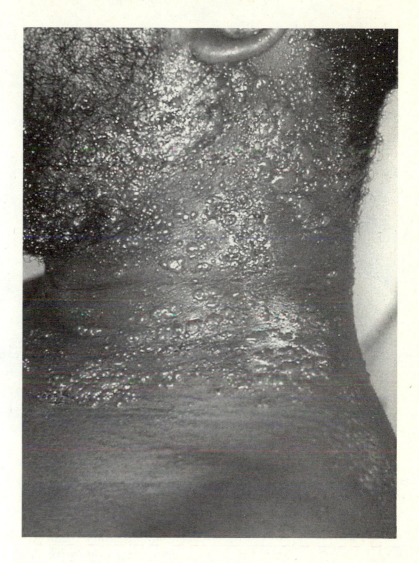

Severe seborrheic dermatitis, or seborrhea, may be seen in HIV-positive patients. Many clients may have small area of seborrheic dermatitis, but in AIDS patients the seborrhea may be much worse. Red, scaly patches in all areas of the face, but especially the hairline and ears, are apparent. Severe seborrhea may cause cracks in the skin and bleeding. Oozing lesions may also be present. The scalp can also be severely affected. Again, seborrhea affects many healthy individuals, but in AIDS patients it is much more widespread, inflamed, and chronic. Normal treatment may prove to be unresponsive. More potent topical steroids are often needed to control the disorder (Figure 3-3). Psoriasis may develop or worsen in AIDS patients.

FIGURE 3–3   Seborrheic dermatitis in an HIV-positive patient. *Courtesy Rube J. Pardo, M.D., Ph.D.*

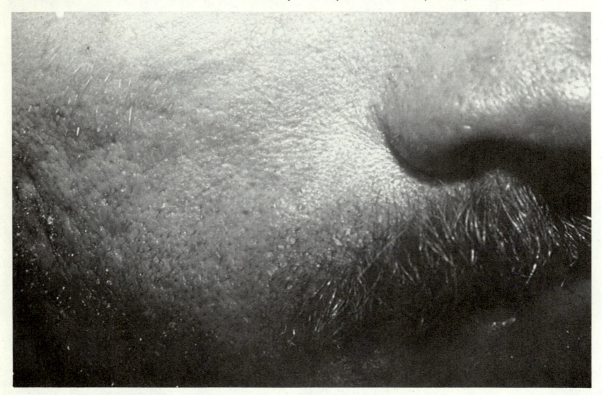

Mouth Symptoms

One of the earliest symptoms of AIDS may be a yeast infection of the mouth called oral thrush. Candida albicans is the name of the yeast that causes thrush. Thrush symptoms include an abnormally thick, white paste covering mouth tissues. It often occurs in HIV-positive patients. It looks like cotton stuck to patches in the mouth. Thrush is often a problem for small children who do not have AIDS. It is not seen often in normal, healthy adults.

Hairy leukoplakia is a tumor-like eruption that can occur on the tongue or the insides of the cheeks. It is hard and scaly looking. Herpes lesions, or "fever blisters," may also affect the inside of the mouth of AIDS patients.

Other Skin Symptoms

Many unusual skin lesions plague HIV-positive patients. Strange skin bumps and lesions may be apparent. Because AIDS patients have lowered resistance to infection, physicians constantly see new and strange lesions on the skin of patients.

Skin Cancers Associated with AIDS

Kaposi's sarcoma is a frequent symptom of AIDS. It appears as purple-brown lesions. It is a rare form of skin cancer, but since the AIDS patient's body is immunosuppressed, is often seen in AIDS patients. Kaposi's sarcoma can also infect internal organs as well as the skin (Figure3-4).

Other skin cancers are also seen in AIDS patients. While not as prevalent as Kaposi's sarcoma, basal and squamous cell carcinomas have been detected in AIDS patients and seem to spread much faster. Malignant melanoma may also be seen and also has a tendency to spread faster in immunosuppressed patients.

The Mental and Emotional State of AIDS Patients

It is possible for an AIDS patient to experience many different emotions concerning the illness. Because it is a relatively new disease, much is still to be learned about AIDS. While we basically understand its transmission and its effect on the immune system and the body, we still have much to learn concerning management of the HIV-positive individual. Because of these uncertainties, AIDS patients may have great difficulty coping with their situations. There is no cure for AIDS. Although the medical community is learning more and more each day about AIDS and management of HIV-infected patients, the disease is still fatal at the time of this writing.

AIDS or HIV-positive patients may feel anger towards others or themselves about the disease. They may also deny having the disease. They experience many of the same emotional conflicts felt by cancer patients. The stigma originally attached to AIDS, a so-called "gay disease," is decreasing, but many people are still not educated about its transmission. This, again, is where the esthetician can play a part in helping to educate the public. If a client says something incorrect about AIDS, tactfully correct the client. Only by getting the right word out can the many misunderstandings about this illness can be clarified.

FIGURE 3–4 Kaposi's Sarcoma in an AIDS (HIV-positive) patient. *Courtesy Rube J. Pardo, M.D., Ph.D.*

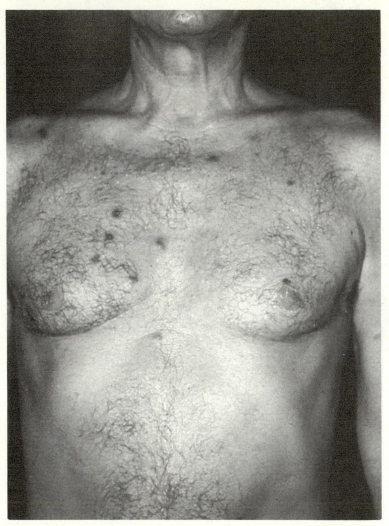

AIDS and the Future

At the time of this writing, there are about 1.5 million HIV-positive individuals in the United States. This number will likely increase. Likewise, the cases of AIDS, ARC, and related diseases will also increase. We hope that a cure or at least a vaccine is on the horizon. Until then, all we have is prevention and education. A client may come to you for advice concerning his or her exposure or illness. You of course should refer the patient to a physician. When talking to HIV patients, use the same caring attitude you would use with any client. These people need lots of help and an understanding, listening ear.

1. Why is it possible for an HIV-infected person to show no symptoms?

2. Discuss the medical management of the HIV-infected person.

3. What can be done to prevent the spread of AIDS?

4. Why is it important that AIDS often affects the skin?

5. Why are skin infections in AIDS patients so much more severe than in healthy individuals?

6. Discuss the future of the AIDS epidemic.

4

Hygiene and Sterilization Techniques

Sterilization, aseptic techniques, good hygiene, and disinfection methods are essential for every health and personal-care practice. Esthetics is no exception. You will learn techniques for disinfecting many salon implements, as well as the importance of aseptic techniques. You will learn to protect yourself and your clients from exposure to pathogenic organisms.

Germs are microorganisms that literally cover almost every surface, including the skin of the human body. Because this is true, it is important that we learn how to control microorganisms through proper sanitation and sterilization.

Let's take a minute to review some of the various types of microorganisms. Bacteria are one-celled microorganisms. There are both pathogenic (disease-causing) and nonpathogenic (non-disease-producing) bacteria. In fact, our bodies need certain types of bacteria to help process foods. However, this chapter will not focus on "good guy" bacteria. We are concerned here about disease-producing, pathogenic bacteria (Figure 4-1).

FIGURE 4–1 Bacterial shapes

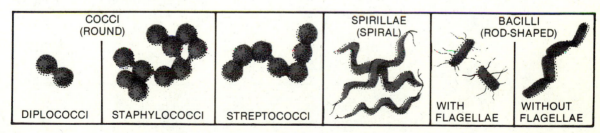

COCCI (ROUND)		SPIRILLAE (SPIRAL)	BACILLI (ROD-SHAPED)	
DIPLOCOCCI	STAPHYLOCOCCI	STREPTOCOCCI	WITH FLAGELLAE	WITHOUT FLAGELLAE

There are basically three types of bacteria:

1. **Bacilli** are rod shaped bacteria that cause a variety of diseases. Among these diseases are tuberculosis and tetanus.

2. **Cocci** are round bacteria that often occur in groups. There are three types of cocci. Staphylococci grow in small groups. Pustules are an example of an infection caused by staphylococci. Staphylococci can produce various systemic infections, which are those that affect the entire body. Localized infections are confined to one area. A pustule is an example of a localized infection. If an infection spreads into the bloodstream, then it is said to be systemic. Staphylococci infections are sometimes called staph ("staff") infections. Streptococci infections cause strep throat. They are another form of cocci. Diplococci, still another form of cocci, cause pneumonia.

3. **Spirilla** are a third form of bacteria. Spirilla are also called spirochetes. They are spiral in shape. Syphillis is probably the best known disease caused by spirilla.

Bacteria can be active or inactive. In their inactive stage, they form cocoon-like shells called spores. Spores are much harder to kill than active bacteria. This is important to know when we discuss sterilization later in the chapter.

Viruses are another form of microorganism. As we discussed in a previous chapter, viruses are not really cells, in that they do not have membranes. They are more like pieces of DNA proteins and are very small.

There are various types of fungi. Mold and mildew are examples of fungi. Fungal infections in humans are known as **mycoses**. Many, many illnesses are caused by microorganisms. The variety of bacteria, viruses, and fungi, and the various diseases they can cause, is much too extensive to discuss in this book. We touch on the basics in order to understand the importance of hygiene and sterilization.

Sterilization

Sterilization is the process of killing all microorganisms, including good and bad ones. Sterilization also kills spores—bacteria that are in their inactive stage.

True sterilization is performed by a process called autoclaving. An **autoclave** is a machine that sterilizes equipment, utensils, and other materials through a combination of steam heat and pressure. It works similarly to a pressure cooker. Microorganisms cannot survive in an autoclave.

Autoclaves have a large metal chamber, in which can be placed metal surgical instruments, sponges, gauze, and other materials. After the chamber is filled with the materials to be sterilized, a heavy-duty door is shut, locking and forming an air-tight seal. The autoclave then heats up, at the same time building pressure inside the chamber. The temperature of the heat goes above the boiling point of 212 degrees Fahrenheit. Articles are sterile when they have been exposed to very high heat (usually about 260 degrees), and sufficient pressure has built up inside the autoclave. Once the autoclave has reached a sufficient temperature and pressure, materials are left to sterilize for about 20 minutes. The autoclave is then vented, allowing the pressure and temperature to drop. The pressure is so high that it is impossible to open an autoclave during the sterilization cycle.

Items placed in the autoclave are placed in sealed plastic or paper envelopes so they remain sterile once the autoclave has completed sterilizing. It is important to read the manufacturer's instructions well before operating an autoclave, because different manufacturers will have different instructions for sterilizing procedures.

Some materials cannot be autoclaved. Glass, for example, cannot withstand the high pressure. Check manufacturers' instructions to see what items cannot be autoclaved.

An autoclave is a very important tool for the esthetician, as well as any other personal-care or health-care professional. In this age of AIDS, it is very important to protect your clients and yourself from exposure to any pathogenic microorganisms. The AIDS epidemic brought great attention to sterilization procedures. However, the AIDS virus is relatively easy to kill through sterilization. Hepatitis viruses, tuberculosis bacteria, and other microorganisms actually pose a much greater health risk in terms of sterilization procedures.

Disinfection is the process of killing the majority of pathogenic microorganisms. Disinfection is the general procedure that is usually followed in the cosmetology industry. Because we do not perform **invasive** procedures, or procedures that enter the body, we do not have to concern ourselves with the types of sterilization that are used in hospitals. However, we do perform procedures such as extraction, waxing, and tweezing that sometimes expose blood on the surface of the skin. Because of this exposure to blood, we must be very careful to use excellent hygiene and sterile or disinfected materials.

Disinfectants are chemicals that kill pathogenic microorganisms. The most popular disinfectant chemical used in the cosmetology industry is quaternary ammonia. Seventy percent isopropyl alcohol is another commonly used disinfectant.

Disinfectants are also used in maintenance, such as disinfectant floor detergents and aerosol sprays, to kill bacteria in the air and control the odors they cause.

Antiseptics are a weaker form of disinfectant. They are usually mild enough to use on the skin. Hydrogen peroxide and other first-aid chemicals are examples of antiseptics.

Aseptic procedure is the term scientists use to describe proper handling techniques of sterilized and disinfected equipment. Placing a sterile comedone extractor on a dirty towel is a violation of aseptic procedure. Handling sterile equipment with other sterile materials is good aseptic procedure.

Theoretically, nothing is completely sterile once a seal has been broken on an envelope of an autoclaved utensil. Because bacteria, viruses, and other microorganisms are in the air, they land on the sterile equipment. But, we cannot sterilize a building or a room, so we must do the next best thing in handling disinfected and sterile equipment with the best hygienic techniques possible.

Hospital disinfectants are somewhat stronger than quaternary ammonia and are being used more frequently in salons, particularly in esthetics and electrolysis practices.

Popular stronger disinfectants are glutaraldehyde, formaldehyde solutions, and sodium hypochlorite (household bleach). These types of disinfectants are very strong. If they are not thoroughly removed by lots of rinsing, the residue can cause allergic and irritating reactions to the skin.

Glutaraldehyde solutions are excellent for disinfecting mask brushes, metal instruments such as tweezers, and other implements that cannot be autoclaved. Glutaraldehyde is available from medical and esthetic supply houses under a variety of trade names.

Glutaraldehyde often comes in concentrated form. It is mixed with water to form a solution that is potent in killing many microorganisms for three weeks. Read the label well and follow all manufacturer's instructions. Household bleach can be diluted 1:10 with water and serves as a good disinfectant for many articles. Besides being used for laundry, bleach can also be used to disinfect sponges and other linens. Do not use bleach to disinfect metal instruments. Chlorine is extremely corrosive to metals!

Disposable Materials

The best way to insure aseptic procedure is to use disposable materials. These materials should be used once and discarded. There is no way to transfer microorganisms from one client to another if you are using disposable materials.

Popular disposable items include:

- cleansing pads made of sheet (roll) cotton.
- disposable one-use lip brushes.
- one-use mascara wands.
- disposable eyeshadow sponges.
- inexpensive cellulose sponges.
- cotton swabs.
- wax strips.
- disposable spatulas for wax or junior size tongue depressors.
- paper towels and sheets.

Lancets should always be presterilized for one use and disposable. Never use a lancet more than once! Electrolysis needles and filaments are also available in disposable types.

Disposables should be discarded in sealed plastic bags. Sharp items such as lancets and electrolysis needles should be disposed of in a "sharps box." A sharps box is a plastic box with a hole in the top in which you place used lancets and needles. The plastic box helps to prevent you or any other persons handling the refuse from accidentally injuring themselves with used lancets or needles. Even though blood is a rarity, it is best to protect everyone by using these precautions.

Nondisposable Items

Some items must be used more than once. Because of expense and practicality, items such as brush attachments, high-frequency electrodes, mask brushes, suction apparatuses, comedone extractors, and other items must be either sterilized or disinfected.

When cleaning utensils you must be careful not to cross-contaminate the utensils. Cross-contamination means that utensils are accidentally re-exposed to microorganisms during handling. Examples of cross-contamination are rinsing utensils in a non-disinfected bowl, handling clean brushes with dirty towels, and re-dipping used spatulas into the same jar of cream.

You must use extreme care not to ever contaminate any item used in treatment by touching it with something that is dirty or has been used on a client. The following are instructions for properly disinfecting implements, utensils, or equipment pieces.

Mask brushes should be autoclaved if possible, but most brushes do not hold up well in the autoclave. The high temperature melts the glue that holds the brush together. Soak brushes well in a disinfectant soap solution. The soak will help loosen mask materials from the brush. After soaking the brushes, put on a pair of gloves and rinse them well in a bowl. After they are thoroughly rinsed, place them in a solution of glutaraldehyde or other medical disinfectant. Let brushes soak for 20 minutes in the disinfectant. Remove them, rinsing well in a different rinsing bowl. It is best to label your rinsing bowls so that you don't rinse disinfected brushes in the soap-rinsing bowl. Remember to rinse very well so that you do not have disinfectant residue on the brushes. Store the disinfected brushes in a large jar until dry. After they are dry, they should be kept in a clean, closed container, a clean drawer, or a UV sanitizer. UV sanitizers are good for storing clean, disinfected items. They kill some types of microorganisms with ultraviolet light. They do not sterilize. Utensils still must be disinfected before they are stored in a UV sanitizer.

Machine brushes should be washed well or soaked in a soap solution to remove all debris. They should then be soaked in a disinfectant solution, similar to mask brushes. Rinse machine brushes well and store in a clean, dry place.

High-frequency electrodes should be carefully cleaned with 70 percent isopropyl alcohol. After initial cleaning immerse the bulb part of the electrode (not the metal part) in a disinfectant solution for 20 minutes. Rinse the glass well with cool water, being very careful not to get the metal part of the electrode wet. Gently dry with a clean towel. Because high frequency is performed after extraction, it is possible that small amounts of blood or bacteria may be present on a used electrode. You should have more than one electrode so that one may be used while another is being disinfected. Do not attempt to autoclave electrodes! Galvanic desincrustation attachments should be thoroughly cleaned with 70 percent isopropyl alcohol after each use. Using cotton covers over desincrustation attachments will also help to reduce contamination.

Iontophoresis rollers should be thoroughly cleaned with 70 percent isopropyl alcohol. The metal rollers can be detached and soaked in a disinfectant solution for 20 minutes. Follow manufacturer's directions for cleaning, as attachments may differ. Be careful not to immerse any electrical parts of the machine.

Again, it is advisable to have additional machine attachments so that one can be used while another is being disinfected.

Suction attachments should be thoroughly cleaned with 70 percent isopropyl alcohol, then allowed to soak in a disinfectant solution for 20 minutes. Store in alcohol or in a clean, dry place.

Comedone extractors are very likely to contain small amounts of blood or debris after use. Clean them well with 70 percent alcohol. It is important to autoclave comedone extractors! If an autoclave is unavailable, soak the clean comedone extractor in a glutaraldehyde solution for 20 to 25 minutes. Rinse thoroughly. Never use an extractor on more than one person without sterilizing!

Tweezers should be cleaned well with 70 percent isopropyl alcohol after each use. Metal tweezers can be autoclaved or disinfected. Store tweezers in a bowl or jar with quaternary ammonia and rinse well before each use.

It cannot be stressed enough that it is important to have additional implements of all types available. It is also very important to be extremely systematic about cleansing and disinfecting all materials at all times. Your entire staff should be aware of salon sterilization procedures so that all staff members follow the same techniques and cross-contamination does not occur (Figure 4-2).

Cleaning Sponges

Ideally, cleansing sponges should be used once and discarded. Many salons include the price of the sponges in the service and then give the used sponges to the client so that they may be used at home between salon treatments.

If disposable sponges are not a possibility, sponges should be washed in the washing machine with chlorine bleach. After washing they should be removed from the washing machine and autoclaved. If an autoclave is not available, the following disinfecting procedure is recommended. Collect several dozen sponges after they have been washed in the washing machine. Place the sponges in a garment washing bag (the kind used for hosiery). Place the bag in the washing machine. Fill the washer with cold water and mix in about a gallon of household bleach. Allow the sponges to soak for 15 to 20 minutes in the bleach solution. Depending on the size of your washing machine, more or less bleach may be added. The bleach solution should be 1 part bleach to 10 parts cold water. After allowing sponges to soak for 15 to 20 minutes, put the washing machine on the rinse cycle. It may be necessary to run the sponges through two rinse cycles to remove all the bleach solution. The spin cycle will remove most of the water. Allow the sponges to dry in a clean place. It is best to store sponges in a UV sanitizer.

FIGURE 4–2 Commonly used disinfectants and antiseptics

COMMONLY USED DISINFECTANTS

Name	Form	Strength	How to Use
Quaternary Ammonium Compounds (Quats)	Liquid or tablet	1:1000 solution	Immerse implements in solution for 20 or more minutes.
Formalin	Liquid	25% solution	Immerse implements in solution for 10 or more minutes.
Formalin	Liquid	10% solution	Immerse implements in solution for 20 or more minutes.
Alcohol	Liquid	70% solution	Immerse implements or sanitize electrodes and sharp cutting edges 10 or more minutes.

COMMONLY USED ANTISEPTICS

Name	Form	Strength	Use
Boric Acid	White crystals	2–5% solution	Cleanse the eyes.
Tincture of Iodine	Liquid	2% solution	Cleanse cuts and wounds.
Hydrogen Peroxide	Liquid	3–5% solution	Cleanse skin and minor cuts.
Ethyl or Grain Alcohol	Liquid	60% solution	Cleanse hands, skin, and minute cuts. Not to be used if irritation is present.
Formalin	Liquid	5% solution	Cleanse shampoo bowl, cabinet, etc.
Chloramine-T (Chlorazene; Chlorozol)	White crystals	1/2% solution	Cleanse skin and hands, and for general use.
Sodium Hypochlorite (Javelle water; Zonite)	White crystals	1/2% solution	Rinse the hands.

Other approved disinfectants and antiseptics are being used in beauty salons. Consult your state board of cosmetology or your health department.

General Cleaning

The facial room should be cleaned between each client. Utensils and equipment should be thoroughly disinfected. All towels and linens should be replaced between clients.

At the end of each day, the room should be very thoroughly cleaned.

The following are instructions for room "shut-down" procedures at the end of each day-

1. Put on a pair of latex gloves.

2. Remove all dirty laundry from the hamper. Spray the hamper with a disinfectant aerosol spray or wipe down with disinfectant. Mildew grows easily in hampers.

3. Remove all dirty spatulas, used brushes, and other utensils. Most of these should have been removed between clients during the day. Thoroughly disinfect all materials.

4. Wipe down all counters, the facial chair, machines, and other furniture with 70 percent isopropyl alcohol or other disinfectant. The magnifying lamp should be cleaned on both sides in the same manner.

5. Replenish the room with fresh linens, spatulas, utensils, and other supplies so it is ready for the next day.

6. Change disinfecting solution as necessary.

7. Maintain vaporizer as necessary.

8. Check the room for dirt or smudges on the walls, baseboards, or dust in corners or on air vents.

9. Vacuum and mop the room with a disinfectant.

10. Spray the air in the room with a disinfectant aerosol spray.

11. Replenish any empty jars. If you are reusing jars for dispensing creams from a bulk container, always use up the entire content of the small jar before replenishing. Never add cream to a partially used jar. Rinse the empty jar well with hot water and then disinfect with alcohol, rinsing thoroughly. Allow to dry before refilling the jar.

Following these procedures on a daily basis will serve three purposes:

- Your room will always be ready the next morning.
- Cleaning at night cuts down on the number of microorganisms that can breed overnight.
- Your room will always be spotless, making your clients confident and reassured that they are being treated in a hygienic environment.

Laundry

Anyone handling dirty laundry should always wear thick rubber or latex gloves during the entire laundry procedure. Dirty lancets, sponges, and gauze may be contaminated and can accidentally get mixed in with the laundry. Sheets and towels should be washed well with chlorine bleach and immediately dried in the dryer. Headbands, turbans, smocks, and labcoats should also be washed in the same manner.

Linen service is an alternative to washing. Linen services are familiar with hospital sanitation procedures and are a good choice if you have little space in your salon.

Protecting You and Your Clients From Disease

Besides the many sanitation, disinfection, and sterilization procedures already discussed, it is important that you personally carry out personal sanitation procedures on a routine basis. You must be careful not to reuse disposable items or to contaminate your products by using a spatula more than once. To avoid cross contamination while removing creams from jars, there are several good techniques to use:

1. Always remove creams from jars with a disinfected spatula. Use spatulas only once before discarding or disinfecting.

2. When removing creams from jars, remove enough for the entire service. It is better to remove too much product than to have to re-dip into a jar. If you need more cream, use a fresh spatula. Place used spatulas in a soaking bowl for later cleaning and disinfecting. You should have at least six spatulas for each client you see per day.

3. It is a good idea to use small, disposable paper cups for dispensing creams. You may prepare measured portions of various products early in the day before clients arrive. Because you have measured the correct amount, this procedure eliminates all chances of contamination because you never touch a client's skin during preparation. Store cream portions wrapped in plastic wrap, or use small portion cups with plastic lids, like the kind used in restaurants for ketchup or sauces.

4. Pumps are another great idea, because they prevent contamination. Cleansers, fluids, and moisturizers can easily be dispensed from pumps. Squeeze bottles with flip-tops are another good type of dispenser. Using these types of dispensers also saves time in the treatment room.

5. Tubes or pumps are by far the most sanitary method for retail client use products. Your clients should also be instructed to use spatulas for jars at home. Using tubes or pumps eliminates this problem.

6. Wax should also be dispensed using one spatula per dip. Again, a larger amount of wax may be removed and placed in a paper cup for application.

Use of Antiseptic Washes

Always wash your hands between clients with a good antiseptic soap or wash. Dispensers are the most sanitary method of accomplishing this. Bar soap is not appropriate because you touch and retouch the bar each time you wash your hands.

Gloves

You absolutely must use latex gloves when performing waxing, or any service that might involve exposure to blood or body fluids. It is strongly suggested to use gloves from start to finish of all facial treatments, electrolysis, and waxing (Figure 4-3).

Gloves will protect your hands from exposure to many microorganisms. If you don't use gloves for the entire facial treatment, at least wear them during and after extraction, through the remainder of the treatment. If you have any cuts, abrasions, or irritations on your hands, you must use gloves at all times!

The best type of glove to use is latex examination gloves. They conform much better to the hands than vinyl or plastic gloves and are much more comfortable for both the esthetician and the client. Many estheticians think that gloves take away the "personal touch" from the client. The truth is that most clients think that gloves feel smoother than hands for massage, and they appreciate your efforts to use sanitary procedures.

Gloves need not be sterile. Nonsterile, disposable, latex gloves usually are available in small, medium, and large sizes from a medical, dental, or esthetic supply house.

Techniques for Avoiding Blood Exposure During Treatment

Always begin extractions from the chin and work upward on the face. If you should encounter blood, gravity will pull the blood down the face and away from areas you will be extracting next. While wearing gloves, try to avoid touching anything but the client's skin. Prepackaged, portioned products discussed earlier will help to prevent you from touching any bottles, jars, or other utensils while extracting.

Using a magnifying lamp during extraction helps protect your eyes from exposure to debris. While masks and eye goggles are necessary for many health-care workers, they are not necessary for estheticians. If you work with an assistant, the person should also wear gloves. Blood may accumulate under a mask in an acne treatment, for example. Wear gloves when removing masks or finishing the treatment. It is generally not necessary to wear gloves during makeup application unless you are working with an acne patient or performing paramedical makeup on a client with open abrasions or incisions. Makeup brushes should also be washed and disinfected between uses. Makeup brushes are damaged much more easily during disinfection than mask brushes. Be careful to use a mild disinfectant for makeup brushes.

FIGURE 4–3 It is important for estheticians to wear gloves during many procedures, including facial treatments, extraction, waxing, and electrolysis.

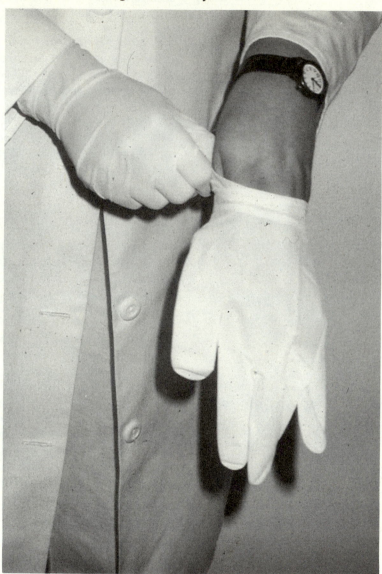

Other Diseases

Most states have cosmetology laws that prevent cosmetology professionals from working on clients with infectious diseases or on clients who have open sores suggestive of infectious disease. Taking a good client history on all new clients will help inform you of diseases that the client may have. Clients with infectious diseases such as conjunctivitis (pinkeye), impetigo, herpes infection, and other infectious diseases should not be worked on until a doctor certifies that they are well.

In Conclusion

The esthetician is at relatively little risk of infection with most microorganisms. However, it is important to take precautions to always avoid contact with blood or other body fluids. Always wear gloves and use the disinfection and sterilization procedures outlined in this chapter. Most important, use common sense. Always be aware of your professional hygiene techniques. Constantly practicing good techniques will become a habit.

TOPICS FOR DISCUSSION

1. What is the difference between disinfection and sterilization?
2. What is an invasive procedure?
3. What is aseptic procedure?
4. Discuss various methods for disinfecting equipment and materials.
5. Discuss general cleaning procedures.
6. Why are gloves important?

CHAPTER

5

Hormones

OBJECTIVES

Every esthetician needs to be familiar with the endocrine system and hormones. Hormones have very definite effects on the skin, and their functioning is directly related to many skin problems. This chapter will familiarize the esthetician with the major glands of the endocrine system and their function. You will also learn about the menstrual cycle, pregnancy, menopause, and diseases and disorders of the endocrine system. How hormones affect the skin will be discussed in depth.

Hormones are special chemicals that are manufactured or **secreted** by glands within the body. As you have previously learned, many glands are present in the body. **Exocrine** glands such as the sebaceous glands and the sudoriferous glands have ducts through which chemicals move. **Apocrine** glands are present in the groin and armpit. **Endocrine** glands secrete hormones. The endocrine glands empty hormones directly into the bloodstream. While most people think of hormones in terms of sex hormones, sex hormones are only a few of the hormones that the endocrine system produces.

Hormones work by transmitting chemical messages to the various body cells. The hormones have special "keys" that fit the "locks" on the cell membranes that they are intended to affect. The key fitting the lock causes the cell membrane to produce enzymes that stimulate other chemical reactions within the cell. The "locks" on the cells are called **receptors**. Each hormone affects specific cells in different ways, and each endocrine gland produces different hormones.

The Endocrine Glands

There are eight major endocrine glands in the human body (Figure 5-1).

61

FIGURE 5–1   The endocrine system

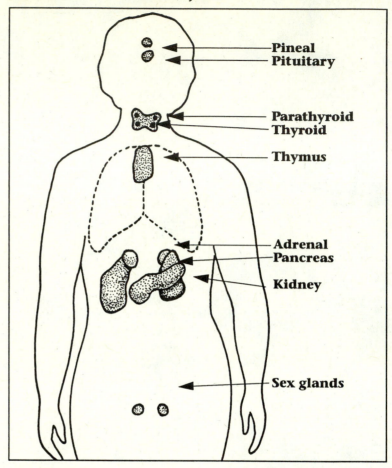

The **pituitary gland** is found in the center of the head. It serves as the "brain" of the endocrine system. It is connected to the brain by another endocrine gland called the **hypothalamus gland**.

The pituitary gland secretes many hormones called **trophic** hormones. Trophic hormones are chemicals that cause other glands to make other hormones. Trophic hormones are "signal hormones." Trophic hormones secreted by the pituitary gland include FSH (Follicle Stimulating Hormone), which is the pituitary hormone that causes production of sex hormones in the glands present in the sex organs. The pituitary gland also produces special hormones that cause regulation of the amount of fluid retained by the body, hormones that control growth, and special hormones that cause the female breast to produce milk.

The **hypothalamus** controls some involuntary muscles, such as the muscles in the intestines that help move food through the gastrointestinal system. The hypothalamus also manufactures a variety of hormones that cause stimulation of the pituitary gland to make other hormones. You might say that the hypothalamus is the "interpreter" between the brain and the pituitary gland. The hypothalamus is able to detect needs of various parts of the body by chemically monitoring the blood that flows through it.

The **thyroid gland** is located in the neck. It regulates both cellular and body metabolism and produces hormones that stimulate growth. One of the hormones secreted by the thyroid gland is called **thyroxin**. Without thyroxin dwarfism occurs in children.

The thyroid gland uses a lot of iodine in its manufacture of hormones. This is why it is important to have some iodine in the diet. Iodine is present in fish, meat, and some vegetables.

Behind the thyroid gland lies a related glandular structure called the **parathyroid gland**. The parathyroids are responsible for regulating calcium and phosphates in the bloodstream, which are necessary for proper bone growth. Vitamin D is an important element in the regulation of calcium also.

The **adrenal glands** are located just above the kidneys. Like hair, they have an inner part called the medulla and an outer core called the cortex. The medulla makes two main hormones, called adrenaline and noradrenaline. These two hormones are needed by the nervous system to transport nerve impulses.

Adrenaline is also secreted when the body is under stress. We have all experienced an "almost accident" when a car pulls out right in front of us. That feeling immediately after an "almost accident" is caused by adrenaline. You could call adrenaline the "emergency hormone." No doubt you have heard stories of people having almost super-human strength during emergencies. This is also caused by the adrenal hormones. When a large amount of adrenaline is secreted suddenly into the bloodstream, the body responds by preparing for an emergency. The heartbeat increases, pupils of the eyes dilate, the bronchi in the lungs expand, and the body generally focuses all its attention on the impending emergency. The cortex of the adrenal glands manufactures steroids, which are very small hormone molecules that are able to penetrate cell membranes and enter cells for specific reasons. The steroid hormones produced by the adrenal cortex are called corticoids. The corticoids help regulate the metabolism and the body's use of carbohydrates, proteins, and fats. They also help to maintain water balance in the body and regulate sodium and potassium levels.

The **pineal gland** is located in the brain, like the pituitary gland. It is very small and is funnel-shaped. Its function is not well understood, but it is theorized that it is related to the sex hormones.

The **pancreas** is located in the abdomen. It has several functions. It secretes pancreatic enzymes that are delivered into the intestine. These enzymes help digest foods taken into the body.

Within the pancreas are a group of specialized cells called the Islets of Langerhans. These cells manufacture a hormone called insulin, which regulates blood sugar or glucose levels. **Diabetes** is a disease that results from the pancreas not secreting enough insulin. Diabetics must take synthetically produced insulin.

The **thymus gland** has already been discussed in the immune system chapter. As you know, it produces specialized lymphocytes to help the body fight disease. The thymus gland grows during childhood and begins shrinking in later years.

The last, but not least of the major endocrine glands are the sex glands. These are the **ovaries** in females and the **testes** in males. The ovaries are located above the uterus and are connected to the uterus by two hollow tubes called the fallopian tubes (Figure 5-2). The testes are present within the scrotum. The testes are connected to another tube called the vas deferens, which leads to a holding sac called the seminal vesicle, which holds sperm manufactured by the testes. This series of tubules continues and eventually joins the urethra, which is the tube that leads to the outside of the penis (Figure 5-3).

Hormones Produced by the Ovaries and Testes

The sex glands of both men and women produce hormones. The testes secrete testosterone. Testosterone is the male hormone responsible for development of typical male characteristics such as a deep voice, broad shoulders, body hair, and other male characteristics. Male hormones are called androgens.

The ovaries produce three hormones. Estradiol is one of the female hormones, better known as estrogen. Estrogen is the hormone that gives a woman female characteristics such as breasts and also helps with the development of the menstrual cycle. Another hormone secreted by the ovaries is progesterone, which is a steroid hormone that helps prepare the uterus for pregnancy and is an important hormone in the menstrual cycle. A third

FIGURE 5–2 Female reproductive organs

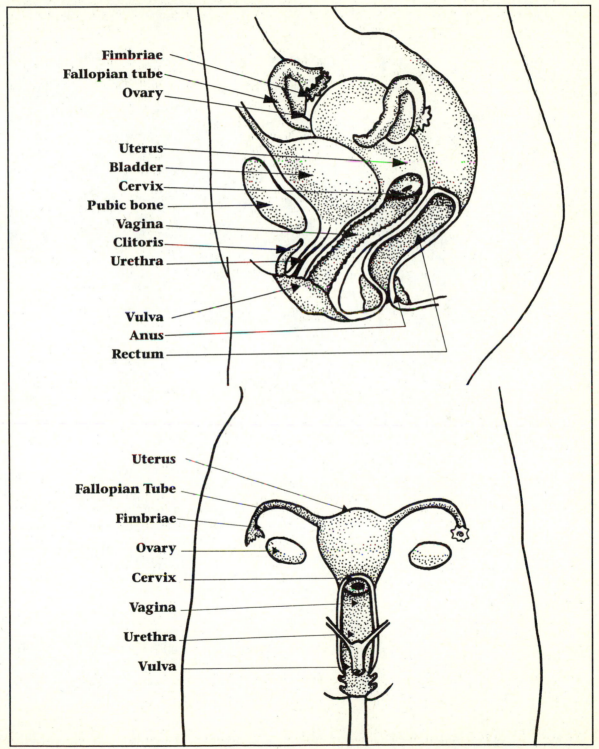

FIGURE 5–3 Male reproductive organs

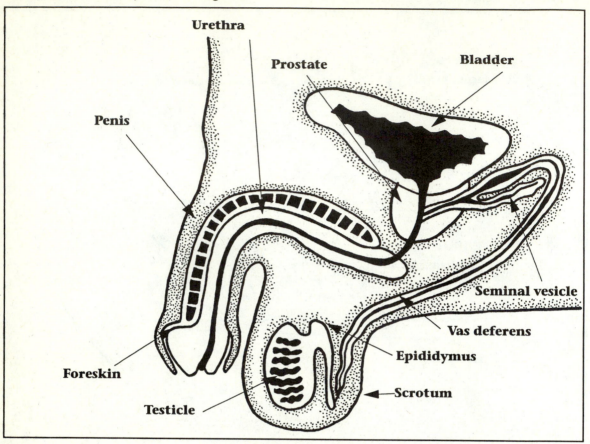

hormone manufactured by the ovaries is relaxin, which helps enlarge the pelvic opening during childbirth.

Both male and female sex glands receive many of their "cues" for hormone production from the pituitary and the hypothalamus. The pituitary makes a hormone called follicle stimulating hormone, referred to as FSH. FSH from the pituitary gland causes the testes to produce sperm. Another pituitary hormone called luteinizing hormone, or LH, causes the testes to manufacture testosterone.

The same types of pituitary hormones cause production of female hormones in the ovaries. The FSH produced by the pituitary causes the development of the ovum, or egg. Luteinizing hormone (LH) causes the actual process of ovulation or the release of the egg (ovum) from the ovary.

Hormonal Phases of Life

There are several phases of life in humans that are dramatically influenced and caused by the presence or lack of hormones. While we produce hormones to some extent throughout life, there are several stages during which pronounced changes occur.

Puberty

Puberty is the stage of life when physical changes occur in both sexes and when sexual function of the sex glands begins to take place. Sexual reproduction is physically possible at puberty.

At the beginning of puberty, which is usually about 12 to 14 years of age (females may be earlier than males), the hypothalamus begins producing a hormone called luteinizing hormone releasing hormone, which in turn stimulates the pituitary gland to manufacture much larger amounts of FSH and LH.

The FSH and LH are trophic hormones. They cause the ovaries and testes to secrete more hormones, specifically estrogens and androgens. The sudden production of these hormones starts a number of drastic changes in physical appearance. Girls begin developing breasts, fat deposits form around the hips to provide feminine curvature, and the sweat glands begin producing body odor. Androgen production in females gives rise to pubic, leg, and underarm hair. In males, these changes in appearance include muscle development, development of the masculine form, broader shoulders, deeper voice, body and facial hair, and general physical growth. Puberty, of course, also triggers sexual attraction to the opposite sex.

It is interesting to note that just when sexual attraction begins, the maintenance of attractiveness gets more difficult! Many changes happen within the skin at puberty. As hormone production of the sex organs begins at puberty, many hormone changes occur that affect the skin. Probably the biggest change is related to the production of androgen, the male hormone, which is produced by both males and females. As the production of androgen begins, the sebaceous glands produce more and more sebum. Androgen is a sebaceous gland stimulant. As androgen enters the bloodstream, it carries its hormonal messages, resulting in appearance changes such as body hair growth and the development of body odor. At the same time androgen also affects the sebaceous glands.

The increase in sebaceous gland activity and production causes dilation of the follicles. This is when "pores" are first easily visible. You may notice that small children have no easily visible pore structure on the skin's surface. The pores become dilated due to increased sebum production. As the sebum fills the follicle, it begins pushing against the follicle walls, stretching them and making the pores on the surface appear larger. The nose is usually the first to develop visible pores. This development of the pore structure will continue into the bridge of the nose, then the forehead, and then the chin. You may notice that a 12-year-old client has visible follicles only in these areas. The scalp also becomes oilier due to androgen production. This is the beginning of what many refer to as the "T-zone," so named because of its pattern (Figure 5-4).

FIGURE 5–4 Developing of the "T-zone" pore structure during puberty

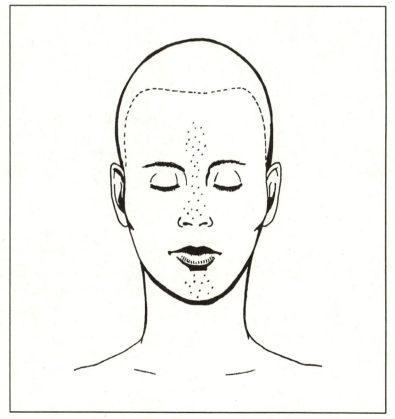

Puberty is also for many teenagers the beginning of acne and break-out tendencies. You may see a young client with large comedones in the nose, chin, and forehead areas, or occasionally only very small comedones in the nose only. The smallness of the comedones at this age is because the follicle walls have yet to stretch out much. The androgens have not yet had their full effect on the sebaceous glands.

Mothers often bring in their young teenagers with all of these problems. The young client should be advised of proper home care, but it is extremely important to keep it simple! Children of this age are often not used to daily skin care. While it is important to instruct them in proper care, they cannot be expected to perform a seven-step regime twice a day! They should be instructed to use a washable, foaming cleanser twice a day, followed by a gentle, low pH toner.

Sunscreen should be used daily. It is important to convince young clients to start using sunblocks on a daily basis. This is the best way to prevent future sun damage. Teaching good health habits at a young age will help the client maintain good skin for a lifetime. Emphasize the dangers of excess sun and give helpful hints about using sunscreens at the beach. Moisturizers are really rarely needed by pubescent teenagers, except in very cold climates. Make sure you always recommend products that are non-comedogenic (see the chapters on comedogenicity and acne).

Treatment in the salon should follow these steps:

1. Cleanse the face well with a cleansing milk for oily or combination skin. Do not use toner or astringent at this point in treatment—the follicles are usually already tight and small. Using toner on this skin at the beginning of treatment will only make extractions more difficult.

2. Presoften the clogged areas by using a desincrustant solution or pre-mask. Steam with this solution on the face for about eight minutes. It is very important that the skin is hydrated for this type of treatment.

3. Remove the pre-mask or desincrustant solution. Gently pat the skin dry.

4. Begin extraction, being careful to explain to the young client what you are doing. Explain to the client that extraction should always be performed by a professional. You may have difficulty extracting these tightly-packed comedones. Be gentle, and take your time. Remember, this is the young client's first experience with extraction!

5. After extraction is complete, apply a toner or antiseptic astringent.

6. Apply a light hydrating fluid and use high frequency.

7. Apply a clay-based drying mask for oily skin.

The first facial treatment for a teenage client should be an educational experience, rather than a "feel-good" treatment. You should help the young client understand (in simple terms) what is happening to the skin and the need for consistent hygiene.

Explain the use of noncomedogenic cosmetics and the need for professional advice in choosing the right products.

Acne development should also be explained to the teenage client so that the client is aware of possible future occurrences and their prevention.

If the young client already experiences acne flareups, you should make the proper treatment recommendations. (See the chapter on acne.) Treatment for most pubescent teens is only necessary bimonthly until further development of the pore structure or the beginning of acne flareups occurs.

Another problem associated with puberty is the development of a condition called **keratosis pilaris**. Keratosis pilaris appears as small pinpoint bumps, usually on the cheeks, accompanied by generalized redness. This condition often seen as "rosy-cheeked" children. In this condition, the androgens have affected the growth of either terminal or lanugo hairs, which have started growing but are not strong enough to push through the follicle opening. The hairs remain trapped inside the follicle and as a result irritate the follicle and the surrounding skin. While this condition is usually treated by a dermatologist, who uses mild retinoids or other exfoliating agents, it is sometimes seen in the salon. You should treat this condition very gently by using mildly abrasive scrubs and light extraction. The routine use of a mild abrasive, such as granular scrubs that are not excessively drying, will help open the follicle and allow the hair to come out, cutting down on irritation. The use of low concentrations of glycolic acid are also indicated and are usually very helpful.

Appearance Changes in Adolescence

As the teenager gets older and further into the teenage years, the client will usually experience more problems with acne. Salon treatments should then be administered on at least a monthly basis, except in cases of more severe acne, when they should be more frequent.

The Menstrual Cycle

With puberty and adolescence comes the onset of **menarche**, the beginning of the menstrual cycle in females. Menarche is the girl's first "period." **Menstruation** is the correct name for the "period." Menstruation is actually the body getting rid of an unused ovum and accompanying endometrium, which is the lining of the uterine wall, that occurs each month in females. The endometrium is formed by the uterus in response to the hormone progesterone. The menstrual cycle is a 27 to 30 day cycle in which the female's ovaries manufacture an ovum and hormonal changes take place that prepare the uterus for pregnancy in case the ovum is fertilized by sperm. When the ovum is not fertilized, the uterus sheds the lining (endometrium), which is menstruation (Figure 5-5).

FIGURE 5–5 The menstrual cycle

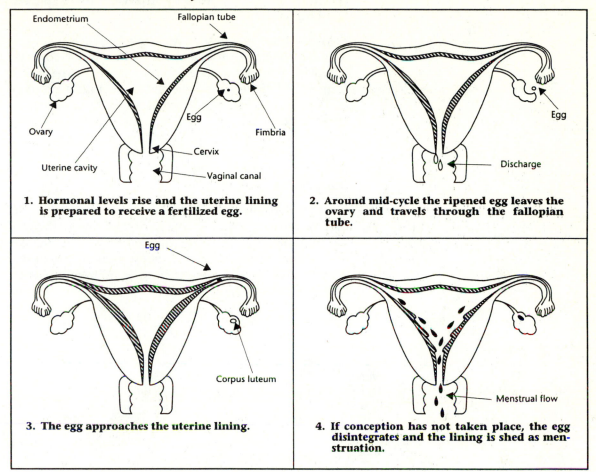

1. **Hormonal levels rise and the uterine lining is prepared to receive a fertilized egg.**

2. **Around mid-cycle the ripened egg leaves the ovary and travels through the fallopian tube.**

3. **The egg approaches the uterine lining.**

4. **If conception has not taken place, the egg disintegrates and the lining is shed as menstruation.**

There are actually six phases to the cycle:

Phase 1 occurs during the first five days of the cycle. The hypothalamus senses low levels of estrogen and progesterone and signals the pituitary gland to secrete FSH and LH. The ovaries then begin producing larger amounts of estrogen and progesterone, which create the ovum.

In Phase 2, the hypothalamus detects that the ovaries are secreting the right amount of estrogen necessary for ovulation, shuts down the pituitary gland's large production of FSH, and begins producing more LH. This occurs during days 6 to 12 of the cycle.

In Phase 3, the hormone levels of estrogen and progesterone are adjusted again. The estrogen level reaches a high point, which signals the pituitary gland to release a very large amount of LH, which then causes the release of the egg from the ovary. The surge in LH occurs in the 12th and 13th days of the cycle.

Phase 4 is on the 14th day, when the egg (ovum) is released from the ovaries and begins its journey down the fallopian tube to the uterus. What is left of the follicle from which the egg was released turns into a hormone producing structure called the corpus luteum, which produces large amounts of progesterone. The progesterone produces the uterine lining or endometrium, which is the "nest" that the uterus builds for a fetus. This 14th day is when a sperm can fertilize an egg and the woman becomes pregnant.

Phase 5 is essentially the last two weeks of the 28-day cycle. If fertilization of the egg has not occurred, the pituitary hormones FSH and LH drop substantially. The corpus luteum shrinks, substantially lowering its production of progesterone. This decrease in progesterone causes the breakdown of the endometrium.

Phase 6 begins menstruation, or the "period." The whole cycle begins again on the 28th day.

Many women experience differences in the actual days on which different phases of the menstrual cycle take place. Stress, obesity, anorexia, and other endocrine system disorders can all affect the cycle.

Pregnancy

If the ovum is fertilized by a sperm on the 14th day of the cycle, the female becomes pregnant. The corpus luteum continues to produce progesterone, and the endometrium becomes much thicker. The fertilized egg goes through a series of transformations, begins mitotic division, and forms a mass of cells. The embryo begins to form, surrounded by a capsule-like structure called a trophoblast. The trophoblast, in simple terms, provides nutrition for the embryo. The membrane of the trophoblast eventually evolves into the placenta, which is a thick layer of hormone-producing cells that serves as the nutrient, oxygen, and waste exchange system between the growing embryo and the blood system of the mother.

The placenta manufactures many hormones, including those that affect the corpus luteum, the growth of the embryo, and the production of milk in the mother's breasts.

Skin and Appearance Changes During Pregnancy

A vast number of obvious changes take place in the human body during pregnancy. Many of these changes affect the skin. Hyperpigmentation is often seen in pregnant women. The skin often tans much more easily than normal. Pregnancy mask is a condition in which the face develops significant hyperpigmentation, resembling a dark facial mask (Figure 5-6a and b). Light

FIGURE 5–6a Mask of pregnancy with hyperpigmentation. *Courtesy Timothy G. Berger, M.D.*

FIGURE 5–6b Melasma in a male patient is very unusual. *Courtesy George Fisher, M.D.*

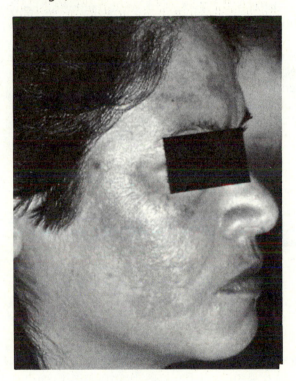

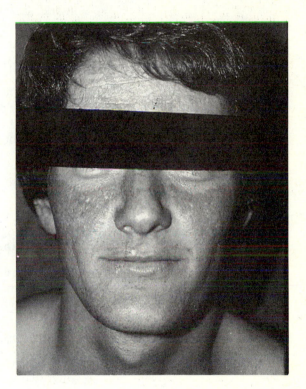

areas surround the eye areas, and the rest of the face is dark with pigment. Pregnancy masks and pregnancy-related hyperpigmentation are caused by a hormone secreted by the placenta, which stimulates the melanocytes, in the skin. Normally hyperpigmentation subsides after the birth of the child, but sometimes the condition will need to be treated in the salon after childbirth. Treating hyperpigmentation during pregnancy is not advisable. Even if there is a bleaching effect achieved by the use of skin bleaches such as hydroquinone, the placenta continues production of the melanin-producing hormone, only to result in more hyperpigmentation. It is best to wait until the pregnancy is over. Observe whether the hyperpigmentation decreases significantly with the shutdown of placental hormones. If the hyperpigmentation does not fade within several months, it can then be treated. Avoiding exposure to the sun will help cut down on the amount of pigment produced during pregnancy. Stretch marks, or striae, are marks that occur in pregnant women. These stripe-like lines may be red or brown-tan in appearance and are the result of rapid weight gain during pregnancy. The skin simply stretches quickly, and the marks occur in the areas of the abdomen, breasts, buttocks, and legs.

Unfortunately little can be done for stretch marks. Many stretch marks fade after childbirth. The use of good, hydrating body creams and lubricants during the pregnancy seems to keep some women from developing stretch marks or at least lessens the severity. The creams must be applied on a daily, consistent basis for best results. In some women creams seem to have no effect. Some theories indicate that the development of stretch marks may be hereditarily or genetically connected. Research is currently being conducted using retinoids, electrical stimulation, and other methods to treat post-pregnancy stretch marks.

An increase in blood flow and blood pressure during pregnancy may lead to the development of **telangectasias,** or small, red, enlarged capillaries on the face and other areas of the body. Avoiding sun and hot temperatures will help lessen the possibility of telangectatic development. Telangectasias are sometimes called **couperose** by European estheticians.

Telangectasias usually fade rapidly after childbirth. If there are still obvious red lines after several months, they may be treated by a dermatologist or plastic surgeon using a special type of current called **diathermy**, or they can be treated by injecting saline or using a laser.

Varicose veins may also develop on the legs during pregnancy, due to weight and pressure on the legs. Resting with the legs elevated helps to prevent their occurrence. Use of support hose is also helpful in preventing varicose veins. Most varicose veins, again, fade after pregnancy, but those that do not can be treated by a dermatologist, plastic surgeon, or vascular surgeon.

Waterproof leg makeup may be used to conceal varicose veins or telangectasias. Pregnant women may also have problems with their facial skin. Fluctuations in hormones may make problem skin worse, or significantly better. In many cases, acne-prone skin will become worse in the beginning of pregnancy, then become much better in the third or fourth month, resulting in clear skin for the rest of the pregnancy. This is the result of the abundant female hormones present in the bloodstream during pregnancy. Acne will often flare up again after the baby is born, or just after the mother stops nursing. This, of course, results from a dramatic drop in female hormones in the bloodstream.

Acne in the pregnant woman should be treated as you would any case of acne (see the chapter on acne), except that therapy with galvanic and high-frequency current should be eliminated.

Precautions for Treating the Pregnant Woman

No type of electrical therapy, specifically galvanic or high-frequency therapies, should be administered to a pregnant woman, except with written permission from her physician. Physicians will often approve of electrolysis treatment, but it is important to get a written note from her doctor and keep it on file with the client's record for legal reasons.

Most routine procedures may be performed on pregnant women. Special courses in body massage therapy for pregnant women are available from certified massage therapy schools. Make sure you have taken such a course before performing body massage on a pregnant woman.

Pregnant women may sometimes develop strange reactions to otherwise well-accepted treatments. Waxing, for example, may suddenly be very irritating to the skin. The only way to predict these types of reactions is to start slowly and patch-test areas for treatment. The woman's physician should supervise any internal or external drugs she takes during pregnancy. Pregnant women need lots of esthetic help during pregnancy. Pedicures may become a necessity, rather than a luxury service. Changes in the nails, skin, and hair may occur. It is also very important to be sensitive to a pregnant client's needs, as pregnancy is a wonderful, but sometimes emotional, time for some women.

Premenstrual Syndrome

Premenstrual syndrome is a condition in which some women experience uncomfortable physical changes before menstruation. These changes are caused by the fluctuating levels of hormone in the bloodstream. Increased estrogen levels may lead to water retention that can cause bloating, swelling of the breasts, swelling of the hands and feet, and general heaviness. The increase in hormones can also cause mood swings and may make the woman more susceptible to stress.

Controlling stress is one of the best ways to deal with premenstrual syndrome, frequently referred to as PMS. Stress-reducing techniques such as deep breathing exercises, aerobic workouts, massage, or general relaxation techniques may help reduce the symptoms. Esthetic care plays an important role in helping women with PMS feel better, both physically and psychologically. Wearing looser clothes may help constricted feelings associated with water retention.

In severe cases, hormones and other therapy administered by a physician may be warranted. Physicians may use drugs for high blood pressure or hormone-suppressing drugs to treat women with severe PMS.

PMS and Acne Flareups

Women frequently experience acne flareups seven to ten days before menstruation. The specific days in the cycle associated with acne flareups may vary in some women. The cause of premenstrual acne is not completely understood. It is theorized that large levels of progesterone, present in the bloodstream during the cycle days normally associated with premenstrual acne, somehow cause the flareups.

Premenstrual acne should be treated in the same manner as any acne flareup. Administering a good deep-cleansing facial treatment one week before the normal monthly breakout seems to help many women reduce or eliminate the flareups. Use of non-comedogenic products also can help control the breakouts, as can other therapies recommended in the chapter on acne. Increased stress during PMS can also cause breakouts or sudden acne flareups. Help your client choose some stress-reducing techniques or suggest that she treat herself to a body massage or other special pampering salon service to reduce stress and make herself feel better.

Birth Control Pills

Birth control pills work by regulating hormones normally associated with the menstrual cycle. They interfere with the normal development of the ovum by preventing or obstructing ovulation.

There are two basic types of birth control pills. One type contains both estrogen and progesterone and works by preventing the egg from maturing, therefore preventing ovulation. The other type is mainly progesterone. These are often called "mini-pills." The mini-pills work by exposing the bloodstream to extra amounts of progesterone, which causes thickening of the uterine fluids, keeping the egg from becoming fertile.

Skin Problems Associated with Birth Control Pills

The biggest problem associated with birth control pills that affects the skin is the tendency of some women to have acne flareups that are caused by hormone fluctuations due to increased levels of particular hormones present in the pills. Mini pills, because they contain little or no estrogen, tend to be more aggravating to acne conditions. Estrogen-dominant pills tend to make acne-prone skin get better.

Starting and stopping birth control pills may have a dramatic effect on acne. Starting an androgen-dominant or progesterone-dominant pill may make acne immediately worse, while starting an estrogen-dominant pill may make acne-prone skin immediately better.

Stopping the pill may have like effects. Because the pill has a tendency to suppress natural hormone levels, discontinuing the pill may throw off natural hormone levels, making acne worse. It may take some time for the body to adjust to not having the hormone "supplement" present in the birth control pills. Some women take much longer to adjust.

Hyperpigmentation and the Birth Control Pill

The other appearance problem related to birth control pills is that of hyperpigmentation, or **melasma**. Splotchy, pigmented complexions may be present after use of birth control pills. This hyperpigmentation usually is located in the forehead and cheeks. The upper lip is also often affected by melasma. Some women can develop a full-scale pregnancy mask associated with birth control pills.

Sunlight, especially deliberate exposure such as sunbathing, can make melasma much worse. Advise a client with melasma to stay out of the sun, and if she must go in the sun to use a strong sunblock. Sometimes the doctor can adjust the client's pill to reduce the possibility of melasma resulting from its use.

You should treat hyperpigmentation with hydroquinone and glycolic acid. See the chapter on retinoids for more information on treating melasma. Paramedical camouflage cosmetics can also be used.

Menopause

Menopause is the time in a woman's life when the ovaries stop producing ova. The pituitary gland secretes FSH and LH, but the ovaries stop responding. The drop in hormone levels in the bloodstream causes a variety of physical symptoms. Hot flashes, rapid heartbeat, decreases in vaginal secretions, emotional irritability, bloating, and other signs may occur.

Esthetlcally, a woman may have thinning hair, or excess hair growth on the face or other body areas, or even experience an increase in oiliness or acne development.

The same symptoms may be produced after a hysterectomy. If a woman has a hysterectomy early in life, the gynecologist often will leave the ovaries and remove only the uterus. The presence of the ovaries will help secure hormone levels in the bloodstream, at least until true menopause takes place. Medical science has discovered that women who lose their ovaries early in life are much more likely to develop **osteoporosis,** a weakening of the bones associated with aging that is predominant in women. Many women have hormone replacement therapy after menopause or after a hysterectomy. Use of synthetic estrogen and progesterone, taken in the sequence of the normal menstrual cycle hormone secretions, helps to prevent many of the symptoms associated with menopause. It, of course, will not make them ovulate again. Estrogen is thought to have a positive effect on lessening the chances of osteoporosis development, a decreased chance of cardiac problems, and may help to prevent rheumatoid arthritis.

About Hirsutism

Hirsutism refers to excessive hair growth. Women who have hormonal fluctuations may experience hirsutism. Excess hair growth, primarily on the face may happen at any time in a woman's life, but especially after menopause. The dominance of the androgenic hormones after menopause is the main cause.

Hirsutism may be treated by waxing or electrolysis in the salon. Excessive facial hair growth is often best treated by electrolysis because the electrolysis is eventually permanent. Waxing may provide temporary relief in minor cases. Stiffer hairs in the chin and lip areas are best treated by electrolysis. Estheticians and electrologists should be aware of other symptoms that may require referral to a physician. While most excessive hair is mainly a cosmetic nuisance, accompanying symptoms such as thinning of the hair, deepening of the voice, and loss of menstruation should be referred to a gynecologist.

Obesity, Anorexia, and Hormones

Women who are extremely obese may experience a loss of hormone activity resulting in menstrual irregularity, hirsutism, and acne. Women who are anorexic may have hormonal fluctuations and irregular menstrual cycles.

Women athletes who have a very low body fat percentage may also experience similar hormonal problems. Many estheticians have observed a correlation in avid female athletes between low body fat, hirsutism, and acne.

Other Hormonal Disorders that Affect the Skin

While it is not the esthetician's job to diagnose illnesses, you should be aware of some symptoms that you may connect with certain skin problems or be able to discuss a client's skin symptoms related to an endocrine illness. You should always refer suspicious skin problems to a physician. If you have a client who has multiple symptoms of any kind of illness, always refer the client to a doctor.

Hyperthyroidism is a condition in which the thyroid gland secretes too much thyroid hormone. Physical symptoms may include heart palpitations, weight loss, and fatigue. Esthetic symptoms include thinning of the skin, hair loss, and rapidly growing nails. **Hypothyroidism** is just the opposite of hyperthyroidism. The thyroid gland does not produce enough hormone. Puffy eyelids, facial swelling, and coarse skin that is very dehydrated are esthetic symptoms of hypothyroidism, if they are also associated with weight gain, poor balance, or hearing problems.

Adrenal gland disorders can also result in skin symptoms. Cushing's syndrome is a disease of the adrenal glands. Persons with Cushing's syndrome secrete too much hydrocortisone. Too much medicinal hydrocortisone can also cause the disease. Symptoms are thinning of the skin and bruises that occur easily. Addison's disease is the exact opposite of Cushing's syndrome. The adrenal glands do not produce adrenal hormones. Skin symptoms include severe hyperpigmentation on the face, dark freckles on the torso, as well as hyperpigmentation on the palms of the hands. Addison's disease is easily treated with hormonal therapy.

TOPICS FOR DISCUSSION

1. What are the major endocrine glands?

2. What is puberty, and what hormonal changes take place with puberty?

3. What precautions should the esthetician take when treating a pregnant woman?

4. What are some esthetic side effects of birth control pills?

5. What are some esthetic problems associated with menopause?

6. Name several endocrine disorders and discuss their effects on the skin.

6

Allergies

OBJECTIVES

While allergic reactions are the domain of the dermatologist and the allergist, it is important that estheticians be very familiar with allergic reactions, sensitive skin, and cosmetic ingredient allergens. This chapter will inform you about sensitive and allergy-prone skin. It will discuss ingredients that frequently cause allergic reactions. The esthetician will learn how to handle allergic reactions and how to help pinpoint ingredient allergens.

Allergies can affect any area of the body, but the skin is probably most susceptible to being affected by an allergy. An allergy is, clinically, the body's immune system rejection of a particular substance. The immune system, for some reason, sees a particular substance (or cosmetic ingredient) as a foreign invader. It reacts by sending out T-cells to fight off the allergy. This immune response is what causes the redness and irritation associated with an allergic reaction on the skin. This is the definition of a true allergy. However, a number of similar reactions may be present on the skin that are not "true allergies."

Sensitive Skin

Sensitive skin is very thin, fragile-looking, pink-colored skin. People with red hair, or of Celtic or Irish, Scottish, or British descent will be more likely to have sensitive skin than other ethnic groups. Because of the sensitive skin's thinness, the blood vessels and nerve endings are much closer to the surface of the skin. This is why this type of skin reddens so easily, but it is also why it becomes irritated by cosmetics more easily.

Sensitive skin will often react to internal factors such as eating spicy foods, stimulants such as caffeine or tobacco (nicotine), or niacin (vitamin B^3). These substances are called **vasodilators**. Vasodilators dilate the blood vessels, making more blood flow through the arterial systems. This dilation will often show up on the skin of a sensitive-skinned person as red, blotchy patches.

They may be isolated on the face, may appear in other localized areas, or may be all over the body. Some clients may tell you that their skin gets red after drinking wine or eating Mexican food. Although this could be an allergy, it is probably just sensitive skin, due to heredity.

Sensitive-skinned clients should be told to avoid spicy foods, alcohol, tobacco products, and any other stimulating foods or consumables. Hot water and any extremes in temperature should be avoided. Aerobic exercise should be done indoors in air conditioning for these individuals. Heat, both body and infrared (sun), can cause sensitive reactions in this skin type. Long-term exposure of sensitive skin to heat, sun, stimulants mentioned previously, saunas, steam baths, or any irritating or hot environmental conditions can cause telangectasias, or dilated capillaries, referred to by European estheticians as couperose.

Symptoms of Sensitive and Allergy-Prone Skin

As we discussed earlier, redness and pinkness is typical of sensitive skin. You will usually observe this, along with skin thinness, telangectasias, and blotchiness, during routine analysis.

Other symptoms may be observed during a reaction. Some of these symptoms are:

- Rash—a splotchy, red, usually flat area, sometimes associated with itching. The area is seldom raised.

- Wheal (also called a welt)—a raised red lesion associated with sensitivity or allergy.

- Hives—a group of wheals with surrounding redness. They often itch or sting. Hives are caused by the release of a hormone-like chemical called histamine. Hives are medically known as *urticaria*.

- **Antihistamines** are drugs that are produced to combat the formation of histamines. Nasal allergies are often treated with antihistamines, but skin reactions can also be treated with the same drugs.

Generalized redness, also called **dermatitis**, which just means inflammation of the skin, may be seen in isolated or general areas.

Sensitive skin is almost always more likely to develop reactions and allergies to cosmetics. Many reactions to cosmetics on sensitive skin may not actually be "true allergies." Irritations develop much more easily on sensitive skin.

Avoid any stimulating treatments such as scrubbing granules, products with large amounts of alcohol, extremely fragrant products, and stimulating masks.

Treating Sensitive Skin

When treating sensitive skin, a few basic rules should be followed:

1. First and foremost, keep the treatment very simple! Do not overcomplicate by trying a large number of techniques. The simpler the better is the rule of thumb when treating sensitive skin. If the client reddens during a simple treatment, it will be much easier to isolate the particular treatment technique that may have caused the irritation.

2. Use unfragranced products. Fragrances may aggravate sensitive skin.

3. Keep heat to a minimum. Prolonged steam, heat masks and paraffin treatments should be completely avoided. Extremely cold compresses should also be avoided.

4. Massage should be very gentle. Use only effleurage, shiatsu, or gentle tapotement. Petrissage should be completely avoided, as should any rapid or deep manipulation.

5. Extraction should be very gentle, at least until you know how sensitive your client is.

6. Avoid enzyme treatments, chemical or mechanical peelings, or scrubs. For home care, follow the same recommendations for allergy-prone skin found later in this chapter.

Suggested Treatment for Sensitive Skin

1. Gently cleanse the skin using a cleansing milk with little or no fragrance or a rinseable cleanser, preferably a product designed for sensitive skin. Follow with non-alcohol, low- or nonfragranced toner. The toner should be extremely gentle and nonstimulating.

2. Steam the skin at a distance of at least 18 to 20 inches for only a few minutes (three to five minutes). You can increase this time slowly as you treat the client in the future and have a better view of her sensitivities. Applying a lightweight hydrating fluid before steam may help cut possible irritation from steam. Hydrating fluid must also be nonstimulating and fragrance-free.

3. You may use galvanic desincrustation at a very low setting (0.2mA) for a very short period of time. Desincrustation should be limited to clogged or acne-flared areas, and should only be performed for about two to three minutes. Again, this can be slowly increased as you progress through the weeks with the client. Dry skin should not have galvanic desincrustation treatment.

4. Brushing and vacuuming should be completely avoided on sensitive skin. Both of these procedures are very stimulating.

5. Proceed with gentle extraction, using the cotton swab technique described in Chapter 14. Avoid using a comedone extractor on sensitive skin. If the skin begins to welt,

redden severely, or swell, stop extraction immediately. Extraction on sensitive clients should be limited to about three to four minutes, particularly during the first visit.

6. Spray the skin with a mild toner solution.

7. If the skin is very red after extraction, allow the skin to calm down before proceeding. Allow the skin a five to ten minute "cool-down" period after extraction. Cool (not cold) wet cotton compresses may be helpful in reducing redness and sensitivity.

8. After the skin has sufficiently "cooled down" and is not swollen or severely red, apply a light, nonfragranced hydrating fluid and gently massage for a short period of time. Remember to use only gentle manipulations. If redness develops or increases, discontinue massage immediately. Massage should be limited to three to four minutes on the first visit.

9. Apply high frequency at its lowest setting for one to two minutes. Ionization may be used instead for one to two minutes, again at a low setting (0.2mA). A cool compress mask or cool "globes" may be used as another alternative. Remember, any treatment should be cool, not cold!

10. Apply a non-setting gel or cream mask. Setting, drying masks should be completely avoided. If you prefer you may use more lightweight, nonstimulating fragrance-free hydrating fluid instead of a mask.

11. Allow the mask to sit for 10 to 15 minutes. Check frequently with the client to make sure it is not burning or irritating.

12. Remove the mask by spraying with a toner solution, then remove the treatment with a wet, cool, cotton pad or a cool, soft cloth.

13. Allow about three minutes before applying protectant or day cream.

It is highly advisable for sensitive clients not to wear makeup immediately after a facial treatment. A waiting period of two hours is recommended before makeup is applied.

Irritations

Irritations are inflammations of the skin that are caused by outside sources. Irritations may be caused from scrubbing the skin too hard, shaving, or certain exfoliating cosmetics or drugs.

Mechanical irritations are caused by things continually rubbing against the skin. They, too can cause skin reactions such as urticaria. Clothing, bras, belts that are too tight, helmets, chin straps, eyeglasses, and even playing the violin can cause skin reactions and dermatitis.

Exfoliants, including scrubs and roll-off type peeling treatments, are examples of possible mechanical irritants. These should be avoided on sensitive skin.

Exfoliating or keratolytic agents such as resorcinol, salicylic acid, glycolic acid, phenol, lactic acid, retinoic acid, and benzoyl peroxide are examples of chemical exfoliants that may be irritating. The reaction they cause is an irritation, due to the way the chemicals work on the skin, but it is not a true allergic reaction.

"While allergic reactions can happen while using all of the above-mentioned chemical agents, they actually exfoliate by irritating the skin. Clients may experience slight redness from these agents, particularly when the client first starts using them. The client may panic because they are slightly red or peeling. The best way to keep the client from panicking is to educate clients about the possible side effects of the treatment. While explaining that peeling and slight redness may be a side reaction to the use of these products, hives, rashes, and excessive itching and burning are not normal. If clients experience these more severe symptoms, they should discontinue use of the product.

Consulting with the Allergy-Prone Client

Clients who have sensitive or allergy-prone skin tend to be cosmetically "gun-shy." Often the new client will have had an unpleasant reaction to a cosmetic years ago and assumes that all cosmetics are bad. The blame is placed on the cosmetic, when it is almost always the person's immune system that is the problem.

There are two ways to help calm the client's concerns. First, you must know what you're doing with allergy-prone skin, and second, you must convince the client that you know what you're doing!

It is important to be honest with the client. Promise to do your best to help the client find usable products. Try to discuss past problems. Ask the client to be specific about what products caused problems in the past. Often you will find that the client experienced an irritation reaction rather than an allergic reaction. The client may have peeled from benzoyl peroxide or retinoic acid, and assumed it was an allergic reaction, when it actually was a normal reaction.

On the other hand the client may have had an actual allergic reaction. Get a description of the symptoms. Minor redness and peeling is usually just an irritation. Hives, rash, wheals, swelling, and itching are usually symptoms of an allergy (Figure 6-1). Another common misconception that many clients have is confusing an allergic reaction with acne. They might say, "I tried this brand of moisturizer, but I was allergic." Upon further investigation, often you will find that she experienced an acnegenic reaction to a product rather than an allergic reaction. It is important to tactfully explain the difference. If the client has a tendency to develop acne, the problem may have been **comedogenic** products. After reading Chapter 12 and 13, you'll be able to help with that too.

Common Cosmetic Allergies

Allergic reactions to cosmetics are in a category of allergies known to dermatologists as **contact dermatitis**, which simply means that when an allergic person comes in contact with a particular substance, a reaction occurs. Not all contact dermatoses are cosmetic, but cosmetics often do cause allergic reactions. It is important that we be aware of the cosmetic ingredients that are most likely to cause allergic reactions (Figure 6-2).

Hypoallergenic cosmetics are cosmetics that have had removed from them many well-known allergens. These ingredients have a history of causing allergic reactions in many people. Hypoallergenic does not mean nonallergenic. There is no such thing as a nonallergenic cosmetic! Somewhere in the world there is a person who is allergic to every cosmetic ingredient! More and more companies now claim that their products are designed for sensitive skin. This usually means that the product is fragrance-free and is free of many common allergens. Basically this is the same thing as being hypoallergenic.

Fragrances

Fragrances and perfumes are the biggest source of cosmetic allergies. Many different fragrances are used in cosmetics, derived from various sources. Some are natural, having been extracted from plants, such as essential oils. Turpenes extracted from trees are another variety. Some musks are derived from animal byproducts, and synthetic fragrances are developed.

There is no real advantage of using natural over synthetic fragrances, except perhaps in the actual odor. Plant extract fra-

FIGURE 6–1 Urticaria (hives). *Courtesy Rube J. Pardo, M.D., Ph.D.*

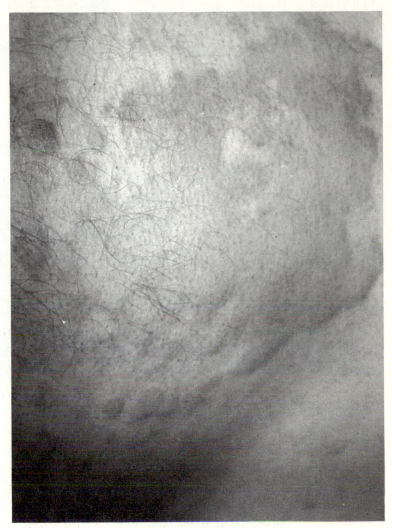

grances, including essential oils, may produce frequent allergies, especially in individuals who are very prone to allergic reactions.

While essential oils are widely used in esthetics, and certainly have their place in facial therapy, they are also capable of producing allergic reactions. Plant extracts of any type are made up of a variety of chemicals, from salicylic acid to water to glucose. They may also contain very small amounts of insecticide or other contaminants. Remember that earlier in the chapter we discussed keeping sensitive and allergy-prone clients' treatments very simple. Unfortunately, when we add a large number of plant extracts, we add many new chemicals. It is best to stay

FIGURE 6–2 Severe contact dermatitis as a reaction to cosmetics. *Courtesy Rube J. Pardo, M.D., Ph.D.*

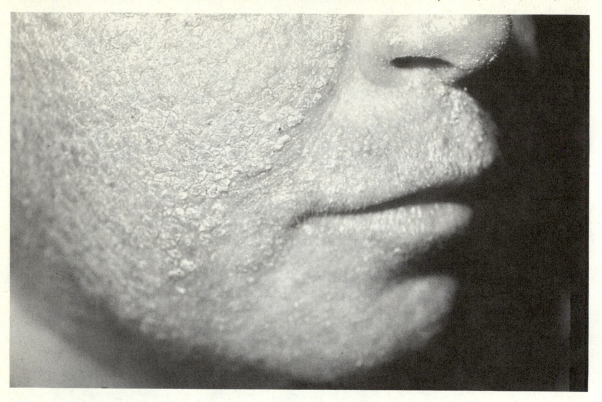

with known chemicals when dealing with ultrasensitive skin. If the client experiences an allergic reaction, it will be much easier to isolate the responsible ingredient.

It is generally accepted by the medical community that fragrances cause most cosmetic reactions. If you have a client who is allergy-prone, it is always best to stick to fragrance-free products, or at least to use a cosmetic that is scented with only one plant oil.

Preservatives

The next category of cosmetic allergens is preservatives. Preservatives are necessary in cosmetic, drug, and food products. They keep harmful bacteria from contaminating these products.

The most frequently used preservative complex in the cosmetics industry is the parabens. Methylparaben and propylparaben are used in literally thousands of cosmetic formulations. It has been estimated that 1 percent of the United States' population is allergic to these preservatives.

Imidazolidinyl urea is the next most commonly used preservative. It is often used with methylparaben and propylparaben, because the three agents work well together against a large number of microorganisms.

Many preservatives work by emitting minute quantities of formaldehyde. Unfortunately formaldehyde is a well-known skin irritant. Used in small quantities, these preservatives do not cause problems for most individuals. However, there will always be some people who are sensitive.

Other frequently used preservatives include quaternium 15, DMDM hydantoin, citric acid, and 2-bromo-2-nitropropane-l,3-diol. A relatively new preservative complex, methylchloroisothiazolinone and methylisothiazolinone, was introduced fairly recently to the cosmetic market. This complex has been found to cause problems when it is put into products that stay on the face, such as creams. It is widely used, successfully, in rinse-off products such as shampoos. For more on preservatives, see Chapter 8.

Color Agents

Color agents are another source of allergies. Color agent allergies are often associated with lipstick and eyeshadow allergies. Lipstick allergy is characterized by swollen, peeling lips after using a particular lipstick. Eyeshadow allergy shows up as red, flaking upper, and sometimes lower, lids. While it is possible to be allergic to any color agent, many people are allergic to the D & C yellow colors and D & C red colors.

Sunscreen Allergies and Sensitivity

Many clients are allergic to sunscreen ingredients. Para-amino benzoic acid, better known as PABA, has caused many allergic reactions. While PABA is an excellent UV-B sun filter, there seems to be a lot of people allergic to PABA. PABA has "cousin" ingredients such as padimate-O, padimate-A, and amyldimethyl PABA. PABA may be present not only in sunscreens, but also in lipsticks, foundations, day creams, and moisturizers. Many cosmetic manufacturers put sunscreen ingredients in day creams routinely. Many do not make a sunscreen claim for the product, but it is nevertheless present in the product.

Salicylates

Many people are also allergic to the salicylates, a group of chemicals related to salicylic acid. Salicylic acid in its oral form is aspirin. Be careful to screen products carefully if your client tells you she is allergic to aspirin.

Salicylic acid is used frequently for treating acne and clogged pores. It is an excellent gentle exfoliant for these skin types. However, it should not be used on clients who have aspirin or other salicylate allergies. Octyl salicylate and phenyl salicylate are excellent sunscreens and may be used in conjunction with other screens in a sunscreen product or day cream.

Other Sunscreens

The two most popular sunscreens at the time of this writing are methoxycinnimate and benzophenone. These two chemicals are often used in combination to screen a wider range of ultraviolet rays. There seem to be fewer reactions to these screen agents. However, some people are allergic to these as well.

Two of the least allergy-prone screening ingredients are zinc oxide and titanium dioxide. Zinc oxide is the white cream that surfers use on their noses to prevent sunburn. These sunscreens work by reflecting the sun, rather than absorbing it.

The good thing about these two ingredients is that few people are allergic. The bad thing is that they are opaque and can be seen, to some extent, while they are being worn. For esthetic purposes, they are rarely used on the whole body. Zinc oxide and titanium dioxide are also often used in foundations because they provide excellent coverage. The sunscreen benefit in these foundations is just an added benefit!

Tips About Using Sunscreens and Allergies

Many clients complain that sunscreens burn their eyes. This occurs when the client gets hot and perspires while wearing the screens. Often the client has applied the sunscreen haphazardly, getting the product too close to the eyes or applying too much at once.

Advise the client to apply the screen about 30 minutes before going out. This will allow the screen to absorb better into the skin and avoid running into the eyes. Using a cream-based screen rather than a gel seems to work better for many of these clients.

Another helpful tip for clients is not to apply sunscreens on hot skin. Many clients will wait until they are already outside to apply sunscreen. Any irritating factor will be more pronounced when applied on skin that is at an elevated temperature. Again, advise the client to apply the screen before going outside.

Gel screens are lighter-weight products and are in general much better for oily, clog-prone, and acne-prone skin types. They are, however, not very waterproof. They often have a base that is an alcohol called SD alcohol, which may irritate some sensitive skins when applied.

Nail Products

Many nail products contain formaldehyde or a formaldehyde derivative. Many people are allergic to nail products. Nail polish, hardeners, conditioners, top and base coats, as well as other nail chemicals, often contain these allergens.

Acne Products and Allergies

Because many acne products are also exfoliants or peeling agents, two factors must be considered to help allergy-prone or sensitive skin. Irritation caused by acne products is often necessary for the product to work. Slight redness, minor irritation, and flaking, peeling skin is a fairly normal occurrence when using peeling agents to treat acne and oily skin.

This built-in irritant can be a problem for ultrasensitive skin. You may find that your client cannot tolerate every-night use of a particular acne product. For these clients, recommend that they apply the product every other night. On the alternate night suggest that they use a noncomedogenic, fragrance-free, hydrating agent. Alternating these two products seems to work well for many sensitive oily skins. The theory is that you are peeling one night and hydrating the next. Therefore you are reducing the amount of irritation and soothing the skin on alternate nights.

Another solution for clients sensitive to acne peeling agents is to have the client use them daily, but only for short periods of time, slowly building up to longer exposure. For example, a sensitive-skinned client may only use benzoyl peroxide for 10 to 15 minutes the first night of treatment. If this short treatment is tolerated successfully, on the next night the client can leave the product on for 30 minutes, and so on. This will slowly build the client's tolerance for the treatment. Your client will learn her tolerance level.

Benzoyl peroxide, an excellent acne treatment, is available in several strengths. The standard strengths are 2 $\frac{1}{2}$ percent, 5 percent, and 10 percent. Sensitive clients may tolerate low strengths much better than higher ones. Unfortunately some clients develop allergies to benzoyl peroxide and have to choose another acne treatment.

There are three alternatives for clients who are allergic to benzoyl peroxide. They are glycolic acid, sulfur combined with resorcinol, and salicylic acid.

Salicylic acid has already been discussed. It is a generally a milder treatment, but cannot be used by clients with salicylate allergies. It is a good treatment, though, for sensitive clients who are not allergic to salicylates.

Sulfur, which is combined in many treatments with resorcinol, is a standard alternative to benzoyl peroxide and is one of the oldest acne treatments. Unfortunately, again, some clients are also allergic to sulfur or resorcinol, or both.

Glycolic acid is a fairly recent addition to the spectrum of acne treatment products. Glycolic acid seems to cause few allergies; however, it does burn when applied and may cause irritation in sensitive clients. Many clients develop a tolerance for the burning sensation when using glycolic acid regularly.

In general, you need to be very careful when treating oily, sensitive skin. Many clients see better results with slow, nonaggressive treatments. Using gentle, rinseable cleansers, toners, and low-strength peeling agents is almost always a better solution for these clients. Try to avoid using a peeling agent in more than one product for these clients.

Other Noncosmetic Allergies

Frequently, you will have clients who are allergic to products other than cosmetics, but these allergies will result in cosmetic skin symptoms. Many clients are allergic to nickel, which is frequently used in laundry detergents and jewelry. Dryer sheets or fabric softeners cause problems for some individuals.

Clients with nasal allergies will sometimes have skin reactions related to their nasal allergies. These clients should be referred to an allergist.

Eyelid Dermatitis

A frequent problem the esthetician sees is eyelid dermatitis. The eyelid skin is the thinnest skin on the human body and is also the most sensitive to irritants and allergens.

Red, flakey, swollen upper and/or lower lids are the signs of eyelid dermatitis (Figure 6-3). If a client comes to you complaining of eyelid dermatitis, you need to check the following:

1. Has the client started any new eye treatment, eyeshadow, liner, mascara, false eyelashes, or any other new eye products?

2. Is the client wearing nail polish? If so, is it a new color or brand?

FIGURE 6–3   Eyelid contact dermatitis from cosmetics. *Courtesy Rube J. Pardo, M.D., Ph.D.*

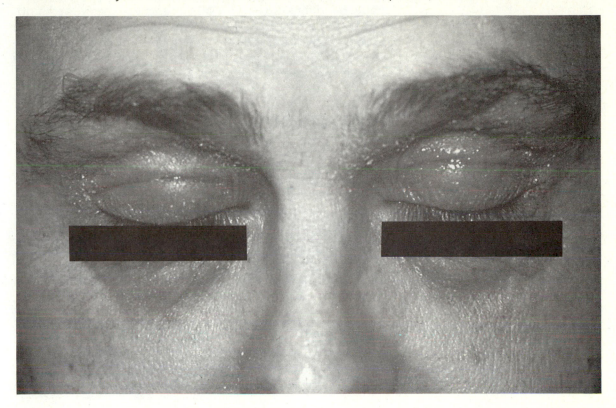

3. Has the client had nail service recently?
4. If *yes* is the answer to question 3, did the nail technician use any new treatment?
5. Does the client have new hand cream?
6. Does the client have a history of nasal allergies?
7. Has the client had an eyebrow waxing recently?
8. Is the client taking any new prescription drugs?
9. Does the client wear contact lenses and therefore use contact lens cleaning solution?
10. Does the client use eyedrops?

All or any of these factors can cause eyelid irritation and dermatitis. If the reaction is severe, the client should be referred to a dermatologist or an allergist.

Besides cosmetic and other products used directly on the eye, nail and hand products seem to cause many of these lid reactions. Suggest that the client remove all nail products until the reaction has cleared. If the reaction clears, the nail products were probably the culprits! Clients experiencing lid irritation should be told to discontinue all treatment to the eye area until the reaction has cleared. If the client must use some product on the area, petrolatum (petroleum jelly) and mineral oil are two of the least allergenic products available. They are very unlikely to cause or worsen allergic reactions.

Treatment for Cosmetic Allergies and Contact Dermatitis

Standard treatment for cosmetic allergies is topical hydrocortisone creams. These hormone-based creams relieve the symptoms. Their effect is in some cases almost immediate. Dermatologists prescribe a variety of strengths of chemical steroidal treatments for skin allergies. In more severe cases, an oral steroid, or antihistamine may also be used.

Estheticians are not qualified to treat allergic reactions. Always refer the client to a dermatologist. You may, however, help the client and the doctor pinpoint the allergic substance. Help the client trace back her cosmetic rituals over the past several days to see if the client used anything that was new or out of the ordinary routine.

In severe cases of allergy, the dermatologist will test the client for individual cosmetic reactions. These tests are usually done on the client's back or forearm. The doctor paints on various cosmetic ingredients in small patches across the back and covers each with a small bandage. Either 24 or 48 hours later, the doctor removes the bandages and checks the client's "patches" for redness, swelling, urticaria, or other signs of allergy (Figure 6-4). The dermatologist can often pinpoint the offending allergic ingredient. Once this has been established, you can help the client by checking any present or future use cosmetics for the allergen ingredient.

This is the standard procedure for dermatological testing for cosmetic allergies. Estheticians can patch test different products on the client as well. If your client has very sensitive or allergy prone skin, patch test new products on the client's back before trying them on the face. The procedure is simple:

1. Check the client's past allergy history. Does the client have any known ingredient, drug, or cosmetic allergies? If she does, you can eliminate using any cosmetics that have those known allergenic ingredients.

FIGURE 6–4 (a) Dermatologist-administered patch tests for various contact allergies; (b) positive patch test indicating allergy to nickel. *Courtesy Rube J. Pardo, M.D., Ph.D.*

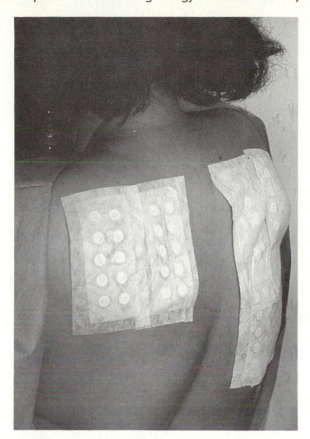 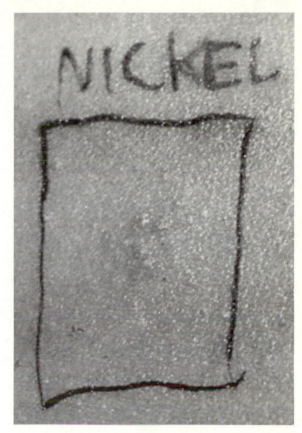

2. Type and analyze the client's skin as you normally would.

3. Select the proper home-care program for the client, taking special precaution to avoid fragranced products as much as possible and avoiding products with long ingredient lists. Also avoid essential oils and other stimulating ingredients.

4. Paint a small amount of each product on the client's back. Each application should be about the size of a nickel. Cover each patch with a bandage and write the coded number of the product being tested. Record the number and the corresponding product on the client record. For example, the test cleanser is #1, the toner is #2, and so on.

5. Instruct the client not to wash her back for the test period.

6. After 48 hours has elapsed, remove the bandages and check each patch for irritation, redness, swelling, itching, urticaria, or flaking. If you see any of these signs, avoid that product.

7. Notice what ingredients are in the offending product and compare the ingredients with the ingredient list of a product to which the client did not react. What do the two lists have in common, or more importantly, what is different about the two lists? For example, if the client reacted to her day cream, which contained a preservative like one of the parabens, but did not react to her night cream, which contained the preservative DMDM hydantoin, you may find that the client is possibly allergic to a paraben.

It takes time and experience to be good at isolating allergic ingredients. An essential knowledge of cosmetic chemistry and ingredients is also essential. If you do not feel comfortable with these procedures, refer the client to a dermatologist for patch testing.

Unfortunately, sometimes what occurs on the back does not occur on the face! The facial skin tends to be more sensitive than the body skin on most people, and occasionally a product that did not react on the back will react on the face! Again, it is important that both the esthetician and the client realize that allergic reactions are seldom predictable, unless it is known what specific ingredients are the allergens.

External Factors that Influence Allergic Reactions

Besides general cosmetic allergies, other factors can influence allergic reactions, and possibly worsen their severity. Climate is one of these factors. Hot, humid weather or extremely cold weather can play a part in allergy. Hot, humid weather is often accompanied by a high pollen or mold count in the air, which can make persons allergic to pollen or mold more susceptible to both nasal and skin reactions. Heat alone can aggravate sensitive skin, enlarging capillaries and making the skin more reactive than normal. Extreme cold can have similar effects. Cold weather and wind tend to dehydrate the skin and make it dry and flakey. Dehydrated, thin skin is almost always more reactive to irritants and allergens. Severely dehydrated skin may burn or tingle when moisturizers are applied. Sunburned skin can also react to cosmetics or other topicals more easily.

The general rule of thumb with all these climatic effects is to stick to simple hydrating, nonfragranced products. Avoid any stimulation of the skin during these weather-induced conditions. Some drugs may make skin more sensitive. The retinoids, such as Retin-A™ and Accutane™ can have side effects of extreme sensitivities to cosmetics and other topical substances. See Chapter 17 for more information on these possible reactions.

Other drugs such as tetracycline, which make the skin more sensitive to sun, may also make the skin more reactive to cosmetics. It is very important to take a health history, including prescription medications. Advise the client to consult a doctor or pharmacist about possible skin reactions to internal medications.

Late Onset Allergies to Cosmetics

Occasionally a client will develop an allergy to a cosmetic after years of use. This is called a **late onset allergy**. Constant exposure to a particular product or ingredient has caused the body to develop an allergy to that product. This may be very confusing to a client who does not understand why the product suddenly causes a reaction. While acute reactions or immediate reactions are more likely to occur with cosmetics, delayed reactions do occur. Try to help the client pinpoint the allergic ingredient, and, after the reaction has cleared, try to help the client find a good alternative. You may need to patch test products to find the right one to use.

Sudden Reactions

A client will sometimes come into the salon complaining of a sudden rash or other allergic reaction or sensitivity. See if you can specify any recent changes in cosmetic habits or lifestyle. Always check for new cosmetics, nail products, and other possible topical contact allergens. If the client has not changed anything about the home care, you must try to find the allergy cause.

Have the client discontinue all home products, preferably including makeup, until the reaction has stopped and all the redness and allergy symptoms are gone. Then, one by one, have the client use products on the skin, each day adding another product. When and if the allergenic product is added, the client will know what it is.

Often a client has actually experienced some allergic reaction other than cosmetic, but because of skin symptoms it appears to be cosmetic. Sometimes these symptoms disappear, never to return. Again, as always, a dermatologist should be consulted for chronic or severe allergic reactions.

What To Do If a Client Has a Reaction in the Treatment Room

Occasionally a client will experience a reaction in the treatment room. Most of these reactions are mild, and many are actually sensitivities rather than true allergies. A client may complain of a particular product burning or stinging. Some products, such as glycolic acid, are supposed to cause a mild burning sensation. Most of the time these minor sensations quickly dissipate.

Red, rashy, swollen skin, however, is not normal. Severe burning and stinging are not normal. If a client experiences extreme burning, redness, or swelling, remove whatever is on the face immediately. Apply cool, wet compresses or spray atomized water on the skin to soothe it. Many times simply removing the offending allergen greatly reduces the irritation. It is always best to end a treatment if a client has such a reaction. Applying further products may only aggravate the reaction. Wait until the reaction has completely subsided for a couple of days before consulting with the client about the problem. As always, severe reactions should be immediately referred to the dermatologist.

The following list of common cosmetic allergens may help you pinpoint possible allergic ingredients for allergy-prone clients or may help you pinpoint possible allergens if your client is experiencing chronic allergies or sensitivities. Remember, no ingredient is nonallergenic. These ingredients, listed by type, are simply some of the more frequent allergens.

Fragrances	Preservatives	Sunscreens
Clove oil	Methyl, propyl, ethyl, or butyl paraben	PABA
		Padimate-O
Eucalyptus	Imidazolidinyl urea	Padimate-A
Jasmine	Quaternium-15	Methoxycinnimate
Sandlewood oil	Benzalkonium chloride	Benzophenone
Cinnamics	Triclosan	Methyl salicylate
Essential oils	Methylchloroisothiazolinone	Octyl salicylate
Geraniol	Methylchlorothiazolinone	**Other ingredients**
Musk ambrette	2-Bromo-2-nitropropane-l, 3 diol	Propylene glycol
Other plant extracts	DMDM hydantoin	Salicylic acid
		Benzoyl peroxide
		Sulfur
		Resorcinol
		Tocopherol
		Triethanolamine
		Formaldehyde
		Hydrolyzed animal protein
		Lanolin

All of the above ingredients are extremely useful in cosmetics, and they all are needed in order to manufacture good cosmetics. Do not arbitrarily eliminate these ingredients as unacceptable.

TOPICS FOR DISCUSSION

1. What is an allergy?
2. What is the difference between a true allergy and a sensitivity?
3. Describe sensitive skin.
4. Discuss some rules for treating sensitive or allergy-prone skin.
5. What is the difference between a reaction and an irritation?
6. Name some common cosmetic allergens and their functions in a cosmetic formula.

7

Essential Knowledge of Chemistry

The esthetician is not really a chemist. The esthetician specializes in applying cosmetic chemicals and teaching clients about their uses. However, it is extremely important that the esthetician have a working knowledge of basic chemistry to better understand the biochemical functions of both the skin's cells and the cosmetics and products used in the practice of esthetics. This chapter will focus on basic principles of chemistry, providing the practicing esthetician with the basic knowledge needed to communicate better with clients about skin care and cosmetic products.

Principles of Chemistry

Chemicals make up our whole world, from the ink on this page to the tip of your finger. Everything is made of chemicals. In the practice of esthetics, estheticians handle many chemicals on a daily basis. When you prescribe a product, or use galvanic current, or clean a steamer with vinegar you are dealing with chemistry. Because our lives, as well as our jobs, involve a series of chemical reactions and procedures, it is important that the esthetician understand the basics of chemistry.

An **element** is a chemical in its simplest form. In other words, it cannot be changed to be any purer by practical purposes and means. There are about 110 elements that make up all chemicals and all matter.

Matter is anything that takes up space and has substance. You are matter. This book is matter. Your products are matter. Essentially everything is matter! And therefore everything is chemicals!

Examples of elements are silver, gold, carbon, oxygen, nitrogen, silicon, hydrogen, sodium, chlorine, etc. Remember, these chemicals (elements) cannot be broken down by ordinary means. The chart of all of the elements is called the **periodic table** (Figure 7-1).

FIGURE 7–1 Periodic Table of the Elements

ACTIVE METALS NONMETALS

1A	2A	3B	4B	5B	6B	7B	8B			1B	2B	3A	4A	5A	6A	7A	8A
																1 H	2 He
3 Li	4 Be	TRANSITION METALS										5 B	6 C	7 N	8 O	9 F	10 Ne
11 Na	12 Mg											13 Al	14 Si	15 P	16 S	17 Cl	18 Ar
19 K	20 Ca	21 Sc	22 Ti	23 V	24 Cr	25 Mn	26 Fe	27 Co	28 Ni	29 Cu	30 Zn	31 Ga	32 Ge	33 As	34 Se	35 Br	36 Kr
37 Rb	38 38	39 Y	40 Zr	41 Nb	42 Mo	43 Tc	44 Ru	45 Rh	46 Pd	47 Ag	48 Cd	49 In	50 Sn	51 Sb	52 Te	53 I	54 Xe
55 Cs	56 Ba	57 La	72 Hf	73 Ta	74 W	75 Re	76 Os	77 Ir	78 Pt	79 Au	80 Hg	81 Tl	82 Pb	83 Bi	84 Po	85 At	86 Rn
87 Fr	88 Ra	89 Ac	104 Rf	105 Ha													
LANTHANIDE SERIES				58 Ce	59 Pr	60 Nd	61 Pm	62 Sm	63 Eu	64 Gd	65 Tb	66 Dy	67 Ho	68 Er	69 Tm	70 Yb	71 Lu
ACTINIDE SERIES				90 Th	91 Pa	92 U	93 Np	94 Pu	95 Am	96 Cm	97 Bk	98 Cf	99 Es	100 Fm	101 Md	102 No	103 Lw

The smallest measurable unit of an element is called an **atom**. An atom is made up of a **nucleus,** which is the center of the atom, and **electrons** which orbit around the nucleus. An atom resembles planets orbiting the sun. The "planets" are the electrons and the "sun" is the nucleus. The nucleus of an atom is made up of **protons** and **neutrons**. Protons are very small positively charged particles, while neutrons are very small particles with no real charge.

Electrons, which orbit the nucleus, are negatively charged. Remember from basic science how positive and negative charges are attracted to one another? This principle is what keeps electrons orbiting around the nucleus. The electrons, which are extremely light (it takes about 1,800 electrons to equal the mass of one proton), are attracted to the nucleus because they are negative. The nucleus, of course, is positive, since it is made up of positive protons and neutrons that have no charge. Electrons orbit the nucleus in circular patterns. These patterns are called electron shells or energy levels. We refer to these orbital patterns as shells or levels. There may be one shell or many shells, depending on the size of the particular atom (Figure 7-2).

FIGURE 7–2 Sodium and chlorine atoms

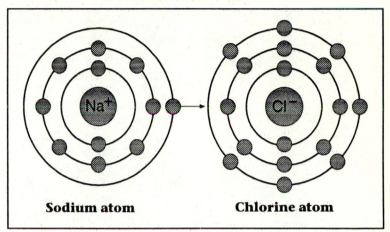

Sodium atom   **Chlorine atom**

All atoms of the same element are exactly alike. They are the same size, weigh the same, and have the same number of protons. Atoms also have the same number of protons and electrons. The atomic weight of an element is the number of protons in one of that element's atoms. So if the number of protons in an atom is the same as the number of electrons in that atom, and you know the atomic weight of that element, you know exactly how many protons and electrons an atom of that element has. For example, hydrogen is a very small atom. It has a molecular weight of 1. That means that it has one proton in its nucleus and one electron orbiting the nucleus. Carbon is a bigger atom. It has an atomic weight of 6. Therefore, it contains 6 protons orbited by 6 electrons.

It takes a certain number of electrons to fill one of the shells, which are also called energy levels. The bigger the element, the more levels of electrons will be present. The first energy level holds two electrons; the second level holds 8 electrons; the third level holds 18 electrons. The reason this is important is because each level has a certain capacity of electrons it can hold, sort of like the capacity of a room. Atoms have a physical need to have full outer levels.

What this means is that if an outer level of electrons is almost full, the level will "want" to fill itself up. If the outer level is almost empty, it will "want" to get rid of its few outer electrons. For example, chlorine has seven electrons in its outer level. It needs eight to complete the level. Chlorine will have a tendency to "want" to fill that level. Sodium, on the other hand has only one electron in its outer level, it will have a tendency to "want" to get rid of that one electron, so its next level will be full. Remember, the normal configuration of atoms is to have "full" outer levels of electrons. Where can the chlorine atom find that extra electron it needs to fill its outer level? Maybe it can get one from the sodium atom that wants to get rid of its outer electron! So chlorine "steals" the electron from sodium, which sodium is glad to get rid of. Both atoms now have full outer levels of electrons. However, remember that we said earlier that each atom had the same number of positive protons in its nucleus as negative electrons orbiting the atom? Now that chlorine and sodium have exchanged electrons, doesn't that change their positive-negative electrical charges? Now that chlorine has an extra electron, it has one more electron than it has protons. That means that it has one more negative charge than it did before. Sodium has lost an electron, so it now has one more proton than it has electrons, giving it a positive charge. It has one more positive charge (protons) than it has negative charge (electrons).

When atoms "steal" or "give away" electrons to each other, the resulting atoms with new charges (and numbers of electrons) are called **ions**. Ions are charged atoms. The chlorine is now negative, and the sodium is now positive (Figure 7-3).

FIGURE 7–3 Sodium and chlorine ions

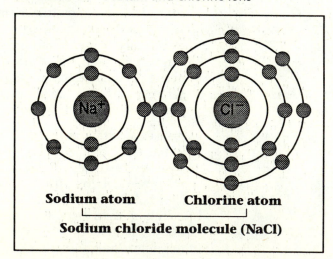

Positive and negative charges are attracted to one another. So chlorine, with its negative charge, will be closely attracted to sodium, with its positive charge. They are so closely attracted they become "locked" together because of their charges. When two or more atoms become "locked" together in this manner, they become a **molecule.** A molecule is two or more atoms joined together. Molecules have completely different properties than individual atoms. Chlorine is a gas, and sodium is a solid. Together in this molecule they are called **sodium chloride**, which is actually table salt! When two ions form a molecule by being attracted to each other's charge, the bond is said to be an **ionic bond**.

Therefore the way atoms are joined together has a lot to do with how many electrons are present in the outer electron levels. The number of electrons in the outer level is known as that atom's or element's **valence**. Low valence atoms are, in general, attracted to high valence atoms.

What happens if an atom has a medium number of electrons in its outer shell? In other words, if the shell is half full, will the atom try to get more electrons or lose outer electrons? Elements with a medium-filled outer level of electrons share electrons, rather than trade electrons like ionic bonds. When atoms share electrons, the bond between the atoms is called a **covalent bond**. For example, carbon has four electrons in its outer level. It needs four more electrons to fill its outer level. So it shares electrons with other atoms. Often it shares with four other carbon atoms (Figure 7-4).

Let's go back and look again at the periodic table of the elements. The elements in vertical columns are called families of elements. The elements that are in the same horizontal column are called a period. The elements are listed from left to right in order of their atomic numbers, or the number of protons in each element's atoms. Also listed is the atomic mass, which for the purposes of this discussion is the weight of an atom of that element.

Each element has its own abbreviation, or symbol. Some symbols are the first letter or the first two letters of the element. Some abbreviations are taken from the Latin word for that element. For example, the symbol for carbon is C, but the symbol for iron is Fe, which stands for *ferrous*, the Latin term for iron.

When atoms join together to form molecules, the number of atoms of each element in the molecule is listed beside the symbol for the element. For example, H_2O is made of one atom of oxygen and two atoms of hydrogen. Hydrogen atoms need one electron to fill the outer level. Oxygen needs two electrons to fill its outer ring. Each hydrogen atom shares an electron with the oxygen atom (Figure 7-5).

FIGURE 7–4   Carbon atoms "sharing" electrons with other carbon and hydrogen atoms

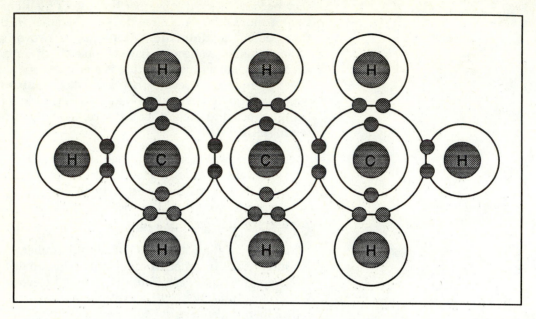

FIGURE 7–5 H_2O molecule "sharing" electrons between hydrogen and oxygen atoms

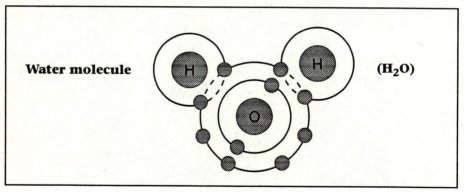

When a molecule joins two different elements together, the reaction produces what is known as a **compound**. A compound is two or more elements joined chemically to produce an entirely different substance. The new substance has completely new chemical and physical characteristics.

A **mixture** is produced when different elements or compounds are mixed together physically, but still retain separate characteristics. Most cosmetic formulas are mixtures. In other words, the ingredients do not change when mixed with other chemicals. We will discuss cosmetic formulations in more depth in Chapter 8.

A **solution** is a mixture of other chemicals. It is an even mixture, which means the various chemicals are evenly dispersed throughout the mixture. An example of this is saltwater. If you mix salt in water, the salt will distribute itself evenly throughout the water. If you keep adding more salt to the water, the salt will begin to pile up on the bottom. This means that no more salt can be dispersed evenly in that amount of water. The point at which mixtures no longer mix evenly is known as the point of saturation.

The liquid part of a solution is called a **solvent**. A **solute** is the solid part of the solution. So, in the example of saltwater, salt is the solute, and water is the solvent. Saltwater is a mixture, not a compound. The salt has not changed chemically, it is simply dispersed through the water. Salt (sodium chloride) is compound, and so is water (H_2O). The two compounds are mixed together but do not react chemically with one another (Figure 7-6). Many cosmetics are solutions. Makeup is a good example of pigments evenly distributed through a solvent of oil or water or both. This, too, is a solution.

pH, Acids, and Bases

When water is added to certain compounds like acids, the water (H_2O) breaks up and restructures, with certain atoms joining the acid chemicals. Hydrogen chloride (HCl), for example, becomes hydrochloric acid when mixed with water. The hydrogen ions float separately in the acid. The measurement of these hydrogen ions is known as the pH of the substance. pH is an abbreviation for the negative logarithm of hydrions (positively charged hydrogen ions). Acids have a low pH, which actually means that they have a large number of hydrogen ions. Alkaline substances, or **bases**, have a low concentration of hydrogen ions. They have high pH values. Acids all have similar chemical characteristics. Bases, or alkaline substances, are also similar to each other.

The pH scale ranges from 1 to 13. The lower the pH, the more acidic the substance. The higher the pH, the more alkaline the substance. Figure 7-7 gives examples of various substances and their pH values.

Why pH Is Important in Cosmetics

The skin has an acid mantle on its surface, made of a mixture of lipids, sebum, and sweat. This acid mantle has a pH of about 5.5. Therefore it has a slightly acid pH.

Cosmetics should also have a slightly acid pH. Higher pH values tend to swell the skin and make it more permeable. This can be

FIGURE 7 – 6   NaCl solution

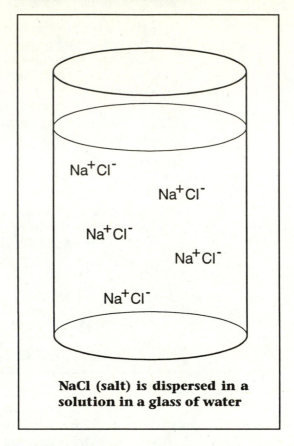

**NaCl (salt) is dispersed in a
solution in a glass of water**

good or bad, depending on the circumstances. For example, desincrustant solutions and "pre-masks" used for treating clogged pores and oily areas need to have a slightly alkaline pH to slightly dilate the pores for easier extraction. They also help to conduct electricity (galvanic current) better for desincrustation.

Cleansers for oily skin may also have a slightly higher pH than that of the acid mantle. This enables these cleansers to perform a more efficient job of cutting the sebaceous secretions of oily or problem skin. Most of these high pH cleansers are followed by low pH toners. A cleanser with a pH of 6.5 or 7.0 is often followed by a toner with a pH of 4.0 or 4.5. High pH values, however, can be harmful to the skin also, particularly if they are not controlled. High pH increases the permeability of the skin, making it easier for bacteria, microorganisms, and other harmful substances to enter the body. Harsh, high pH soaps can be very irritating and can severely overdry the skin.

FIGURE 7–7 Average pH values

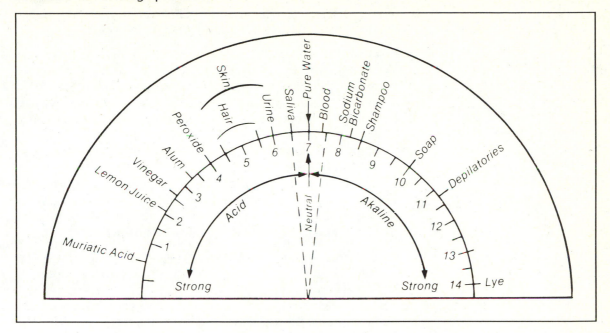

How Chemical Reactions Take Place

Reactions between two elements or two compounds that result in chemical changes are called **chemical reactions.** During a chemical reaction, electrons of the elements or compounds involved begin either to share energy levels in a covalent bond, or to form ionic bonds.

Some chemical reactions take place simply by mixing two chemicals together. Sodium, for example, is very reactive with water. In fact sodium is violently reactive with water. The sodium bonds with hydrogen and oxygen to form sodium hydroxide (lye) and allows hydrogen gas to escape. In the process much energy is given off in the form of heat. The reaction is as follows:

$$2Na + 2H_2O = 2NaOH + H_2 + energy\ (heat)$$

Let's talk about this equation, or symbol, for the chemical reaction taking place. Remember the chemical symbols from the periodic table. Na is the symbol for sodium; O is for oxygen; and H is for hydrogen. The number in front of each chemical stands for the number of molecules of each chemical. Numbers below a chemical symbol stand for the number of atoms of that element in a particular molecule. So, getting back to the reaction, 2Na stands for two atoms of sodium, and 2 H_2O stands for two molecules of water, which equals 2NaOH, two molecules of sodium hydroxide, plus H_2, 1 molecule of hydrogen.

Notice that the same number of atoms are present before and after the reaction. Before the reaction, there were two sodium atoms, four hydrogen atoms, and two oxygen atoms, $2Na + 2H_2O$. After the reaction there are the same number of atoms, only with a different chemical structure. Because of the electron change-overs, we now have two totally new chemicals, lye and hydrogen. Hydrogen, of course, is a gas, and generally escapes into the air. 2NaOH, or 2 molecules of sodium hydroxide, have two atoms of sodium, two atoms of oxygen, and two atoms of hydrogen. The other two hydrogen atoms are given off as H_2 (hydrogen gas). So, equal numbers of the same atoms are on either side of the reaction. This is why the reaction is called an **equation**.

Some reactions such as the one discussed above occur very naturally, by simply combining two chemicals. Other reactions do not happen as naturally. These types of chemical reaction require what is called a catalyst. A catalyst is a substance that helps to cause the reaction, or speed up the reaction, without its atoms becoming a direct part of the reaction's products.

Another condition required for some chemical reactions is heat. Heat can trigger chemical reactions. Some reactions require exposure to ultraviolet light or pressure to take place.

Chemicals Found in the Skin and Body

When we discuss chemicals and chemical reactions within the body, we are talking about a subject called **biochemistry**. Biochemistry is a highly complex subject that we will barely touch. So many complex chemical reactions take place in the body. Many reactions are still not fully understood.

As discussed in previous chapters, almost every body function involves chemical reactions. The hormones that tell our cells what to do are chemicals that react with receptor sites. The pituitary hormones that signal other glands to manufacture other hormones is another example of chemical reactions within the body.

Most of the chemical reactions within the body are called organic reactions. Organic chemistry does not mean natural chemistry. Organic chemistry is the chemistry of compounds containing carbon atoms. Carbon is an element that is a large constituent of almost all the many chemicals in the body. The chemicals that the body uses most are oxygen, carbon, hydrogen, and nitrogen. Carbon and hydrogen frequently bond together in chains. These chains of carbon-carbon and carbon-hydrogen bonds are known as **polymers**. Polymers are found in many of the body's chemicals. Proteins, DNA, sugars, carbohydrates are just a few of the examples of polymers in the body's chemistry.

Protein is made of carbon, oxygen, nitrogen, hydrogen, and sulfur. The basic unit of a protein molecule is called an **amino acid**. Think of amino acids as modules or cars of a toy train. When many different modules are placed together, a protein molecule results. Simple proteins are groups of amino acids linked together. Sometimes the amino acids will have another chemical linked to them that is not an amino acid. These proteins with a non-amino-acid group are called conjugated proteins. Conjugated proteins make up most of the substances found in intercellular cement. Glycoproteins are amino acid chains with a carbohydrate group attached to it. Lipoproteins are amino acid chains with lipids or fats attached to the chain. Phosphoroproteins have a phosphorus or phosphate group attached to the protein chain.

The bond between two amino acid groups is called a **peptide bond**. When many amino acids are in long chains, there are obviously many bonds. A chain of amino acid molecules is known as a **polypeptide**.

Simple proteins make up basic materials for the body's tissues. The skin, hair, and connective tissue are made up of a protein called schleroprotein. The protein that makes up the blood and lymph are called globulins. Albumin is another type of simple protein used in the blood. Nucleic acids within protein DNA structures are another type of simple protein product. The carbohydrate groups include sugars and other compounds. Carbohydrates are formed by a chain of carbon atoms united with oxygen and hydrogen. They form units, similar to protein and amino acid units. A simple unit of a carbohydrate is called a **saccharide**. One saccharide by itself is called a monosaccharide. Two saccharides together are called a **disaccharide**. Many saccharides bonded together are called a **polysaccharide**. Examples of the various carbohydrates are illustrated (Figure 7-8).

Monosaccharides are simple sugars like glucose (blood sugar) Disaccharides include sucrose or table sugar, and maltose, the sugar used to make malted milk.

Polysaccharides are the more complex carbohydrates. They include the sugars in starch and the carbohydrates that make up vegetables and cellulose type substances.

FIGURE 7–8 Examples of (a) monosaccharide, (b) disaccharide, (c) polysaccharide

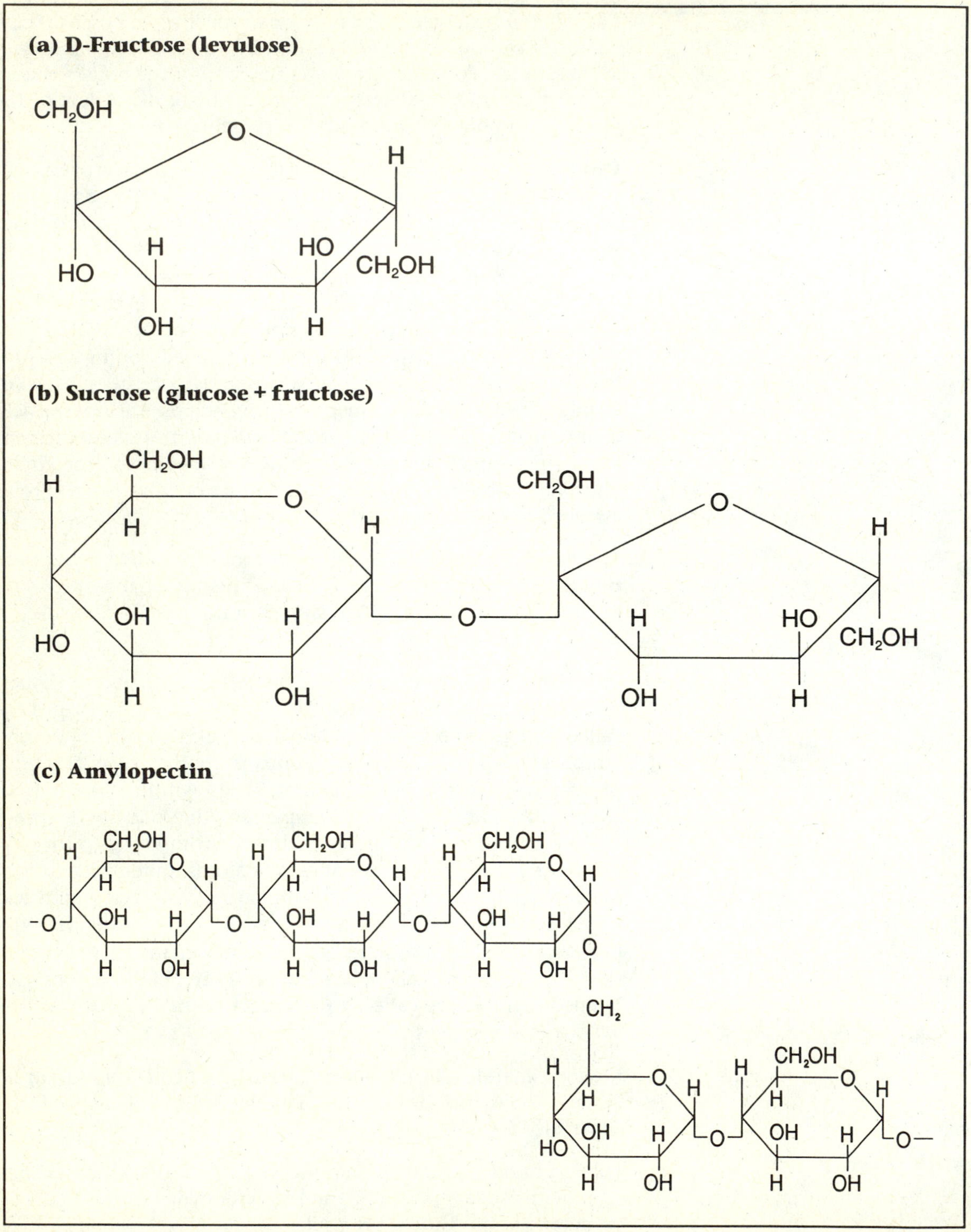

(a) D-Fructose (levulose)

(b) Sucrose (glucose + fructose)

(c) Amylopectin

Lipids are basically fats. They are a third major chemical group within the body. Lipids are made up of carbon, oxygen, and hydrogen. Lipids do not form in units like proteins and carbohydrates. They are more complex. Triglycerides are the best known type of lipid. Other lipids include waxes, fats, and steroids.

Again, lipids are very important chemicals in cosmetology. They can bind with proteins to form proteo-lipids, which are a major part of the intercellular cement. Phospholipids and glycolipids are two examples of lipid-protein compounds found in the intercellular cement.

Chemical Terms Estheticians Should Know

There are a variety of chemical terms besides those already mentioned that estheticians should know to better interpret ingredient labels and understand more about cosmetic chemicals. Some of these words are actually suffixes or prefixes that you will see attached to different chemical names. Most of these are derived from Latin.

Proteo—refers to protein. *Proteolytic*, as in proteolytic enzyme peelings, means protein-dissolving.

Lipo—refers to fats, lipids, or waxes. Examples are lipoproteins, found in the intercellular cement, or liposuction, the surgical procedure used to remove fat.

Saccharides—can refer to any carbohydrate group. An example is mucopolysaccharide a popular moisturizing ingredient.

Saturated—can either mean that a solution has absorbed as much solute as possible, or that a molecule has taken on as many hydrogen atoms as it can hold, as in saturated fat.

Aqueous— water-based, as in an aqueous solution.

Aerobic—refers to a reaction that takes place in the presence of oxygen. *Anaerobic* means without oxygen.

Hydration—water is added.

Homogenous—a mixture that is even. The solute is evenly dispersed throughout the solvent.

Suspension—the solute is suspended throughout a solvent. Suspension is usually not homogenous. A separating makeup foundation is an example of a suspension.

Alcohol—is a molecule that has a hydroxy (OH) group bonded to it. The molecule must be a hydrocarbon made of carbon and hydrogen atoms.

Amino—(prefix) refers to compounds that have an amino acid group attached. May also indicate protein derivation.

Mono—(prefix) means *one*. Example: Monosaccharide, which is a simple sugar with one saccharide group.

Di—(prefix) means *two*. Disodium means two sodium atoms that are included in a molecular structure.

Carbo—has carbon as a base in the molecule. Example: carbohydrate.

Distilled—heating to remove one chemical from another. Water, for example, is distilled by boiling water and allowing the gas to condense back into liquid, separating the water from impurities and other contaminant chemicals.

Enzyme—a protein that is involved as a catalyst in a chemical reaction. Enzymes in cosmetics are often used to break down substances, as a proteolytic enzyme breaks down keratin protein in dead cells. The chemical names of enzymes generally end in the suffix *-ase*. Examples are *lipase* (fat-dissolving enzyme) and *maltase*, which breaks maltose, a disaccharide into two simple glucose (sugar) molecules.

Ionized—substance has been charged by changing atoms to ions. *Deionized* means that ions have been neutralized and do not have a charge.

Poly—means many. Example: *polymer, polysaccharide*.

Tri—means three. Example: *tridecyl trimellitate*, an emollient.

Cyclo—(prefix) means that the molecule is in a ring structure. The carbon atoms are joined in a ring formation.

Aldehyde—a compound made of carbon and hydrogen, with a carbon, hydrogen, and oxygen group on the end of the molecule.

TOPICS FOR DISCUSSION

1. What is an element?

2. Explain why electrons orbit the nucleus.

3. What is the difference between an element, a compound and a mixture?

4. Describe pH. Give some pH values for various substances.

5. Explain how variations in pH affect the skin.

8

Cosmetic Chemistry

It is very important that the esthetician be well-informed about cosmetic ingredients. This chapter is an overview of common types of cosmetic ingredients. Discussion of their chemical functions in formulations will also be included. The esthetician will learn about vehicles, including surfactants, emulsifiers, and emollients. We will also discuss preservatives, coloring agents, and other chemicals necessary to produce cosmetics.

Cosmetic chemistry is a highly complex field. Cosmetic chemists work very closely with cellular function and must be well-versed in medicine, biology, chemistry, pharmacology, and cosmetology. They must be aware of the beauty needs of people, but at the same time be well-trained in chemistry in order to make beauty products.

Making cosmetics is not as simple as many people think. Cosmetics vary greatly in formula. One slight variation in chemical makeup can create a whole new product texture, color, or other property. Cosmetic chemicals are divided into two basic groups. The first group is the **vehicle** group. Vehicles are spreading agents and other chemicals necessary in the formulation of a cosmetic, but they do not necessarily cause the cosmetic to alter the skin's appearance. Chemicals that cause physical changes in the skin's appearance or alter the appearance in any way are called **active agents**. The next chapter will discuss active agents. In this chapter we will primarily discuss vehicle chemicals. Vehicles include a large number of types of cosmetic ingredients.

Surfactants

Surfactants are chemicals in cosmetics that cause the cosmetic to be able to slip across or onto the skin. Surfactants lower surface tension on the surface of the skin to allow cosmetic products to slip across and adhere to the skin. They are one of the biggest categories of cosmetic chemicals.

Surfactants also include detergents and soaps. **Detergents** are surfactants that are used for cleansing. They break up oils, fats, and other debris, and cause the debris to separate from the skin. When detergents are applied to the skin and are mixed with water, they begin to bubble. This bubbling is a good example of how surfactants and detergents reduce surface tension and allow water to spread more easily across the skin. Bubbling is air that has come between the surfactant and the surface of the skin. The surfactant removes surface oils from the skin, as well as makeup, dirt, pollutants and other agents that have come in contact or adhered to the skin during the day.

Another good example of reduction of surface tension by a surfactant is in your kitchen. You cooked hamburgers for dinner and you left the pan with the hamburger grease on the stove while you ate dinner. During that time the grease, which is fats and fatty acids, has solidified in the pan. After dinner, you add hot water to the pan, which liquifies the fat. It is the temperature, not the water that liquifies the fat. If you leave the water in the pan, the grease will remain nonsolid for the most part. But we know that hot water alone will not remove beef grease from a pan.

So you pour in some dishwashing liquid. If you look closely while you are pouring in the dishwashing liquid, you will notice that the fat has a tendency to "run" from the dishwashing liquid. This "running" is actually the surfactant or detergent improving the water's ability to remove the grease from the pan's surface. The grease will break up much faster with the detergent added to the pan.

During the process of cleaning the pan, you accidentally rubbed grease from the hamburgers on your hand. When you remove your hand from the sink, you discover that your hand is greasy. Dipping your hand into the dishwater seems to loosen the grease from your hand. This is because the surfactant (detergent) works on skin in the same way that it works on the dishes or pan.

Of course, the surfactant used in dishwashing is much too strong a detergent to use routinely on your skin. Similar detergent agents may be used in dishwashing liquids, but the concentration of detergent in the formula is far greater than that used in a facial cleanser. Detergent facial cleansers also may vary in strength and concentration. The four major types of surfactants vary with the pH of the water being used in the formulation. The four basic types of surfactants are:

1. **Anionic** surfactants, which have a negative ionic charge. Anionic surfactants are strong cleansers and are frequently used in household products.

2. **Cationic** surfactants have a positive ionic charge. They are frequently used in cosmetics and hair shampoos.

3. **Amphoteric** surfactants may have either a positive or negative ionic charge. They will adapt to the pH of the water used in the solution. Because they are so adaptable to both acid and alkaline water, they are frequently used in facial lotions and creams. The neutrality of the surfactant is important to the mildness of the cosmetic product.

4. **Nonionic** surfactants are used in heavier creams such as hand creams.

Some surfactant ingredients are very frequently used in cosmetic cleansers. Some of these are:

Sodium lauryl sulfate

Sodium laureth sulfate

Disodium lauryl sulfosuccinate

Ammonium lauryl sulfate

Cocoamphocarboxyglycinate

Cocamidopropyl betaine

All of these surfactants can help to remove oils, dirt, and other debris from the skin's surface. How much they remove depends on the amount of surfactant in the individual cleanser.

For sensitive and dryer skin types cosmetic manufacturers often add a fatty acid, oil, or wax to cut the contact of the surfactant with the skin. The fatty substance prevents too much of the surfactant from coming in contact with the skin. Too much detergent can be irritating or dehydrating to sensitive, dry, or thin skin.

Cleansers can also vary in strength directly from the amount of surfactant that is in the formula. A cleanser for oilier skin will, in general, contain more surfactant than a cleanser for dry skin. Most cleansers are carefully prepared so that they prevent irritation on most skin types. Surfactants are also added to creams to improve the cream's slip and adhesive qualities. Some surfactants may be very irritating to the skin when used in creams.

Emulsifiers

Emulsifiers are chemicals that keep water and oil solutions mixed well. Let's go back to the kitchen for a moment. Remember that greasy pan? Let's pretend that the grease is in a mayonnaise jar. If you add water to the jar with grease in it, what happens to the oil? It floats to the top. This is because water and oil will not mix under normal circumstances.

If we add some dishwashing detergent to the jar, the oil will start to "break up." If we put a top on the jar and shake it, the oil will be dispersed throughout the water evenly. The water will become cloudy because the oil has saturated the water in small droplets.

The detergent is what made the oil break into small droplets and disperse throughout the water. But didn't we add a detergent to the water? You thought that this section was about emulsifiers? Well, it is. it just so happens that surfactants, detergents included, are also emulsifiers. They reduce the tension of the water in a cleanser and also reduce the tension of the water in a solution, or even a cosmetic lotion!

Emulsifiers work by forming a sort of "shell" around the very small oil droplets, allowing them to remain suspended in a solution of water. When a solution of water and oil is mixed, and it is mostly water, the solution is called an **Oil-in-water** solution. When the solution is mostly oil, it is called a **Water-in-oil** solution (Figure 8-1).

FIGURE 8–1   Types of emulsions

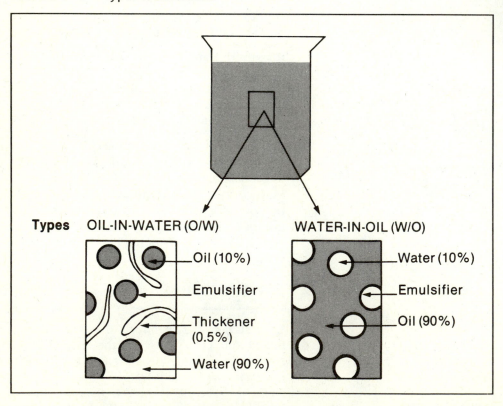

Most lotions available today are oil-in-water emulsions. They are much lighter in weight and texture, feel much less greasy, and are easier to remove. Most bottled moisturizers are oil-in-water (abbreviated o/w) emulsions. O1d fashioned cold creams are a good example of a water-in-oil emulsion. Some heavy night creams are also water-in-oil.

As a general rule, almost anything in a bottle is an oil-in-water emulsion. Almost all water-in-oil emulsions are packaged in jars. They are often too heavy and thick to be poured out of a bottle. Another way to determine a particular product's emulsion type is to check the ingredient label. The FDA requires that cosmetics list their ingredients in descending order. If oil is listed before water, it is a water-in-oil emulsion. If water is listed first, then it is oil-in-water.

Emulsifiers help to provide stability and texture to lotions and creams. They make the cream feel even and smooth. If they were not used in moisturizers the lotion would feel wet and oily when applied! Some frequently used emulsifiers are:

Amphoteric 9

Cateth-20

Beeswax

Polyethelene glycol (PEG)

Polysorbate

Carbomer

Carbopol

Stearamide

"Water-based" generally means that the emulsion or lotion is an oil-in-water emulsion. It does not necessarily mean that the emulsion is oil-free. The main reason cosmetic companies refer to a product as being "water-based" is to appeal to the consumer. Consumers who have oily or problemskin and consumers who do not like greasy products look for products that are watery-textured because they are lighter weight and nongreasy.

How can you tell the difference between the three basic types of surfactants? Surface active agents (which reduce surface tension of water for spreading of cosmetic products), detergents (cleansing and foaming agents), and emulsifiers (which keep water and oils in emulsion state) are all surfactants.

The difference between the three has to do with their molecular structures. The size of the molecule determines the different properties that the particular surfactant will have in a cosmetic solution. Surfactants are polymer molecules. This means that there is a chain of carbon atoms that are connected to one another. Surfactant polymer molecules have two ends. One end is attracted to water; the other end is repelled by water. The end that is repelled by water is instead attracted to fatty substances. **Lipophillic** means *fat-loving*. **Hydrophillic** means *water-loving*. The size of the lipophillic end of the polymer determines which kind of surfactant group the molecule will be. Shorter chain carbon polymers, chains with eight or ten carbon atoms, have a shorter lipophillic end and are surface active agents used in creams to improve slip and spreadability.

Medium-length chain molecules with a medium-size lipophillic end are the detergents used in cleansers that help foam and remove surface debris. Long chain polymers, which have a large lipophillic end, are the emulsifiers. This makes sense, because these molecules must have a strong attraction to fat. Remember, these molecules are the ones that "surround" or form the "shell" around the oil droplets and spread themselves throughout the water solution. The other end of the emulsifier (the hydrophillic end) is attracted to the water in the solution. So the molecule produces a "tug-of-war" between the oil and the water. The emulsifier is attracted to the oil and is more or less wrapped around the oil, but the other end is attracted to the water in which it is floating. This constant "pulling" keeps the oil or fat evenly suspended in the water solution, or vice-versa in the case of a water-in-oil suspension. The oil droplets in an oil-in-water emulsion are referred to as **globules**. They are the dispersed part of the emulsion and are referred to as the **internal phase**. The water in an oil-in-water emulsion is called the **external phase**. A **suspension** is a liquid solution in which the internal and external phases do not stay mixed for any period of time.

We have only talked here about lotions. Many types of cosmetic emulsions are not lotions and contain other components besides water and oils. Makeup, for example, is a solid such as talc that is emulsified in a liquid. The external phase of a makeup base is usually water, possibly mixed with propylene glycol or another solvent. Aerosol hair spray is an example of a liquid that is emulsified within a gas. Mousse is an example of a gas that is emulsified within an external phase liquid.

Emollients

Emollients are ingredients that lubricate the skin and give cosmetics a soft, smooth feeling. Emollients also significantly help adhere cosmetics to the surface of the skin. Because they are so lubricating, emollients are also used as **active agents** in cosmetics. An **active agent** is the part of the cosmetic that actually causes a physical change, which is responsible for the change in appearance that cosmetics create. In other words, it is the active ingredient.

Emollients can sit on the surface of the skin and impede water loss (dehydration.) They are generally made up of large molecules that help prevent water from leaving the surface of the skin. Therefore they help stop water evaporation. Chemists often refer to chemicals that stop water evaporation as **protectants**. Protectants also help prevent other agents from entering the skin. For example, silicone is an emollient that leaves a protective film on the surface of the skin. Silicone foams are used by doctors, dentists, estheticians, other health- and personal-care professionals to prevent constant rubbing of the hands with latex gloves. The foam is applied before gloves are put on. Another good example of how an emollient works as a protectant is applying petroleum jelly to a baby's bottom. The petroleum jelly, also known as **petrolatum,** prevents urine and soggy diapers from irritating the baby's sensitive skin.

Petrolatum is frequently used as an emollient. Because many emollients are good at adhering to the skin, they are also frequently used as vehicles for both cosmetics and drugs. They are often excellent spreading agents. There are many different types and textures of emollients.

Fatty Acids

Fatty acids are derived from plant or animal sources. They are triglycerides that have been broken down by removing glycerin from fat. They help give a soft, firm texture to lotions and creams. They are good lubricants and smooth across the skin evenly. They also add stability to formulations. Fatty acids are a major ingredient of many soaps. When fat is mixed with sodium hydroxide, soap forms.

Fatty acids are also often used in creams, lotions, shaving creams, lipsticks, and are used as pressing agents in pressed powders and blushes. They are also used in foundations and cleansers. Each cosmetic use of fatty acids may be somewhat different.

In lipsticks, for example, the fatty acid may be used to improve creaminess or improve adherability. In shaving creams, **stearic acid** is frequently used because it adheres well to the skin and allows the razor to move smoothly across it. It is also a good protectant against razor burns, and accidental cuts to the skin.

In makeup, it may be used for improving spreadability and texture. In pressed powders and blushes, fatty acids are used to "press" the powder into a cake, which keeps the product in a solid form until it is used.

Common fatty acids used in cosmetic formulations are:

- **Stearic acid**—derived from animal fats and some plants.

- **Caprylic acid**—derived from coconut oil, palm oil, or animal sources.

- **Oleic acid**—from animal fats and vegetable oils.

- **Myristic acid**—occurs in coconut oil, animal fat, palm seed, and other vegetable fats.

- **Palmitic acid**—derived from plant and animal sources.

- **Lauric acid**—derived from laurel oil and coconut oil.

All of these acids are derived from fats (triglycerides) from natural sources.

While fatty acids have many good properties for cosmetic use, many can be comedogenic. (See the chapter on comedogenicity.)

Fatty Alcohols

When most people think of alcohol, they think of isopropyl alcohol, poured on cuts when they were children. They may also think of alcoholic beverages. All of these forms of alcohol have negative connotations. This may explain the notorious (and undeserved) reputation that alcohol has in the cosmetic industry. While isopropyl (rubbing) alcohol can be very drying to the skin's surface, this is only one type of alcohol. The term *alcohol* simply means that an oxygen and hydrogen atom have attached themselves to the end of a carbon chain.

There are many types of **fatty alcohols**, which are fatty acids that have been exposed to hydrogen. They have a slightly waxy feel as a raw ingredient. They are used as emollients. They are less sticky and heavy than many fats. Fatty alcohols are also frequently used to improve the **viscosity** of lotions and creams. *Viscosity* is the thickness and liquidity of a solution. There are many types of fatty alcohols:

- **Cetyl alcohol**—a widely used fatty alcohol. Cetyl alcohol is used as an emollient, an emulsifier, an **opacifying agent** (helps to turn a cream an opaque color, which helps protect the product from light exposure), and as a spreading agent. Cetyl alcohol is derived from animal tallow, but can also be made synthetically.

- **Lauryl alcohol**—derived from coconut and palm seed oils, is used as an emollient and spreading agent.

- **Stearyl alcohol**—derived from stearic acidis used a foam-booster in detergent cleansers, as an emollient, and as a viscosity-opacity builder.

- **Cetearyl alcohol**—a mixture of cetyl and stearyl alcohols; its uses are the same as its parent alcohols.

- **Oleyl alcohol**—derived from oleic acid, is somewhat fattier and greasier than other alcohols. It is often used in superfatted soaps and dry skin emulsions.

Fatty Esters

An **ester** is formed when an organic (carbon chain) acid combines with an alcohol. Fatty esters are used in cosmetics as emollients and conditioning agents. One of their best qualities is that they do not feel as oily to the touch as some other types of emollient fatty ingredients. They can be used to smooth the surface of the skin or hair, to serve as a protectant, to help replace natural esters missing from older, dryer, skin types, and can sometimes be used as an emulsifier.

The easiest way to spot a fatty ester in an ingredient label is that they have the suffix -*ate.* An example is isopropyl palmitate. Isopropyl palmitate is a palmitic acid molecule that has been attached to the carbon chain of an alcohol, propanol.

Fatty esters vary greatly in molecular weight and size. The size can have an effect on how the ester is used in cosmetics. Again, many fatty esters are comedogenic. (See Chapter 13.)

Frequently used fatty acids in cosmetic formulations are:

Isopropyl myristate

Isopropyl palmitate

Octyl palmitate

Octyl stearate

Isopropyl isostearate

Glyceryl stearate

Propylene glycol dicaprate/dicaprylate

Cetyl palmirate

Decyl oleate

Solvents

Solvents have already been discussed in the chemistry chapter. Solvents are used in cosmetic formulations either as vehicles for the product or as vehicles for other ingredients.

Plant extracts used in cosmetics, for example, have to be extracted from the actual plant. The solvent normally used for extraction is propylene glycol. So, if you see "arnica extract" on a cosmetic label, it often means that the arnica extract is present in a solution of propylene glycol or another solvent. Alcohols of various types are also often used as solvents for plant extracts.

Preservatives

Preservatives are chemical agents that inhibit the growth of microorganisms in creams or cosmetic products. Because of the many fats used in cosmetics, formulations are more susceptible to invasion by microorganisms than other types of chemical formulations.

The three main types of microorganisms present in cosmetic formulations are bacteria, fungi, and yeast. Cosmetics may become contaminated because of cross-contamination by the user. The user will apply the cream to the skin, re-dipping the same hand that has touched the skin into the jar of cream. When the fingers touch the cream, bacteria and other microorganisms come in contact with the product in the jar.

Preservatives must be added to cosmetics to kill these contaminating bacteria. Bacteria are also present in small amounts in the raw ingredients used to make the cosmetic. In the making of cosmetics, preservatives are usually the first or one of the first ingredients used in the production process. This is because, if the preservative is already in the mixing tank, any bacteria introduced into the formula will be killed as ingredients are added.

Preservatives work by either directly poisoning bacteria or releasing other chemicals that poison the microorganisms. We have already discussed the allergy possibilities associated with preservatives. It is important that enough preservative be used in the cosmetic formulation to kill microorganisms without adding so much preservative that allergies will be more likely to flare.

The most commonly used preservatives are methylparaben, propylparaben and imidazolidinyl urea. Other paraben groups such as ethyl and butyl paraben are also used.

There are many preservative agents besides those already mentioned used in cosmetic formulations. Some of the more frequently used preservatives are:

Methylparaben

Propylparaben

Ethylparaben

Butylparaben

Imidazolidinyl urea

DMDM hydantoin

Methylchloroisothiazolinone

Methylchlorothiazolinone

Quaternium-15

Diazolidinyl urea

Preservatives are used in very small quantities so they do not cause unnecessary irritation. Because they are present in small quantities, they are almost always some of the very last ingredients to be listed on an ingredient label. Remember, federal law says that ingredients must be listed in descending order of their presence amount.

Other Types of Preservatives

Besides microorganisms, chemical reactions can take place that can alter or even ruin cosmetics. **Oxidation** is one of these chemical reactions. Oxidation is the process by which oxygen is exposed to certain ingredients, which results in a breakdown of the ingredient. Fats and fatty substances are particularly vulnerable to oxidation. Have you ever been to a picnic and noticed that the potato salad is a yellowish color on the top, but when you spoon some onto your plate, noticed that the potato salad below the surface is lighter?

This is oxidation. One of the main ingredients in potato salad is mayonnaise, which is mainly oil. The oil in the mayonnaise oxidizes very quickly, causing the yellow color on the top of the potato salad.

The exact same reaction takes place in the fats, fatty acids, and esters in cosmetic products. Oxygen constantly comes in contact with the cream during the manufacturing process. After the product is opened by the consumer, the product is exposed to more oxygen. Every time the consumer opens and shuts the container, the product is exposed to oxygen.

Antioxidants are chemicals that are added to cosmetic formulas to prevent oxidation. They also keep creams and other products from developing color and odor changes caused by oxidation. A bad odor may develop in creams that do not contain enough antioxidant. An oxidized cosmetic product that has discoloration and/or odor due to oxidation is said to be **rancid**. Commonly used antioxidants are:

> Butylated hydroxyanisole (BHA)
>
> Butylated hydroxytoluene (BHT)
>
> Tocopherol (Vitamin E)
>
> Benzoic acid

Chelating Agents

A **chelating agent** is a chemical that is added to cosmetics to improve the efficiency of the preservative. Chelating agents work by breaking down the cell walls of bacteria and other microorganisms so that the preservative is more easily absorbed by the microorganism.

Common chelating ingredients are disodium EDTA, trisodium EDTA, and tetrasodium EDTA. EDTA stands for the chemical name *ethylenediamine tetraacetic acid*. Again, you will see these ingredients further down on the ingredient list because they are not used in large quantities.

Buffering Agents

Buffering refers to adjusting the pH of a product to make it more acceptable to the skin. Sometimes, when products are made, the pH of the end product may be too high or too low. These pH levels may be irritating to the skin if they are not adjusted.

To remedy this problem the chemist will add a small amount of an acidic or basic chemical to bring the pH up or lower it appropriately. Citric acid is commonly used to lower the pH of a product. Tartaric acid is another acidic agent used in small quantities to bring the pH down to an acceptable acid level.

Some products have the opposite problem. The product turns out to be too acid for the skin. Ammonium carbonate or calcium carbonate is sometimes added to a product to raise the pH. Both of these buffering agents are added in very small quantities and again will be seen lower on the ingredient label, indicating their small concentration in the product.

Gellants and Thickening Agents

A **Gellant** is an agent that is added to a product to give it a gel-like consistency. It improves the appearance of the product and gives it more body, making it stiffer and less runny. Thickening agents make the product thicker, so that it spreads more easily, is easier to handle, and is more acceptable to the eye.

Examples of thickening and gellant agents are methyl cellulose, xanthum gum, beeswax, and carbomer. Many thickening agents can also be used as emulsifiers.

Coloring Agents

Colors are added to products to make them more appealing to consumers. There is no other legitimate reason to use color agents in skin-care products.

In makeup of course, color agents are extensively used. Color agents will appear on the ingredient label as a variety of different names. There are two types of regulated colors, certified and noncertified colors.

Certified colors are pigments, also called **lakes**, that are certified and regulated by the Food and Drug Administration (FDA). They are named by listing the color name, the number assigned to that color agent by the FDA, and the metal associated with the chemical structure. An example would be *D & C* (stands for Drug and Cosmetic) *Red No. 4 Aluminum Lake*. On food packages, you may see listed on the ingredient label *F, D & C Yellow*, for example. Some colors are approved for use in drugs, cosmetics and foods. However, in general, you will rarely see *F, D & C* listed on a cosmetic ingredient label.

The colors certified by the FDA are blue, green, orange, red, and yellow. Noncertified colors are not metal salts. Most of these are natural plant or animal extracts, mineral pigments, and sometimes synthetic colors. While these colors are regulated by the FDA, they do not have a specific certification number. They include a variety of common cosmetic color agents, including iron oxide, zinc oxide, carmine, beta-carotene, chlorophylin-copper complex, annatto, ferric ferrocyanide, mica, the ultramarine colors, henna, and others.

Iron oxides are used extensively in the development of foundations. Iron oxide is frequently used to give makeup its color. There are various shades of iron oxide, and of course they can vary with the amount used in a particular solution. Iron oxide is actually rust, but is used in scientific formulations in makeup production.

Color agents are used extensively in the formation of foundations, mascara, eyeshadows, eye pencils, lip pencils, powders, blush, lipstick, and contour and camouflage products. Certified colors are not permitted by the FDA to be used in any cosmetics intended for the eye area. Chemists must use noncertified colors in eyeshadow, eyeliner, and other cosmetics intended for the eye area.

When the FDA first began regulating colors, there were about 116 certified colors. Over the years the FDA has determined that many of these colors are not safe for continual use, and therefore the list has dwindled to about 35 certified color agents. Some individuals are allergic to certain of the color agents. You must be careful to notice if a client tells you she is allergic to a particular color. You must check the ingredient labels of any products you wish to use on her or sell her for that particular color agent.

As discussed previously, the reason is no reason other than esthetics to put color agents in skin-care products. The one exception to this rule would be a moisturizing bronzer, designed to moisturize or protect and still give a slight hint of color to the skin's surface.

Many cosmetic companies now totally eliminate color from their skin-care products, because the public is becoming more aware of the lack of need for these chemicals in skin-care formulations. Also, because color agents can occasionally cause allergic reactions, eliminating the coloring agents from skin-care products cuts down on the likelihood of allergic reaction to the product.

If you use imported cosmetics, you must check to see if the import company has complied with FDA rules concerning color. Some countries do not have strong laws governing the use of color agents, and therefore may use color agents that are not permitted in cosmetics in the United States. The European Economic Community (ECC), Germany, and Japan all have regulations regarding color, but even they may differ significantly from those of the United States.

About Water

Water is the number one ingredient used in cosmetic formulations. Because most skin-care products on the market today are oil-in-water emulsions, water is extensively used, and in a lotion makes up most of the product.

Water must be prepared before it is used in cosmetics. Cosmetic factories have large tanks that prepare the water by filtering, distilling, deionizing, and sterilizing the water that is used in cosmetics.

You will notice that deionized water is almost always used in cosmetic and skin-care formulations. By deionizing the water before it is used, the chemist insures a more stable formulation, particularly when using an emulsifier.

Water is both a vehicle and an active agent. It is an excellent spreading agent for creams, as well as a good rinsing product for cleaning. It also works as an active agent in moisturizers, helping to hydrate the skin. Water is, of course, the real magic ingredient in moisturizers, since it binds to the other humectants and moisturizing agents in the moisturizer. We will discuss the use of these agents more extensively in the chapter on active agents.

High-Tech Vehicles

As we learn more about the skin's anatomy and physiology, the intercellular cement, and penetration of the skin, we learn more about formulating products that are more easily accepted by the skin and that penetrate the skin's surface better.

We know, for example, that the intercellular cement is made of various lipids. It is theorized that the closer we can formulate a product to resemble the intercellular cement, the better it will be accepted by the intercellular cement, and therefore it will be a much better vehicle for active agents such as moisturizers and conditioners.

Micelles

If you overemulsify an ingredient, the result is called a **micelle**. When you add emulsifier to a solution of water and oil, the emulsifier surrounds the internal phase of the solution. As the emulsifier lines up around the oil, as an example, there are small spaces between emulsifier molecules (Figure 8-2).

In a micelle, the emulsifier completely surrounds the oil, creating sort of a bubble. The bubble encloses the oil, or whatever internal phase ingredient is being emulsified. A cosmetic that has micelles present in it is said to be micellized.

FIGURE 8–2   Detergent micelle

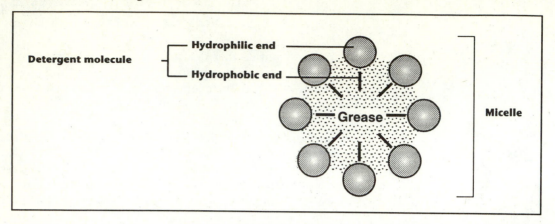

Liposomes

Liposomes are hollow spheres made of phospholipids. You can think of a liposome as a balloon, made out of lipids that are compatible with the lipids making up the intercellular cement.

Liposomes may be used to transport other agents, which may include moisturizers, conditioning agents, or drugs. Drugs, of course, are not used in cosmetic formulations.

The liposome may be **loaded**, which means that the liposome may be implanted with an ingredient. This ingredient, theoretically, will penetrate the skin. Eventually the liposome will begin to dissolve, releasing the ingredient into the intercellular cement, to carry out whatever function it is meant to complete (Figure 8-3).

What you can put into a liposome depends on many factors. These include the size of the liposome, the size of the ingredient to be carried by the liposome, the shape of the liposome, the ionization of any components, and the purpose of the product. Many ingredients are simply too big to put inside a liposome.

Empty liposomes, or unloaded liposomes, are sometimes used in cosmetics, to improve the penetration of a cream or moisturizer. Liposomes are not listed as such on ingredient labels—ingredients of the liposome are listed. These may include soya lecithin, lecithin, phospholipids, ceramides, or others.

The theories behind liposome functions are still being confirmed. While chemists have a good idea of how liposomes work, more is being learned all the time about their value in cosmetics.

FIGURE 8–3   This diagram shows encapsulation methods in the liposome and the nanosphere or microsponge. *Courtesy Francosmetics, Inc.-René Guinot.*

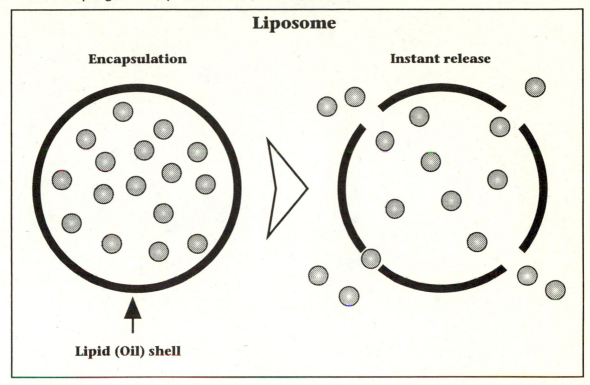

Other Innovative Vehicles

Other new vehicles similar to liposomes are currently being investigated. One type involves a "microsponge" that releases an active ingredient once inside the skin. Another is the nanosphere.

Such innovations may be used for drugs before they are developed for cosmetics. As we learn more about the functions of the epidermis and the ways chemicals react with the surface of the skin, we will learn more about transport mechanisms for various cosmetic as well as pharmaceutical ingredients.

TOPICS FOR DISCUSSION

1. What is a vehicle?

2. Discuss the difference between a surfactant, a detergent, and an emulsifier.

3. What is a suspension? List some examples.

4. How are fatty esters formed? Why are they often used in cosmetic formulas?

5. Why are preservatives necessary in cosmetics? Name some frequently used cosmetic preservatives.

6. Discuss liposomes and their use in cosmetics.

9

Active Agents

The part of the cosmetic that makes appearance changes in the skin is called the active agent. These are by far the most important ingredients in cosmetics. In this chapter the esthetician will learn all about various active agents used in hydrators, moisturizers, and products designed for dry, oily, aging, and sensitive skin.

In Chapter 8, we discussed cosmetic chemistry in terms of vehicles. We defined vehicles as the part of the cosmetic that delivers the active agent. An **active agent** is an ingredient that makes the cosmetic function and changes the appearance of the skin. They are, in essence, active ingredients. However, we will not refer to them as active ingredients because this particular wording is reserved for drugs. An active agent is any cosmetic ingredient that makes a cosmetic do what it is supposed to do to affect the appearance of the skin.

Every cosmetic product has an active agent. Active agents may also be vehicles. For example, an emollient helps to spread the cosmetic, but the emollient also helps to keep water from leaving the stratum corneum. Therefore, this emollient is not only a vehicle, it is also an active agent.

In this chapter we will refer to the properties of various active agents and discuss their use in various products. We need to establish here that some ingredients used in cosmetics are present because of anecdotal data. **Anecdotal** means, for purposes of this discussion, that the ingredient is, supposed to provide certain benefits to the skin, but they have not yet been substantiated, or proven, by scientific means. The main reason you need to know this is because you do not want to make drug claims when you practice esthetics. Cosmetics are products that, by law, change the appearance of the skin, not the physiological function. We will discuss this in much more depth in Chapter 11, on claims for cosmetics.

Cleansing Agents

The active agents in cleansers may be of two types, detergents or emulsion cleansers.

Detergents cause cleansers to foam, as we discussed in Chapter 8. An active agent detergent will be present in any foaming cleanser, most rinseable cleansers, and shampoos. They are essentially **defatting agents** which mean they remove fats and lipids, along with dirt, makeup, and debris, from the surface of the skin.

Soap also defats the skin's surface. Soaps are usually made of salts of fatty acids. There are two basic disadvantages to soap. Most soaps have a high pH, which can irritate the skin. Second, many soaps, because of their fatty acid content, leave a residue or film on the skin that it created by insoluble salts formed when the soap is used. The effect of both the fatty acid salts in soap and detergents in foaming cleansers can be overdrying to dry or dehydrated skin. Therefore, fats or oils are often added to the cleansers and soaps to prevent too much of the irritating active agent from coming in contact with the skin for a prolonged period of time, and overdrying and irritating the skin. You can think of these fats and oils as "bufferzones" set up to keep the product from stripping too much oil from the skin's surface. These products, with fat added, are often referred to as **superfatted**. Of course the fats that are added to these products can also leave a film on the skin. This can be a problem, especially for oily skins.

Common detergent ingredients used in cleansers are:

Sodium lauryl sulfate

Ammonium lauryl sulfate

Disodium lauryl sulfosuccinate

Sodium laureth sulfate

Lauramphocarboxyglycinate

Cocamidopropyl betaine

The ingredients listed above are all detergents. They may be used in any foaming or rinseable type cleanser. Some detergents are stronger than others. Their cleansing action will vary with the amount of active agent detergent used in a particular product, as well as how long it is left on the skin. The amount of fat added to the product will, of course, affect the cleansing detergent's aggressiveness.

These ingredients are frequently used soap salts, used in true bar soaps:

Sodium tallowate

Sodium oleate

Sodium cocoate

Sodium stearate

You will notice that soap ingredients will almost always start with the word *sodium* and end in a fatty ester of one of the main fatty acids listed in Chapter 8: stearic, myristic, oleic, etc. Sometimes potassium will be used as the reactant instead of sodium.

Emulsion cleansers are what most estheticians think of as cleansing milks. They are often used for removing makeup and are often recommended for sensitive skin types because of their gentleness. Most do not have detergents, but detergents can be used in these products to help the product foam slightly or to make the product more rinseable and easier to remove. Cleansing milks are made mostly of water, with an oil or fat mixed in the emulsion; therefore they are an oil-in-water emulsion. The oil or fat is the active agent used to create a slippery surface for removal of makeup or other debris from the skin's surface. The advantage to these cleansing milks is that they are less drying and irritating to the skin and perform an efficient job of removing makeup. The disadvantage is that they generally leave a residue on the skin. This residue is usually an emollient, the same one often used as the active cleansing agent, helping to loosen the debris from the skin's surface.

The emollient film left on the skin can be good or bad. For drier skins that do not make enough oil, it can actually help condition the surface. For oily skins or acne-prone skins, it can be a problem leaving a residue of fat to further clog the problem skin.

Another type of emulsion-type cleanser is cold cream. Cold cream is often made primarily of mineral oil, making it a water-in-oil emulsion. It is certainly a more oily emulsion cleanser, although very effective for heavy makeup. It often leaves a significant amount of oil on the skin after use. Clients often complain about the greasy feeling after using a cold cream cleanser. These types of cleansers are slowly losing popularity. Emulsion-type cleansers should always be followed by using a toner.

Active Agents in Toners

Depending on the skin type the toner is designed for, active agents vary greatly.

For oilier skins, alcohol may be used as an active agent. S.D. alcohol is a drying alcohol, not a fatty alcohol like that used in creams. S.D. alcohol is "specially denatured" ethyl alcohol. It is a strong cleanser, helping to remove oils and fats on the skin's surface. In large quantities, it is also an antiseptic, helping to kill surface microorganisms. It is has an astringent effect on the skin, helping to tighten the skin by causing small amounts of swelling, and from the drying of the skin due to the evaporation of the alcohol from the skin's surface. Astringents with SD alcohol will often claim that their use minimizes pore appearance. Again, this is caused by a slight amount of swelling, as well as an overall drying effect that only makes the pores or follicles appear smaller. As soon as the effects of the swelling wear off, the follicles return to their normal size.

S.D. alcohol will be listed on an ingredient label followed by a number. This number will indicate the technique that is used to denature the alcohol. Denaturing means that the alcohol is not suitable for drinking purposes. This is done as a safety precaution so that small children will not drink the liquid products. Bittering agents are added to the product to make it taste terrible, so if a baby puts the product in his or her mouth, it will taste awful and the baby will leave it alone.

Isopropyl alcohol is also sometimes used in astringents for oily and acne-prone skin. Again, it is used for its strong drying, antiseptic, and astringent effects. Toners or astringents made with isopropyl alcohol are, in general, somewhat stronger than those made with S.D. alcohol.

A Word About Alcohol

Alcohol has an undeserved terrible reputation in the cosmetics industry. Many companies tout that their products are "alcohol-free," referring to the drying effects of alcohol on the skin.

While large amounts of S.D. or isopropyl alcohol can be very irritating or overdrying to dry or sensitive skin types, they are very useful in helping to control oiliness in oily and acne-prone skin types. Do not reject a product simply because it has some S.D. or isopropyl alcohol. Make your decision based on the skin type you are treating. **Witch Hazel** or **hamamelis** extract is an alcoholic extract of the hamamelis plant. Witch hazel also has an astringent or drying effect on the skin, but is generally not as drying as S.D. or isopropyl alcohol. Lemon extract is often also used for its astringent purposes. Lemon contains citric acid, which naturally helps to lower the pH of the toner, which should always have a reasonably low pH. The lemon also leaves the skin feeling refreshed and is used in a water-based toning lotion.

Humectants such as propylene glycol and sorbitol are often added to toners designed for dehydrated skin for their water-binding and softening capabilities. More will be discussed about humectants in the section of this chapter on active agents for dehydrated skin. Alum is an old-fashioned astringent agent still used in some astringents. Alum has a strong tightening and pulling action, but can be irritating to sensitive skin.

pH adjusters are often used in toners to lower the pH. If a cleanser with a higher pH of 6 to 8 is used, a toner with a pH of 4 to 5 will help to lower the pH to an acceptable level.

Various plant extracts are also added to toners for their conditioning properties, depending on the skin type for which they are intended. More discussion on these active agents will follow in the sections on ingredients for various skin types.

Antiseptic and antimicrobial agents such as benzalkonium chloride are also added to toners on occasion to help kill bacteria, particularly for problem skin. Some of these agents will also serve as a preservative.

Active Agents for Dehydrated Skin

When skin is dehydrated, it is suffering from lack of water in the surface. Skin becomes dehydrated from too much sun, weather exposure, harsh cleansers, and aging. Humectants are water-binding agents that are hydrophyllic, or water-loving. They have a strong attraction to water. Many chemically bind water to them, holding many water molecules.

Natural humectants or hydrating agents are found within the cells and within the intercellular cement. These agents are called **natural moisturizing factors**, or NMFs, by scientists and medical doctors. The NMFs in skin help to preserve the water level within the skin layers, which keeps skin soft and supple.

As we age, we tend to lose these NMFs and manufacture fewer of them. This results in an inability of the skin to hold enough water in the surface cells, making the skin dry, flakey, tight, and dull-looking. The natural moisturizing factors in the skin include urea, phospholipids, alphahydroxy acids, and pyrollidone carboxylic acid, better known as sodium PCA.

These natural humectants are present between and within the cells of the stratum corneum, keeping the skin pliable and soft. Fortunately scientists have been able to duplicate many of these natural moisturizing factors in the laboratory. Many are now used as hydrophyllic humectants in cosmetic creams. **Urea** is frequently used in moisturizers. It is an excellent water binder and is also a **keratolytic**, helping to shed loose cells from the surface of the stratum corneum. It is also used in drugs designed for dry and dehydrated skin. Moisturizers containing urea, however, may sting when applied, and some individuals may be sensitive to urea. **Phospholipids** are a relatively new addition to the spectrum of naturally moisturizing humectants. A number of phospholipids are found within the skin. A phospholipid often listed on cosmetic labels is **lecithin**. Lecithin is usually derived from the soy plant. It is an excellent humectant and is compatible with the intercellular cement. Liposomes are often made of lecithin. Many cosmetic scientists believe that the addition of lecithin to a product increases moisturization and hydration, helps to penetrate the corneum better, and holds moisture in the skin for substantially longer periods of time. It is considered one of the most innovative of the newer cosmetic ingredients.

Sodium PCA is an excellent natural moisturizing factor ingredient. It has a tremendous ability to attract and hold water and is readily accepted by the skin. Sodium PCA is frequently used in night creams, day creams, and general hydrators. It is lightweight on the skin and does not cause clogged pores. (See the chapter on comedogenicity.)

The **alphahydroxy acids** include lactic, glycolic, malic, citric, and pyruvic acids. The two most popular are lactic and glycolic acids. These unique acids have the ability to remove and loosen cells from the stratum corneum, helping to make the surface of the skin look more even and smoother. They also have excellent humectant properties.

Lactic acid has been used for some time in cosmetic science, and in larger percentages in prescription moisturizers.

Glycolic acid is, at the time of this writing, beginning to enjoy new prestige in the world of cosmetic science. Glycolic acid is the smallest of all the alphahydroxy acids, and therefore more easily penetrates into the skin's surface. It helps remove dead excess cell layers and also helps retain moisture in the surface layers of the skin. There will be more discussion of glycolic acid in the chapter on therapy for photoaging skin.

Many other humectants and hydrophyllics are excellent water binders. Many of these humectants actually help the natural moisturizing factors perform a better job of hydrating the skin.

Glycerin is a humectant that has been used for many years. It is a very strong water-binder. It is, in fact, so strong that it should not be used by itself. Glycerin can actually make the skin more dry over a period of time because it doesn't just pull water from cosmetics and the atmosphere when applied to the skin. In large amounts, it can pull water from the lower levels of the epidermis, which results in dryer skin. Used in a moderate amount in a good hydrating cream, it is an excellent hydrating agent.

Propylene glycol is another widely used humectant. It penetrates the skin fairly easily, making it a good hydrating agent. In some cases, however, people are allergic to propylene glycol. It is used in literally thousands of cosmetics and drugs. It is frequently used in foundations. **Sorbitol** is another excellent hydrating agent that is frequently used in hydrating lotions.

Transepidermal Water Loss

Humectants and hydrophyllics such as the ones described above help to increase the water level in the stratum corneum by attracting and binding water to themselves. When they are applied to the skin, they either penetrate between cells or lie on the top of the skin's surface. Of course, more and more is being learned about the way these agents penetrate and affect the skin.

Most moisturizers are made mainly of water. Humectants will help to bind some of this water to the corneal cells. The humectants will also, though, pull and attract water from the lower levels of the epidermis. The water must be present in the lower epidermal cells in order for humectant moisturizers to work properly.

A problem arises, however, when humectants are used in too high a concentration (as discussed previously about glycerin). If too much humectant is used, too much water will be pulled up from the lower cell levels. This water will escape into the atmosphere, making dehydrated skin worse instead of better. For example, glycerin should not be used in more than a 50 percent concentration.

This evaporation of excess intercellular water is called **transepidermal water loss** by scientists. Abbreviated TEWL, transepidermal water loss is a serious concern when designing hydrating and moisturizing products. The trick in controlling these active agents is making sure they are present in a well-balanced blend of humectant, emollient, and emulsifier in a cream or lotion product.

Occlusives

An **occlusive** is a heavy, large molecule that sits on top of the skin and prevents moisture loss. Occlusives are exactly what they sound like, forming a barrier on top of the skin to shield the skin from transepidermal moisture loss from the inside out.

A good example of an occlusive is **petrolatum**, or **petroleum jelly**. Petrolatum can either be used by itself or incorporated into a cream or lotion. The amount of occlusion created by the petrolatum depends on the amount of it used in the cream formulation.

The advantages of using petrolatum in formulations are many. It is extremely hypoallergenic, rarely causing a problem with allergies or irritations. Hence it is often used in formulas, both drug and cosmetic, for sensitive or irritated skin.

Petrolatum provides an excellent occlusive barrier both to keep water in the skin and to keep allergens, antigens, and foreign bodies out of the skin. Doctors often recommend that patients who are sensitive to various chemicals apply petrolatum before handling the materials. An example of this is people who are sensitive to latex gloves, such as surgeons, dentists, and estheticians. By applying a small amount of petrolatum before wearing the gloves, a barrier is created between the skin and the latex, reducing contact and therefore reducing the irritation caused by the latex.

Petrolatum is also very inexpensive. Although petroleum products have certainly increased in price over the last decade, petrolatum is still very inexpensive to use.

There are some disadvantages to using petrolatum. First, it is extremely sticky, slippery, and greasy. Most clients do not like this greasy feeling. It is also hard to accomplish any task when your hands are too slippery to handle anything. It is extremely greasy on the face, creating esthetics problems as well. Second, it is disadvantageous to use petrolatum for oily and problem skin. While petrolatum is not comedogenic in its pure state, it is very greasy and heavy. Besides the obvious esthetic problem for oily skin, the occlusive action of petrolatum also blocks the follicles from oil dispersement, as well as from transepidermal water loss. In other words, while it keeps the water in the skin, it does not allow sebum to leave the follicle, therefore causing a "back-up" of sebaceous secretions.

Water and sweat from sudoriferous glands also becomes trapped between the skin and the occlusive petrolatum, which contributes to microbial problems. This is particularly a problem when the occlusive is worn for a prolonged period of time.

Many estheticians do not like petrolatum because it is not "natural." This is simply not true. Petrolatum comes from minerals in the earth. What could be more natural? In short, petrolatum is a useful product, but it should not be used in all cases of dehydration.

Emollients

As the skin ages, it tends not to produce as much of the essential lipids that make up the intercellular cement. This is when emollient ingredients are used in cosmetic systems. **Emollients** are somewhat like occlusives in that they mostly lie on the surface of the skin and prevent water loss. They also help to "fill in the cracks" of dry, dehydrated skin.

Emollients are often used, not only for dehydrated or water-dry skin, but also for oil-dry or alipidic skin.

Alipidic literally means "lack of lipids." These skin types do not produce enough lipids. This could be true of both the intercellular lipids and the sebum produced by the sebaceous gland.

Emollients help to supplement skin that suffers from this lack of lipid production. They serve as a substitute, helping to keep the surface lubricated, and even imitate the natural lipids in the intercellular cement.

These emollients are of several categories. Fatty acids have already been discussed in the previous chapter. They are emollients. Fatty alcohols and fatty esters are also emollients. There are some new types of emollients that are, again, actually a synthetic version of intercellular cement lipids. These include cholesterol, ceramides, lecithin (also a humectant), squalane, and glycosphingolipids.

Lanolin is another good emollient. Lanolin has had much bad press in the past. It was thought to cause many allergies. While this is a problem for some people, it has recently been theorized that most of the old-fashioned lanolin formula creams were also often full of perfumes and fragrances, thought to be a major source of these allergies. Purification processes for lanolin have also improved substantially over the decades, making today's lanolin a useful and relatively harmless active agent.

Mineral oil is another emollient. Like petrolatum, it is a petroleum derivative. It has many of the same advantages and disadvantages as petrolatum. It is hypoallergenic and a good emollient, helping to soothe irritated, dry, scaly skin. But it is also greasy, particularly in its pure state. However, when formulated properly into a cream, it can be an excellent active agent emollient for dry, dehydrated skin, especially when mixed with good humectant active agents.

Other Humectants

Other water binders work very differently than the standard hydrophyllic agents. **Hyaluronic acid** is one of these agents. Hyaluronic acid can hold up to 400 times its own weight in water. The molecule is quite large. It cannot penetrate the skin to any degree. However, because of its excellent water-binding properties, it is a frequently used hydrating active agent. Hyaluronic acid is an expensive active agent. Creams and lotions containing hyaluronic acid may be more expensive than others.

Mucopolysaccharides are carbohydrate-lipid complexes that are also good water-binders. Considered a "mother-molecule" to hyaluronic acid, it is very capable of holding large amounts of water and is an excellent hydrator. It, again, is much too large to penetrate the skin.

Collagen and elastin are large, long-chain molecular proteins that lie on the top of the skin and bind water, also helping to prevent water loss. Collagen and elastin proteins have been used in creams and lotions for some time. They are too big to ever penetrate the skin, but they do a good job of hydrating. Because collagen and elastin stay on top of the skin, they also help to "fill-in" small lines and crevices in the surface, making the skin look smoother.

When collagen and elastin were first introduced as ingredients, it was thought that they helped replace the collagen and elastin fibrils lost from the dermis due to sun damage. This has proven to be untrue. However, collagen and elastin do have good supportive water-binding abilities in the dermis, and these same properties help to hydrate the corneum. Collagen and elastin form a gel-like substance when applied to the skin. They are what cosmetic scientists called **substantives**, which means that they attach well to the skin surface and are a good binding agent.

Ingredients for Aging Skin

While there is no way to completely avoid the aging process, there appear to be steps you can take to slow its signs. Every day more technical information is available about the aging process and measures to help appearance problems associated with aging. New ingredients are rapidly being developed.

Some of these ingredients may be valuable in treating aging skin. However, at the time of this writing many of these active agents are still largely experimental, and scientific substantiation has not been made on many of them. In other words, it appears that these ingredients help aging skin, but scientists are not sure why and if they really work.

Glycolic Acid

Much research has taken place concerning glycolic acid. This ingredient is derived from sugar cane. It gently dissolves the intercellular cement that holds the old, dead, dehydrated cells on the surface of the skin. Getting rid of these cells makes the skin appear much smoother. By reducing the amount of cell buildup on the skin's surface, wrinkles appear less noticeable. Removing the surface skin also speeds the turnover rate of the cells. As we learned in Chapter 1, as cells migrate toward the surface, they break down and produce lipid complexes that make up the intercellular cement. By turning over the cells more rapidly these lipids are replenished. The lipids are not produced in as large quantities by aging skin, due to the slowdown in cell turnover in older people.

Glycolic acid may have additional positive effects on the skin. Glycolic acid is used in larger concentrations as medical peelings and treatments for warts, skin cancers, and precancerous sun damage conditions. Research continues on this new ingredient, which will probably be one of the most innovative ingredients in cosmetics of this age.

Liposomes

We have already discussed liposomes, which are routinely used in modern formulations to help aging skin. As we just discussed, aging skin experiences a slowdown in the manufacture of vital intercellular lipids. Liposomes, lecithin, and other similar lipid ingredients are very helpful in "filling in" these missing lipids, helping to penetrate moisturizing ingredients better, and improving the amount of time that hydrating agents retain water in the skin.

1,3 Beta-Glucan

This yeast cell membrane derivative is better known by its trade name Nayad.® It has been shown to improve wound healing. Scientists theorize that beta glucan works by stimulating the macrophages in the skin, which, in turn, stimulate the fibroblasts, the structures within the dermis that make collagen. Beta glucan is already in several products on the market.

Free Radical Scavengers

We have previously discussed free radicals. Free radicals may be an important factor in the aging process, including aging of the skin. Topical free radical scavengers, called **antioxidants**, help neutralize free radicals before they can attach themselves to cell membranes, eventually destroying the cell.

Antioxidants work by supplying electrons to radical oxygen atoms, who need electrons to be stable. Cell membranes have an excess of electrons, therefore providing a "smorgasbord" for the "electron starving" free radical oxygen atom. Antioxidants also supply electrons, neutralizing the atoms before they have a chance to attach to the cell membranes.

Free radicals occur in normal body cellular and physiological reactions. Free oxygen atoms are given off as a result of various chemical reactions within the body. Smoking, alcohol, stress, and sun exposure also contribute to additional free radical production.

Common ingredients used in cosmetics that are free radical scavengers are:

> Tocopherol
>
> Retinyl palmitate
>
> Ascorbic acid

These agents are better known as vitamin A palmitate, vitamin E, and vitamin C, respectively. In cosmetics, however, they are not called by their vitamin names, because this implies that the product is a drug. If they are included as conditioning agents they are listed by their chemical names. This implies that they are present as cosmetic agents affecting the appearance of the skin.

Another free radical scavenger that is currently being used in cosmetics is **superoxide dismustase**, which is an enzyme that is normally present in the body. Its function in the body is to neutralize free radicals. Superoxide dismutase is synthetically produced for use in cosmetics. The most important ingredients that are frequently used in cosmetics for delaying aging are sunscreens. Sunscreen agents filter and absorb ultraviolet light so that less of it penetrates the skin and causes sun damage. Although most cosmetics do not make sunscreening claims, they often contain sunscreens. Day creams and moisturizers, in particular, often have sunscreen agents added to them because they are worn during the day.

Most cosmetics with sunscreen do not have an SPF listed on the label, because they are marketed as cosmetics, not drugs. Frequently used sunscreen agents are **methoxycinnimate**, **benzophenone** and **oxybenzone**. There are a multitude of sunscreen agents. We will discuss sunscreen agents in much more detail in Chapter 16.

Products for Dry Skin

Most products designed for dry skin contain a combination of humectants and emollients and may contain some of the agents we have discussed that are designed for aging skin. They are normally water-based, or oil-in-water emulsions, although some may be water-in-oil emulsions designed for more alipidic skin.

These creams vary greatly in the amount of emollients and humectants they contain. The more oil-dry the skin is, the more emollient should be used in a treatment cream.

Treatments with large amounts of humectants are designed for oilier and combination skin types. Again, the amount of emollient will depend on the amount of oil being produced by the skin.

Hydrating fluids that are designed for younger skin types or oily adult skin may contain very little emollient. They will usually contain just enough emollient to serve as a vehicle to spread the product onto the skin. Special emollients have been designed to be used in hydrating agents for oily skin. These emollients are specially designed so that they do not clog the pores or occlude the skin. Some emollient creams can cause problems for clog-prone or problem skin. More about these chemicals will be discussed in the comedogenicity chapter.

Plant Extracts

Dozens of plant extracts are used as active agents in cosmetics. Plant extracts are liquids that are pressed or boiled out of different plants.

Most plant extracts are used because of their anecdotal properties.

In other words, they are reputed to cause changes in the skin. Some of these extracts have been shown in scientific studies to be very helpful in treating different skin problems. Some have never had any major scientific research performed on them to determine exactly how they work.

Plant extracts are simply natural complexes of various chemicals. Many estheticians like them because they are "natural." Nevertheless, they are chemicals. Sometimes they are a large number of chemicals together in one extract. Some of these chemicals are very helpful to the skin in helping with appearance changes and conditioning.

Plant extracts are normally used in small quantities in cosmetics. Usually they are listed as an extract, but if they are in a solution of water or alcohol, which most of them are, they may be listed near the top of the ingredient label in words that proceed the extracts, such as "Essence of..." or "Extracts of...." This simply means that water is the main ingredient in the extracts and that the extracts have been prepared before the formula was actually combined.

Special Additives

Special ingredients are often added to humectant and emollient products. Many of these agents are soothing agents that are added because they have the capability of reducing irritation to the skin.

Azulene is a hydrocarbon that is derived from the chamomile flower. It is an intense blue color and is frequently added to products designed for sensitive skin.

Bisabolol is another active agent that is added to cosmetics designed for sensitive skin. Aloe is also known for its soothing properties. Other agents often added for their soothing properties include:

> Allantoin—derived from the comfrey root
>
> Balm mint extract
>
> Calendula extract
>
> Camphor
>
> Chamomile extract
>
> Mallow extract
>
> Zinc oxide
>
> Rice starch
>
> Cornstarch

These ingredients may be added not only to moisturizers and hydrating creams, but also to cleansers, masks, toners, and other cosmetic preparations.

Oily Skin Products

Active agents used for oily skin may be used for several purposes. They may be used as peeling agents to help prevent the buildup of cells that can cause clogged pores and acne breakouts in oily skin. Some agents serve as astringents that help to temporarily tighten enlarged pores, making the skin look smoother. Other ingredients may be added for their soothing properties to help calm reddened skin associated with acne breakouts.

Lemon extract is used frequently in products for oily skin. It has good cleansing and oil removing properties. Lemon extract is less affected by the extraction process than some plant extracts. Lemon contains ascorbic acid, which is a good free radical neutralizer. Scientific inquiry is currently in the process of determining whether ascorbic acid stimulates fibroblasts to produce more collagen.

Many extracts contain **tannic acid**, which is an astringent. Some of these extracts, which are frequently used in oily skin products, are lappa extract, horse chestnut extract, birch extract, and nettle extract. Other extracts with astringent properties are cornflower extract, sage extract, saponaria, chamomile and rosemary extract. Strong astringents may also contain isopropyl alcohol, S.D. alcohol, or potassium alum. These extracts may be used in toners, cleansers, or conditioning creams or lotions.

Treatment products for oily skin are usually oil-in-water emulsions, heavily water-based. They normally contain fewer emollients than those products intended for dry skin, and are often in lotion form rather than cream form, due to their large amounts of water. Other ingredients may be added as general conditioning, soothing, or healing agents. These include panthenol, allantoin, and aloe vera.

Special ingredients may be used in oily skin products to reduce the product's oiliness and heaviness. The **silicones** are good examples. **Dimethicone** and **cyclomethicone** are silicone derivatives often used in products designed for oily and combination skin. These ingredients help to block water from escaping from the corneum cells, but the chemical is lightweight and does not occlude the follicles like heavier emollients. Dimethicone is frequently used in day creams and moisturizers for oily and combination skin. Cyclomethicone is used often in foundations for oilier skin types.

Special Ingredients for Problem and Acne-Prone Skin

Many of the same principles of product formulation are applied for problem skin as for oily skin. Problem skin more often requires the addition of chemicals that are stronger peeling agents and antiseptics. Often these ingredients are added to cosmetics designed for problem skin. However, no claim is made on these products; they are meant to be cosmetics, not drugs. Some ingredients used for acne and problem skin are:

    Salicylic acid

    Sulfur

    Resorcinol

    Benzoyl peroxide

    Glycolic acid

Much more on these ingredients and their uses is included in Chapter 13, "Acne and the Esthetician."

Other Special Ingredients

Clays, such as bentonite, kaolin, hectorite and silica, are used in masks for their tightening and drawing effects and also in drying lotions for acne treatment. Another ingredient used frequently as a drawing agent is magnesium aluminum silicate.

Enzymes are used in treatments to dissolve keratin protein in dead surface cells. These treatment products are often called enzyme peels or peelings. The enzymes are proteolytic, which means *protein-dissolving*. More about enzyme treatments will be discussed in Chapter 18.

Conclusion

Hundreds of chemicals are used as active agents in cosmetics. Some active agents, as you have seen, are also vehicles, and have more than one function in a cosmetic.

We have touched on only a few active agents, but you will be able to use this knowledge to understand ingredient labels and their functions. With additional study, you should eventually be able to pick up a product and, simply by reading the ingredient label, know what kind of product it is and for what skin problem it is intended.

TOPICS FOR DISCUSSION

1. What is an active agent? How does it differ from an active ingredient?

2. What are the two basic types of cleansing ingredients? Discuss the products in which each are used.

3. What are natural moisturizing factors? Name some that are used in cosmetics.

4. Discuss some ingredients used to help aging skin.

5. What are free radicals?

6. Discuss some ingredients used to treat oily skin and problem acne skin.

10

Skin-care Products

After the esthetician graduates from school, he or she will be amazed at the variety of skin-care products available. This chapter discusses various types of skin-care products available, products for different skin types and problems, and the chemical makeup of products for different skin types.

While this chapter provides only an overview of the products available, it will teach the esthetician about factors involved in choosing products for various skin problems and clients' needs.

In the last two chapters you have learned about various ingredients used in manufacturing cosmetics. Now you will learn about practical application of various formulas of cleansers, toners, creams, and other products.

There are literally hundreds and hundreds of different products available to estheticians. These are products that you will both use in the treatment room, and recommend that your clients use at home. It is important to carry a variety of products to sell to your clients for home use. There are many good esthetic product manufacturers, and the most successful skin-care salons carry lines made by at least two or three of them. There is no one line that is the answer to every problem you will see.

A Visit to the Product Stockroom

Let's take a trip to the stockroom of a successful skin-care salon. We will not talk about name brands, but we will talk about various products available in chemical terms. You will be able to use what you have learned. Remember, a primary objective is for you to be able to read ingredient labels and tell what kind of product you are examining, and for what skin type it is intended. As we look into this imaginary stockroom, we will look at various types of products. There are enough types of products in this stockroom to handle most esthetic problems (Figure 10-1).

FIGURE 10–1   A well-organized stockroom full of supplies is important to the esthetics practice.

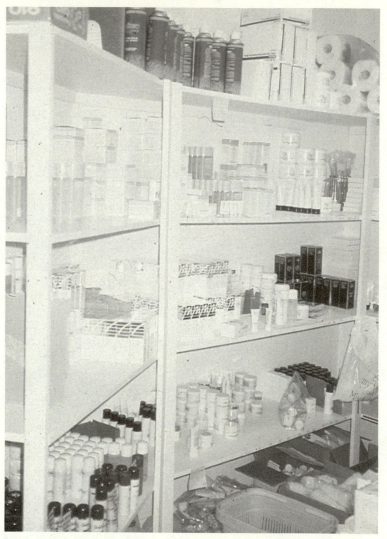

The most important factor in prescribing the right home care for your clients is your education and knowledge of skin analysis. Make sure you receive good training in analysis. It is one of the biggest keys to success in esthetics.

Before we enter the imaginary stockroom, it must be understood that many products are available for the esthetician, and new products are developed every year. We will cover only a portion of the products available, but this will be a representative sampling of what is frequently used in skin-care salons.

Cleansers

As we enter the stockroom, the first thing you notice is the wide assortment of cleansers. There are both milk type cleansers, and rinseable detergent-type foaming cleansers, as well as some specialty cleansers for acne and clog-prone skin.

Let's talk about rinseable cleansers first. Rinseable cleansers usually come in a tube, sometimes in a bottle. They vary in strength and texture. Rinseable cleansers are important to carry because you will find that many clients are used to washing their faces with bar soap, like the foaming action, and do not "feel clean" unless they have "washed" their faces.

Product Profile:
Rinseable Cleanser
for Oily and
Combination Skin

Client and Skin Type: The first rinseable cleanser we will look at is a rinseable cleanser for oily and combination skin. Clients with oily and combination skin are especially fond of rinseable cleansers because these clients need some detergent to help cut excess amounts of oil. However, we don't want our cleanser to overdry them or strip the acid mantle.

Product Characteristics: This particular cleanser is in a tube. The product consistency feels almost like soap. When the client adds water, it begins to foam moderately. It rinses completely, leaving the skin feeling fresh and clean, but not too tight. This clean but not tight feeling is a good sign that the product is pH balanced correctly for the skin type.

Chemical Action and Design: Chemically this product uses disodium lauryl sulfosuccinate as a detergent-surfactant. It also contains smaller amounts of avocado oil and cetyl alcohol, emollient ingredients added to cut the detergent action on the skin's surface so that it will not be stripping. This cleanser is also fragrance-free, a helpful characteristic when treating sensitive skin. This cleanser is a good recommendation for adult oily and combination skin or for clients who are used to heavier moisturizers but really need to switch to a lighter program for oily or combination skin (Figure 10-2a).

Product Profile:
Rinseable Cleanser
for Dry and
Combination Skin

Client and Skin Type: This cleanser is designed for clients who have dry skin, but still want the action of a detergent cleanser. This cleanser will be good for an older client with dry skin, who prefers soap over milk cleanser.

Product Characteristics: This rinseable cleanser is also packaged in a tube. It foams very slightly. It rinses well, but leaves the skin feeling very soft. This cleanser will not be aggressive enough for oily-combination skin. However, for more alipidic skin it is excellent.

Chemical Action and Design: If you look at the ingredient label of this product you will notice that its detergent agent, sodium lauryl sulfate, is listed about halfway down the list of ingredients. This means that the product is not nearly as strong a cleanser as the first cleanser. The ingredients listed after water are different types of emollients, fatty alcohols, and esters. This cleanser contains lots of emollients because it is designed for dry skin. The large amounts of emollients will keep the detergents from stripping too much lipid from the skin's surface. This product is superfatted (Figure 10-2b).

Product Profile: Rinseable Cleanser for Very Oily Skin

Client and Skin Type: This stronger rinseable cleanser is designed for clients who have very oily skin. Their skin is covered with enlarged pores, and they almost never have any dryness or dehydration. This type of client is extremely oily by 10 or 11 o'clock in the morning.

Product Characteristics: This cleanser is a liquid in a bottle. It has almost the consistency of shampoo. It foams quite strongly and rinses thoroughly, leaving the skin feeling very clean. It is much too strong for any skin type except extremely oily skin.

Chemical Action and Design: The active detergent in this rinseable cleanser is a strong anionic surfactant called ammonium laureth sulfate. It is mixed with gelling agents to form shampoo-like consistency. The surfactant concentration in a cleanser such as this is somewhat higher than other rinseable detergent cleansers that are designed for less oily skins. There are no emollients in this product, and therefore the product has no buffer against stripping oil from the skin's surface. However, this is appropriate for a cleanser that is designed for very oily skin.

Product Profile: Rinseable Medicated Cleanser for Acne

Client and Skin Type: This cleanser is made for mild to moderate acne, excessively oily, and chronic acne-prone skin. This type of skin is not sensitive and is fairly thick, due to the accumulation of corneocytes on the surface of the skin. This client may have a currently active acne condition or may tend to develop moderate acne frequently. This product may also be excellent for teenage acne.

Product Characteristics: This cleanser is very similar to the one designed for chronically oily skin, except that it contains an antimicrobial agent to kill bacteria. Medicated cleansers such as this are usually registered as over-the-counter drugs.

FIGURE 10–2 Sample ingredient labels for cleansers

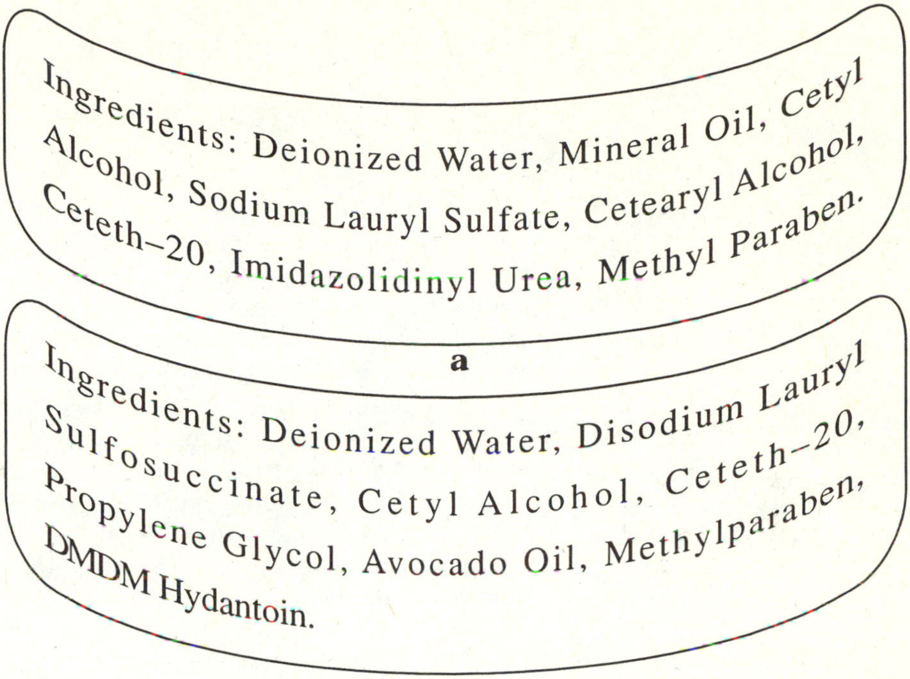

Ingredients: Deionized Water, Mineral Oil, Cetyl Alcohol, Sodium Lauryl Sulfate, Cetearyl Alcohol, Ceteth–20, Imidazolidinyl Urea, Methyl Paraben.

a

Ingredients: Deionized Water, Disodium Lauryl Sulfosuccinate, Cetyl Alcohol, Ceteth–20, Propylene Glycol, Avocado Oil, Methylparaben, DMDM Hydantoin.

b

Which cleanser is stronger? The first one is weaker. The surfactant (sodium lauryl sulfate) is buffered by dominating ingredients cetyl alcohol and mineral oil, which help to prevent too much contact with the surfactant. In the second formulation, the surfactant (Disodium lauryl sulfosuccinate) is diluted only by water as a larger percentage ingredient. The further the surfactant is down the list, the weaker the cleansing action. The first product is designed for dry-combination skin, and the second is for oily-combination skin.

(See the chapter on the FDA and cosmetic claims.) It is a strong foaming cleanser. It may also be made to be an exfoliant, depending on the ingredients.

Chemical Action and Design: Benzoyl peroxide may serve as the antimicrobial in a product like this, or another antimicrobial such as salicylic acid, sulfur, or hexitidine may be used. Benzoyl peroxide (see the chapter on acne) is also a keratolytic agent, as is salicylic acid, which serves to lightly peel away dead corneocytes from the surface of the skin as well as flush the follicular canal. Some products like this cleanser may also contain a mechanical exfoliant such as polyethylene granules. These small, bead-like granules are used in the cleanser because they are gritty and literally "bump off" dead cell buildup.

As you move across the shelf from the rinseable cleanser, you may notice a variety of milk cleansers in several different colors. As you look closer, you notice that these cleansers are designed for a variety of skin types.

Product Profile: Milk Cleanser for Oily and Combination Skin

Client and Skin Type: This cleanser is an emulsion to be used for makeup removal on oily and combination skin. Milk cleanser for acne and extremely oily skin is rarely used, at least not by itself. For acne, a milk cleanser may be used strictly as a makeup remover, followed by a rinseable detergent cleanser for extra cleansing action. This cleansing milk is a good choice for the older person with oily or combination skin who has a tendency towards oiliness and minor but persistent breakout problems. This type of client may find twice daily cleansings with detergents to be too dehydrating. Older skin tends to dehydrate much more easily than younger skin. This skin type may use a rinseable cleanser in the morning and then a gentler milk for nightly makeup removal.

Product Characteristics: This milk is a water-based fluid. It is slightly slippery to the touch and leaves the skin feeling fairly clean when removed. This product should be applied and removed with a room temperature damp sponge cloth or cleansing sponge. It is necessary with all cleansing milks to use a very soft cloth to apply and remove these cleansers, as they do not contain much detergent, if any, and do not rinse as easily as detergent cleansers. This cleanser, however, rinses well when used with a sponge or sponge cloth. Makeup is removed very easily with this product. This product should not be used on the eyes, because it is designed for oily and combination skin and is not chemicallyappropriate for the eye area (Figure 10-3).

Chemical Action and Design: The emollients used in this cleanser are tridecyl stearate, neopentylglycol dicaprate/dicaprylate, and tridecyl trimellitate, which are a complex of emollients designed to be a noncomedogenic oil replacement. They do not clog the skin and are easily removed from the skin. The emollients mix with the dirt, makeup, and oils and work to dissolve these foreign materials so they may be removed from the skin's surface. This product has a pH of about 7.0, typical of a cleanser designed for oily and combination skin. The slightly higher pH helps the cleanser be a more aggressive solvent. The cleansing process should be followed by a lower pH toner to lower the pH and remove any film left from the emollient.

FIGURE 10–3 A soft chamois cloth is used for makeup removal. *Courtesy Correlations, Inc.*

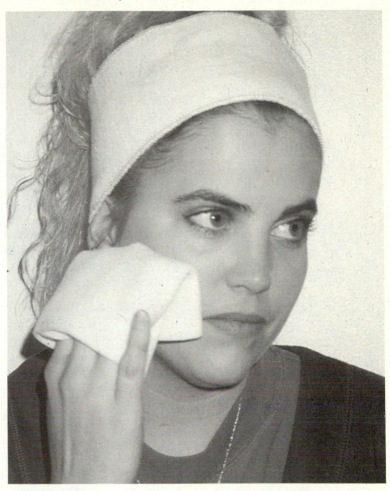

Product Profile:
Cleansing Milk for
Combination Skin

Client and Skin Type: This thicker cleansing emulsion is made for clients who wear heavier makeup and therefore need a more oily cleanser to dissolve the thicker, oilier makeup. This cleanser is often prescribed for older clients with combination skin. It is considerably heavier than many other cleansing milks. This cleanser may also be used frequently by actors and other performers who wear heavier stage makeup routinely.

Product Characteristics: This cleanser is a thicker liquid in a bottle. It absolutely must be used with a sponge or a soft cloth. Otherwise, it would leave a residue on the skin. Its emollients dissolve makeup very readily, making it an excellent product for heavy makeup wearers. This product should be followed by a toner designed for combination skin. The toner needs to be strong enough to remove any residue left from this cleanser.

Chemical Action and Design: Petrolatum and mineral oil are the secrets of the slipperiness of this cleanser. There is enough emulsifier in this product to make it relatively thick. The petrolatum makes the product physically heavy. Mineral oil mixed with petrolatum is an excellent makeup dissolver. Plant extracts have been added to this product for soothing.

Product Profile: Cleansing Milk for Sensitive Skin

Client and Skin Type: This lightweight milk cleanser is designed for sensitive skin. It is designed for the client with thin, fragile skin that reddens easily. It is not specifically designed for oily skin; its emollient content is meant more for dry, irritated skin. The client who has sensitive, thin skin can use this product.

Product Characteristics: This is a lightweight cleansing milk designed to be used with a soft cloth or sponge. It does not leave much residue when rinsed and has very little fragrance. It will remove liquid makeup well.

Chemical Action and Design: This water-based cleanser combines relatively large amount of water with a mixture of emollients to dissolve makeup. It contains azulene, bisabolol, and chamomile extract, which are included for their soothing properties. No fragrance is used because of allergy potentials. The only fragrance is from the plant extract used.

Product Profile: Cleansing Milk for Dry Skin

Client and Skin Type: Dry, mature skin will benefit from the use of this fairly lightweight milk for dry skin.

Product Characteristics: Again, this product should be applied and removed with a damp, soft cloth. This cleanser is slightly richer to the touch than our other milk cleansers. It does leave a residue if not carefully removed and should be used with a toner designed for dry skin.

Chemical Action and Design: The ultra-rich emollient oils in this cleanser are added to help condition the surface of the skin while cleansing, helping to avoid overstripping of the natural oils. It contains no detergents, which can strip older alipidic skin.

Some skin-care companies add expensive conditioners to cleansing product. These conditioning ingredients are normally used in creams, lotions, and fluids that are in the form of day or night treatments. In other words, they stay on the face for long periods of time. Many cosmetic scientists believe that it is useless to include expensive conditioning ingredients in cleansers, because they simply do not stay on the face long enough to do any good. Soothing agents and agents that are meant to strengthen or weaken the action of the cleanser are the only type of these agents that should be added.

Toners

Toners, clarifying lotions, fresheners, and astringents are all basically the same type of product. They vary in strength, drying ability, and alcohol content. They are made for three specific reasons:

1. They remove excess cleanser and residue from liquid cleansers.

2. They have a relatively low pH, helping to adjust the pH of the acid mantle after cleansing so it is not overstripped.

3. It provides a temporary tightening effect to both the skin as well as the individual follicle openings, helping to temporarily shrink "pores."

Product Profile: Toner for Oily and Combination Skin

Client and Skin Type: This toner is designed for oily and combination skin. It is good for the client who develops clogs easily but still needs a hydrating moisturizer. Adult oily and oily-combination skin will benefit from this toner.

Product Characteristics: This toner is a clear, water-based liquid. It should be applied with a pre-dampened cotton pad, a sponge, or a soft cloth after using a rinseable cleanser or cleansing milk. It has a lemon fragrance. After use, the skin feels clean and toned but not dry. Pores do seem to shrink after using this product. Men can also use this product as an aftershave. It is a good product for men, because it is not femininely fragranced and has enough astringent action for after shaving.

Chemical Action and Design: The low pH in this toner is due to a combination of citric acid and lemon extract, which has a fairly strong astringent action. It is blended into a liquid with mostly water, but also contains a glycerin derivative, which is a humectant that helps to restore water to dehydrated skin. It also contains benzalkonium chloride as a preservative, but this chemical is also an antimicrobial, which may be beneficial to oily and combination, slightly breakout-prone skin.

Product Profile: Astringent for Extremely Oily Skin

Client and Skin Type: This toner is made for skin that becomes very oily after only a short period of time and has very large pores that clog very easily. This client never gets dehydrated because the skin is so oily. The client uses a strong, rinseable cleanser for very oily skin; which we discussed earlier. This toner should be applied on a predampened cotton pad or damp sponge.

Product Characteristics: This astringent is a water-based liquid that is used after cleansing milk or rinseable cleanser. It has a strong astringent action. It leaves the skin feeling very clean and tight. Application to dry skin would be too drying.

Chemical Action and Design: This oily skin astringent contains plant extracts for oily skin as well as sulfur, a keratolytic peeling agent, and potassium alum, a strong astringent agent. They are in a base vehicle of water and propylene glycol, a hydrating agent.

Product Profile: Astringent for Acne-Prone Skin

Client and Skin Type: This very strong astringent is made for inflamed acne and extremely oily skin. It is a good product for teenage acne, grades two and three. (See the chapter on acne.)

Product Characteristics: This astringent is a light-colored liquid and has a strong medicinal (alcohol) odor. It is applied with a damp cotton ball after cleansing. It is very stripping, removes lots of sebum, and is very drying to the skin. It may burn or tingle slightly when applied, especially if applied to open acne lesions. Some extremely oily skin needs this much oil removal.

Chemical Action and Design: Isopropyl alcohol and water are the main ingredients in this liquid astringent. The alcohol provides oil-stripping action. Witch hazel distillate provides astringent properties and temporary pore "tightening." Camphor is included as an antiseptic and soothing agent.

Product Profile: Toner for Normal Skin

Client and Skin Type: This toner is a medium-strength tonic designed for normal and sensitive skin. It is for adult skin that basically needs moderate hydrating and has no particular problems.

Product Characteristics: This toner is a liquid and has a very mild astringent action. It does not pull on the skin. It has a moist feeling when applied. It has a slight soothing effect on the skin. It is applied with cool, wet, cotton pads after cleansing.

Chemical Action and Design: This is a very simple formula made with water, rosewater, propylene glycol (as a humectant), cucumber extract for soothing, and allantoin. It contains a smaller amount of witch hazel extract than toners for oily skin.

Product Profile: Toner for Extra-Dry Skin

Client and Skin Type: Dry, mature skin is the type of skin that this toner will help. It has moisturizing properties as well as helping gently remove traces of cleanser from dry, sensitive skin. This type of dry skin can become so dehydrated that the face becomes very tight even after a very gentle cleanser. This toner is designed for dry skin that becomes tender after cleansing. This cleanser should be used after cleansing, applied with a cool, damp cotton pad.

Product Characteristics: This a very moist toner, almost soft to the touch. It has practically no astringent action. It is designed to moisturize the skin with humectants that provide a buffer so that the skin will not become stripped if the toner is used after cleansing.

Chemical Action and Design: A large amount of propylene glycol provides humectant effects for the skin in this water-based, fluid toner. Glycerin also has hydrating action on the surface of the dry skin. Extracts of chamomile, mallow, and cornflower are included for their softening and soothing properties. This is an unusually moisturizing toner.

Day Creams and Treatments

Day creams are made for various skin types. Treatments for everything from acne to extremely dry and aging skin are available. These products vary greatly in texture and thickness, depending on the amount of fats or emollients that are added.

Day creams usually contain either an occlusive agent or some sort of protectant ingredient that helps hold water in the surface layers of the skin. They may also contain various hydrating agents, emollients, or other active agents, depending on the skin type for which they are intended. Many also contain sunscreen to help filter ultraviolet rays. Most of these are marketed as cosmetics. Therefore they do not make strong sunscreening claims. Nevertheless the sunscreen is an added beneficial ingredient.

Product Profile: Day Protection Fluid for Oily and Combination Skin

Client and Skin Type: This product is designed for oily and combination skin. Clients who have oily skin appreciate this product because it does not feel oily or greasy and is noncomedogenic. It is a good choice for 20-to-50-year-old clients who develop clogged pores easily. This product is a good choice for people who need hydrating, but become oily easily. These clients will generally have trouble with their makeup not staying on well and becoming oily during the day. The lack of many emollients in this cream will benefit the client who prefers a light-textured, non-heavy day product. This will also serve well as a daytime moisturizer-protectant for oily skins during the winter months.

Product Characteristics: This lightweight day protection fluid comes in a tube. It is not a thick product and feels very light and non-greasy when touched. It absorbs quickly, helping to hydrate the skin and protect against daytime water loss, and contains sunscreen to shield against routine daily sun exposure during daily activities. In other words, it is not a beach sun product. It is applied with the fingertips in the morning before makeup or alone. It is noncomedogenic, which means that it has been tested and found not to clog pores. This product is unusual because it hydrates, protects, conditions, contains a sunscreen, and is noncomedogenic.

Chemical Action and Design: This fluid is water-based, with small amounts of noncomedogenic emollients added. These emollients are tridecyl stearate, tridecyl trimellitate, neo-pentylglycol dicaprate/dicaprylate, and glyceryl stearate. The active humectants that help to bind water in this fluid are glycerin and sodium PCA. Other conditioning agents include allantoin, cornflower extract, tocopherol, and retinyl palmitate. Methoxycinnimate is the sunscreen ingredient, and dimethicone is used as a water-loss shielding agent, because of its lightweight characteristics.

Product Profile: Daytime Treatment for Oily, Clogged, Adult Skin

Client and Skin Type: This product is designed for oily skin or oily, clogged areas. It is for clients who have a tendency to break out, but find that most drying agents overdry. It is ideal for older adult oily skin, when clients are used to using heavy moisturizers that clog the skin. Adult acne can benefit from this type of product because it incorporates both a peeling agent and a hydrating agent, as well as a protectant. This product is also ideal for an adult oily skin client who is used to using heavy moisturizers that are clogging the skin. It feels like a moisturizer but is actually a very light peeling agent.

Product Characteristics: This lightweight product has an unusual texture somewhere between a gel and a cream. It is very light and dries quickly when applied. It has a matte dry feeling when used. It should be applied in the morning after cleansing and toning. It takes the place of moisturizer and can be used under makeup or alone.

Chemical Action and Design: Salicylic acid is used in a very small quantity in this product to promote some exfoliation. This product contains glycerin and propylene glycol as humectants, and dimethicone provides protection against excess water loss.

Product Profile: Day Oil Controlling Lotion for Extra Oily Skin

Client and Skin Type: This product is for extremely oily skin. It is an astringent day lotion, to control extremely oily skin with very large pores. This type of client's skin gets extremely oily early in the day. This lotion will help to control this excess oil secretion.

Product Characteristics: This lotion is a very liquid product. It is water-based and has the texture of an astringent. When applied, it may sting slightly because of its large amount of S.D. alcohol. It dries quickly; in fact, it may be too drying if the skin is not oily enough.

Chemical Action and Design: This water-based day lotion contains S.D. alcohol as a drying agent and resorcinol and sulfur, both exfoliants. Sulfur also has an antiseptic action on acne-prone, oily skin. It also contains plant extracts for conditioning oily skin.

Product Profile: Day Cream for Dry and Combination Sensitive Skin

Client and Skin Type: Designed for oil-dry (alipidic), dehydrated, sensitive skin, this cream will help the client who becomes dry very easily due to lack of oil production. It is for clients who have a slight amount of oiliness through the T-zone, but the large part of the outer perimeter of the face is dry and dehydrated.

Product Characteristics: This cream is packaged in a tube. It is definitely cream, containing a substantial amount of emollient. It contains a sunscreen and a protective agent. It is not extremely greasy or heavy, so it may be worn by clients who prefer a lighter weight day cream. It is blue due to the azulene content. It should be applied under makeup or alone during the day.

Chemical Action and Design: This cream contains propylene glycol and aloe as hydrating agents. It contains dimethicone as a shielding protective agent and benzophenone, a UVA sunscreen. These active agents are mixed into a water-based blend of emollients, including lanolin, cetyl palmitate, and beeswax. Azulene provides help for soothing, sensitive dehydrated skin.

Product Profile: Day Cream for Dry Skin with Telangectasias (Couperose — Enlarged Capillaries)

Client and Skin Type: The dry, adult, sun-damaged client will appreciate this product. This product is specifically designed to help skin with many enlarged red capillaries seen easily on the face. It helps to soothe the redness and minimizes the appearance of the capillaries.

Product Characteristics: This is a fairly heavy cream due to its emollient content. It is applied under makeup or alone. It comes in a tube. This cream is not for oily skin due to its large amount of emollients.

Chemical Action and Design: The active agent in this cream that helps lessen the appearance of the redness and soothes the skin is horse chestnut extract. Oxybenzone and benzophenone are included as sunscreen agents, and titanium dioxide, a pigment, is contained for both sunscreen and coverage purposes. The main part of the cream is a water-based glycerin emulsion, with isopropyl myristate and glyceryl stearate as emollients. It contains a large amount of coloring agent, designed to cut down on the appearance of redness.

Product Profile: Day Cream for Dry, Dehydrated Skin

Client and Skin Type: This product is meant for clients with very dehydrated and somewhat oil-dry skin. It is rich in emollients.

Product Characteristics: A fairly thick day cream, this product is packaged in a tube. It is somewhat heavy on the skin, providing a good amount of emollient to help prevent dehydration and helping to provide extra fats to the surface of oil-dry areas. It also contains sunscreen. This product should be used under makeup or alone during the day. This cream would be good for dehydrated, dry skin in colder climates.

Chemical Action and Design: Oxybenzone and benzophenone are the sunscreen agents contained in this product. These are mixed with some fairly heavy emollients in fairly large quantities, creating a heavy-textured cream. The emollients are lanolin, jojoba oil, shea butter, and stearic acid, and this cream also contains mineral oil, which helps to prevent dehydration. Sodium lactate is contained as a hydrating agent.

Product Profile: Day Treatment Cream for Mature Skin with Poor Elasticity

Client and Skin Type: This sophisticated moisturizer is for older, very dehydrated skin that has poor elasticity and is sun damaged. It contains liposomes to help hold water in the surface layers for a prolonged period of time.

Product Characteristics: This cream is contained in a jar. It has a light texture when applied and should be used under makeup or alone. Its emollients help protect against surface dehydration, and it contains sunscreen.

Chemical Action and Design: The "magic" in this cream is lecithin, in the form of liposomes, which help to hold water in the surface for much longer periods of time than many other moisturizing ingredients. It contains the humectants sorbitol, propylene glycol, and hyaluronic acid, and the emollients jojoba oil, shea butter, and capric caprylic triglycerides. Sunscreens are benzophenone and oxybenzone.

Night Creams and Treatments

Night treatment creams are normally extra intensive treatment products designed to help hydrate and condition skin during the night, a time when normal tissue repair is taking place all over the body, including the skin. Night treatments are often heavier in consistency and texture than day products. They normally contain more emollient than day cream and are not made for use under makeup. Night creams should be applied all over the skin, according to manufacturer's instructions. It is important that the skin be thoroughly cleansed before night treatment is applied.

About Ampoules

Ampoules are designed to be extra-intensive, concentrated extracts. They often contain larger amounts of active ingredients in a water base. Occasionally they are in an oil base. They are to be applied under a night cream or fluid.

Ampoules are available for a wide variety of skin types and problems. Some are designed to be used in a series once a month or several times a year. Others are designed to be used nightly. The advantage of ampoules is they provide active ingredients in concentration in a measured amount. They generally have positive effects on the skin's appearance. They are native to Europe, where the concept was invented. Many American lines do not have ampoule treatments.

The disadvantages of ampoules are that they are more trouble to use than night cream or fluid and they are generally more expensive to use than night creams and fluids. However, clients who are extremely conscientious about their home care will often take the time to use ampoules, and not mind paying the extra expense.

Product Profile: Night Treatment Fluid for Oily, Dehydrated Skin

Client and Skin Type: This fluid is made to provide hydration to adult oily skin that is also dehydrated. It can be used on oily and combination skin. These clients are normally adults who need to use a hydrating agent, but develop clogged pores and break out easily. This fluid has been laboratory tested and found to be noncomedogenic. It is also ideal for the client who prefers a lighter weight night treatment.

Product Characteristics: Due to its low emollient content, this fluid is very light in texture and feel. It does not feel oily at all because it contains mostly humectants to attract water to the skin, rather than oils and fats that will clog this type of skin. This fluid comes in a tube and should be applied in moderate amounts to the entire skin before bedtime.

Chemical Action and Design: This fluid contains sodium PCA, a natural moisturizing factor (NMF), and glycerin as hydrating agents. It also includes allantoin, retinyl palmirate, and tocopherol in its formula for their conditioning properties. This fluid has been carefully designed without comedogenic ingredients (see the chapter on comedogenicity), to avoid clogging the oily and combination skin for which it is intended. The emollients added are tridecyl stearate, tridecyl trimellitate, and neopentylglycol dicaprate/dicaprylate. This fluid adds hydration to the skin without adding excess emollients that cause buildup of cells, which cause clogs to form.

Product Profile: Night Hydrating Cream for Oily and Combination Mature Skin

Client and Skin Type: Designed for older oily and combination skins that need hydration, but do not need extra oils, this lightweight cream is good for older clients who still have a tendency to break out. It provides hydration without oiliness. This cream could also be used as a night treatment for younger, extra dehydrated skin types. The cream is laboratory tested to be noncomedogenic.

Product Characteristics: The cream is extremely lightweight and is absorbed by the skin easily. After use the skin feels smooth and "plumped up." It is contained in a tube and should be applied to clean skin before bedtime. It contains no color or fragrance, which is helpful for sensitive and allergy-prone skin.

Chemical Action and Design: Sorbitol is the main hydrating agent in this cream and is present in a large concentration. Sorbitol is combined with lecithin, another good hydrator readily accepted by the skin. Lecithin is the material that liposomes are made of, but this cream is not liposomic. It uses the lecithin to retain water in the surface layers, making the cream easily penetrating. It contains the conditioners retinyl palmitate and tocopherol acetate, both reputed to help neutralize free radicals. The cream is constructed to be noncomedogenic.

Product Profile: Night Moisturizing Lotion for Dehydrated Combination Dry Skin

Client and Skin Type: This lotion is constructed to help skin that is both oil and water-dry. This type of skin has a very narrow T-zone with little oil production or visible pore structure. Most clients will be mature women.

Product Characteristics: This treatment is a lotion and is packaged in a bottle. It is slightly oily to the touch, leaving a slight film on the surface of the skin. This characteristic is helpful for drier skin types. It is a light blue color, due to its azulene content. It should be applied before bedtime.

Chemical Action and Design: The lotion contains a mixture of oils, emollients, and humectants, providing both hydration and oils for the oil-dry skin. It contains the humectants urea, propylene glycol, and butylene glycol, and is mixed with sesame oil, peanut oil, and various emollient esters and fats. Because it contains a good amount of both hydrator and oils, it contains sodium lauryl sulfate, used as an emulsifier to keep the oils in the water-based emulsion.

Product Profile: Night Cream for Dry Skin

Client and Skin Type: Oil-dry, dehydrated, mature skin is the target for this heavier cream. This type of client is very dry for most of the year and needs a richer cream.

Product Characteristics: This cream comes in a tube. It is fairly heavy and leaves an emollient residue on the skin when applied. This film stays on skin all night. It is fragranced.

**Product Profile:
Night Cream for
Dry, Dehydrated
Skin**

Chemical Action and Design: This cream is a mixture of humectants and emollients, containing large amounts of the latter. The active ingredient in this cream is the substantive collagen and elastin proteins, which sit on the skin's surface and help hold water. This protein is mixed with the emollients beeswax, isopropyl myristate, and cetyl alcohol. It contains petrolatum in a fairly large amount, giving it an occlusive property.

Client and Skin Type: This night treatment is for adult dry, dehydrated skin.

Product Characteristics: Liposomes are the feature of this cream, mixing a combination of oils, emollients, and humectants in a heavier cream that absorbs well. This fragranced cream comes in a jar. It should be applied nightly for best results. This is a sophisticated treatment complex, with any active agents, making it a more expensive cream.

Chemical Action and Design: Hydrators, emollients, conditioners, and plant extracts are present in this complex night treatment. It is designed to deliver deep hydration through its lecithin (liposome) content, helping to retain moisture for a longer period of time. It contains oxybenzone and benzophenone sunscreens, and urea, mucopolysaccharides, and sorbitol as humectants. This is mixed into a variety of emollients including mineral oil, jojoba oil, cetyl alcohol, shea butter, and capric/caprylic triglycerides. This cream is actually available in two different formulas, one for dryer skin and another for combination dry skin.

Many other types of night treatments are not covered here. Most night hydrators and creams vary in both amounts of hydrating agents and amounts of emollient. Therefore they range in design for oily, dehydrated skin to very dry skin that is both oil and water dry. The oilier the skin, the less emollient. The dryer the skin, the more emollient. Night creams will also vary in price, mainly because of the amount and type of ingredients used. Ingredients such as lecithin, liposomes, beta glucans, and hyaluronic acid are expensive (Figure 10-4).

Special Creams
and Treatments

Many treatment creams are available for special problems or special areas. These treatments should be used in conjunction with other day and night treatments.

Eye creams are specially designed for the skin around the eye area. This area of the skin is usually more oil-dry and more sen-

FIGURE 10–4 Bottle A has more oil and emollient for dry skin. Bottle B has less oil and more hydration for dehydrated, oilier skin.

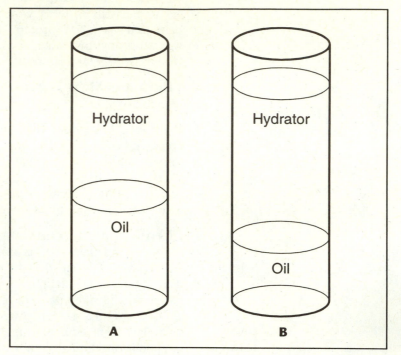

sitive than other areas of the skin. Therefore, creams designed for these areas are generally higher in emollient and lower in humectant content. Because the skin around the eyes is very thin, if you "plump it up" by using lots of hydrating agents, you end up making the eyelid look puffy. More emollient is added to these creams to help supplement the lack of oil production associated with the eye area. Because this area is very sensitive, eye creams must be carefully designed not to irritate. Nevertheless, eye creams often do cause irritation and allergic reactions. Eye creams should be used twice daily.

Neck creams are also made with more emollients and less humectant. The neck area is thinner skin that dries easily. Neck creams should be massaged into the skin twice daily. They are available in a variety of formulations.

Masks are designed to treat a variety of skin problems, from oil-dryness to acne. They are formulated with less water than creams, lotions, and fluids and are considerably heavier than any of these products.

Masks for oily skin generally contain bentonite and kaolin; these clays are helpful in absorbing excess oil and drying the skin. These clays cause the drying of masks designed for cleansing oilier and combination skin types. These masks may contain other conditioning ingredients. For example, for acne-prone skin the mask might contain sulfur, salicylic acid, or benzoyl peroxide. For oily and combination skin it might contain camphor for soothing and antiseptic action or cornstarch for soothing action.

Dry skin masks often do not dry tightly and contain large amounts of emollients. To give substance to the mask, the chemist may use titanium dioxide or may use a gelling agent or thickener to give the mask a thicker texture. These dry skin masks may contain a variety of plant extracts, conditioning agents, emollients, and humectants. They work by adding water to surface layers as well as emollients, helping to temporarily fill in or plump up small lines and wrinkles. They can have a lasting effect on the skin, particularly if preceded by the use of a good humectant or other active agent. The effects may last up to several days.

Exfoliants usually come in the form of scrubs. They are usually water-based products with a humectant, mixed with some sort of abrasive agent such as almond meal or polyethylene granules. They are applied after cleansing and massaged over the skin. The granules literally "bump off" dead cells from the skin's surface. The humectant keeps the product from overdrying the skin. Exfoliants should be used several times a week for best results. They should be followed by a toner and a night or day cream. New treatments are constantly being developed. Improvements in both active agents and vehicle and delivery transport systems for active ingredients constantly help improve the quality of cosmetics and their positive effect on the appearance of the skin. For further information on other new products and developments in cosmetic chemistry, read the chapters on comedogenicity, retinoids and therapies for aging skin, and acne.

TOPICS FOR DISCUSSION

1. What are the differences between rinseable cleansers and emulsion cleansers?

2. What determines the difference between types of rinseable cleansers?

3. Describe some different types of toners.

4. Describe a good day cream for oily or combination skin.

5. Describe some of the various types of day creams you may find in a salon.

6. What is the difference between a day treatment and a night treatment?

11

Claims in Cosmetics

The Food and Drug Administration is a federal agency that regulates the cosmetics industry. In this chapter you will learn about the FDA and how it functions. You will also learn about various claims made about cosmetics, and what the difference is between a drug claim and a cosmetic claim.

You will learn what kind of questions to think about when evaluating claims made by cosmetics companies about their products, which you may be using in your salon.

In 1938 the Food, Drug and Cosmetic Act was passed by the United States Congress. The act called for certain definitions of cosmetics and drugs.

The FDA, which stands for the Food and Drug Administration, is a federal government agency designed to ensure safety of consumer products, namely food, drugs, and cosmetics. They regulate the cosmetics industry. Unlike the regulation of the drug industry, where approval of drugs is necessary before they are marketed, the FDA only controls cosmetics from a disapproving perspective.

This means, essentially, that the FDA only regulates the cosmetic industry when the agency disapproves of a claim or product. This also means that cosmetic companies are not required to list their products or formulas with the FDA. They are required to register only on a voluntary basis.

When a "bad" cosmetic is found by the FDA, the agency begins investigating the cosmetic or claim. If the cosmetic is found to be unsafe, or to be making untrue claims, or to be making drug claims, the FDA will move to warn the company or remove the product from the market.

Drug vs. Cosmetic

The Food and Drug Act of 1938 defines cosmetics and drugs as follows:

- "Drug — Articles (other than food) intended to affect the structure or any function of the body."
- "Cosmetics — Articles intended to be rubbed, poured, sprinkled, or otherwise applied to the human body or any part thereof for cleansing, beautifying, promoting attractiveness or altering the appearance."

Now, we have discussed how active agents work on the skin through the last few chapters. But even if these active agents do affect the function of the skin, we cannot make this claim if the product is a cosmetic. We can, however, say that the product "improves the skin's appearance."

Does this sound silly? Many cosmetic scientists agree, but this is the law as it exists. Cosmetics affect the appearance. If it is claimed that they affect the body or the skin's physiological function, they are considered drugs.

The key words here are *claims* and *intention*. If your product does affect the skin's function, and you do not mention it while selling the product as a cosmetic, you have not broken the law. You are selling the product and claiming that it only improves the appearance.

In other words, what you *intend* for the product to do makes it a cosmetic or a drug. Let's look at a few examples. A toner for oily skin contains an antiseptic ingredient. Killing bacteria is a drug claim because it affects the skin's function and rids the body of possible disease-causing microorganisms. But if the toner contains the antiseptic ingredient and no claim about the antiseptic action is made, then it is not a drug claim. You can say that the toner "helps reduce the appearance of enlarged pores" or "helps remove excess oil" or "improves the appearance of oily areas." These are all claims about the appearance. The fact that the toner also probably kills bacteria is just not mentioned.

Now, if you register the same product as a drug, you can say "This product helps kill bacteria," or "Kills germs that can cause infection." You are permitted to make these physiological claims if the product is registered with the FDA as a drug. "OTC" means over-the-counter drugs. These are drug products for which a physician's prescription is not needed. Prescription drugs require a written prescription from a licensed physician. Dentists and veterinarians are also permitted to write prescriptions. Estheticians use only OTC drugs unless they are working directly under the supervision of a licensed physician. OTC drugs that are used by or sold by estheticians may include sunscreens, acne medications, and hydrocortisone creams.

Let's explore another possibility. A cream is made with good vehicle ingredients that are very acceptable to the intercellular cement, making the probability of deeper penetration of the product higher. The cream includes the free radical scavengers retinyl palmitate and tocopherol acetate. Many cosmetic scientists believe that retinyl palmirate breaks down into retinoic acid when it enters the skin. (See the chapters on retinoids.) The cream also contains beta-glucans, theorized to improve the skin by increasing the production of collagen.

Now these theories may be true, but if the claim is made that "this cream makes cells healthier by reducing free radicals with vitamins A and E, and stimulates the production of new collagen," a drug claim has been made! You are saying that the product (1) contains vitamins, which are known to affect body functions; (2) "makes cells healthier," which is a physiological claim; and (3) "stimulates the production of new collagen," another physiological claim.

So you have made three drug claims in just one descriptive phrase. In order to make these claims, the product would have to be registered as a drug.

Registering a product as a drug means that the product must have had substantial testing to support its ingredient claims, efficacy, and safety. It takes years to have new ingredients approved.

Drug ingredients that have been used for long periods of time safely and effectively are permitted for the uses for which they are approved. Salicylic acid, for example, has long been approved for use in OTC acne products. It is recognized as safe and effective for treating minor acne. Because of its long history of safety, manufacturers may use it in acne products, and must register the product if they are making a drug claim. They do not need to file for "new ingredient" testing, though. Let's go back to your cream. If you claim that the cream makes skin look healthier and helps to smooth the appearance of rough textures, you have made a cosmetic claim. You have simply made the claim that the product improves appearance and have not said anything regarding physiological function.

Verbal Claims

As a licensed esthetician or cosmetologist, you must be careful of what you say to clients regarding claims for products. If you say that a product affects the physiology of the skin, then you intend for that product to have drug effects, and you are therefore making drug claims!

You must be careful never to make a claim about a cosmetic that is a drug claim. Always describe products as "improving the appearance," "reducing the visible signs of wrinkles" (intention: you are reducing the appearance of the wrinkle, not the wrinkle itself), "lessening the appearance of puffy eyes" (you are treating the appearance of puffiness, not the physiological factors that caused the puffiness). Good key words include

- "help to..."
- "reduces the appearance of..."
- "diminishes the visual signs of..."
- "improves the appearance of the skin..."

Any words that imply that the skin looks better are usually appropriate. Remember, a cosmetic cleanses, beautifies, promotes attractiveness, and alters the appearance.

But what about how cosmetics really affect the skin? It is the opinion of this author and many other cosmetic and health scientists that we need a new product classification with the FDA. It has been proposed that a "cosmeceutical" category be established. A **cosmeceutical** would be defined as a product that is designed for appearance improvement, but may have positive physiological effects on the skin, on a cellular level. Because cosmetic scientists, as well as scientists from the medical community, do have evidence that many cosmetic ingredients affect the behavior and function of the skin, it is felt by many that this new category is needed. Cosmetologists and estheticians cannot legally explain the actual chemical reactions that occur in products.

The Labeling Law

In 1977 the Federal Packaging and Labeling Act was instated by the FDA. This package of regulations required all cosmetic manufacturers to list ingredients used in their products. The initial reasoning for this package of regulations was to protect consumers who suffered from allergic reactions to particular ingredients.

In theory, the consumer could check the ingredient label for allergen ingredients and thus, theoretically, avoid a potential allergic reaction.

The ingredients are required to be listed on the outermost part of the packaging. If the product is in a box, the ingredients must be listed on the box. Products that are marketed in jars or containers without using a box or other outer packaging must list ingredients on the container itself. The reason for the requirement for the ingredients to be on the outermost surface of the packaging is so the consumer can easily find the list.

Again, in this author's opinion, this is both helpful and hurtful. It is true that a consumer can check for ingredients to which he or she is allergic. But the consumer often reads other chemical names that he or she does not understand or knows nothing about. As an example, a consumer once said that she did not want to use a particular moisturizer because it contained methylparaben, and she did not like to use products with oils in them! The consumer had mistaken the preservative *paraben* for the oil *parafin*. An easy mistake, perhaps, but nevertheless this illustrates the fact that consumers do not, in general, know enough about chemistry to read an ingredient label, much less know what it means.

The names of the chemicals listed must be registered in the CTFA compendium, which is essentially a directory of generic chemical names agreed upon by the CTFA, the Cosmetics, Toiletries, and Fragrance Association (which is the largest association of cosmetic manufacturers), the FDA, and other interested consumer and manufacturing groups. These names are used so that any two companies who use a particular ingredient will list it in the same way on their ingredient labels. These names are the industry standard. It is not acceptable by the FDA to list chemicals by their trade names or functions.

The ingredients listed on the label must be in the order of concentration that they are present in the product. In other words, a cream that is a mixture of 70 percent water, 10 percent mineral oil, and 5 percent sodium lauryl sulfate must list the ingredients in descending order of concentration such as, "water, mineral oil, sodium lauryl sulfate... ."

The exception to the concentration listing rule is that any ingredient that is less than 1 percent concentration in the product can be listed in any order. In other words, towards the end of the list, after ingredients with 1 percent concentration are listed, any ingredient (at less than 1 percent concentration presence in the product) may be listed in any order.

The sources of the ingredients are also illegal to use on the ingredient label. Some "natural" cosmetics manufacturers will list cetyl alcohol, for example, and then afterwards list in parentheses (*coconut oil*), indicating that cetyl alcohol is derived from a "natural" source. This is an illegal listing, because it may be confusing to the consumer. Secondly, just because a chemical is naturally derived does not necessarily mean that the quality is better.

Extracts from plants are usually listed by the plant name and the word *extract*. The extract may or may not contain a solvent such as oil, propylene glycol, water, or alcohol. The term *extract* implies, according to the industry rules, that there may be solvent ingredients in this plant extract constituent. It is generally accepted that this is an acceptable labeling practice. Sometimes extracts will be listed as "essence of..." or "infusion of...." This means that the extract is in a suspension of water or that extracts have been added to water used in the formulation.

Drug Labeling

On OTC products, the manufacturer must list first the active ingredient(s) and then list the other ingredients used in the vehicle for the cream or topical product. A sunscreen product, for example, may read:

- Active ingredients: Methoxycinnimate, Benzophenone.
- Other ingredients: Water, Propylene Glycol, Carbomer 940, Cetyl Alcohol, Methylparaben, Propylparaben, Fragrance.

The actual active ingredients are listed separately, and vehicle ingredients are listed second. Products registered as drugs must list the active ingredients first on the ingredient label.

Products that contain sunscreen, but do not make a sunscreening claim, may be considered cosmetics. They are not claiming that the product prevents or helps prevent skin cancer or sunburn—simply that the product contains sunscreen ingredients. So a product can be a cosmetic with sunscreen and not be registered as a drug, but cannot be a sunscreen without being registered. Again, the intended use of the product is the main focus.

Once again, the FDA is a disapproving agency, meaning that they only investigate a cosmetic if it is believed that a fraudulent or medical claim is being made, or if the product is unsafe or contaminated. The FDA does not approve cosmetics. Claims that a particular cosmetic is "FDA approved" are false, misleading, and illegal.

Other Cosmetic Claims

Hypoallergenic

A cosmetic that is claimed to be hypoallergenic has generally been manufactured without the use of certain ingredients that are known to frequently cause allergic reactions. Fragrance is generally left out of hypoallergenic cosmetics because fragrance is one of the main causes of allergic skin reactions.

The term *hypoallergenic* does not mean nonallergenic. There is no such thing as a nonallergenic cosmetic. Somewhere in the world there is a person allergic to every single ingredient used by the cosmetic industry. While there is no way to guarantee a product as nonallergenic, hypoallergenic cosmetics statistically cause fewer allergic reactions.

Some companies run sophisticated allergy tests on their products to demonstrate their hypoallergenic status. This unfortunately still does not guarantee non-allergenicity; it simply shows that the company cares and believes in their product enough to have it tested.

The truth is that most cosmetics today are hypoallergenic and are designed that way. Most companies take great care to make sure their products can be used by most people. It is in their financial interest to do so, as well.

Fragrance-Free Cosmetics

As discussed earlier, many cosmetic manufacturers purposely do not use fragrances in their products to reduce the chances of allergic reaction. Such products may still actually have an odor or smell. This is the odor of the actual ingredients used in the product formulation. However, not adding fragrance to a cosmetic is a generally good idea, when possible.

Preservative-Free Cosmetics

This is a crazy claim! Products should never be made preservative-free! The danger of contaminating microbes that would exist in such a cosmetic is a far greater problem than the slight chance of allergy from a preservative. Avoid any company that makes such a claim.

Noncomedogenic

This means that certain ingredients that are known to cause comedone development and acne flare-ups have not been used in these cosmetic formulations. Fats and emollients are the principal agents that cause these reactions.

Unfortunately there is no standard industry definition of the word *noncomedogenic*, and the FDA does not require that testing be performed to make such a claim. Unfortunately, certain companies take advantage of lack of rules and make claims that their products are noncomedogenic without performing the proper testing. For much more information on noncomedogenic testing, see the chapter on comedogenicity.

Nonacnegenic

Often this term is used interchangeably with noncomedogenic, but *nonacnegenic* means that the product has been designed not to cause comedones to develop or follicle irritancy that can cause immediate acne flare-ups. It takes sometimes as much as six months for comedones to form, while follicle irritancy potentially can cause an acne flare-up much more quickly.

Again, a variety of tests for follicle irritancy can be run, but some companies make the claim without proper testing.

Dermatologist Tested

Once again, this can be a very confusing term. Generally, ethical companies mean that the product has been tested for irritancy under the supervision of a dermatologist. One writer asks the question, "Dermatologist tested—for what?"—a good question. This can be a misleading term.

Natural Cosmetics

One of the latest rages in cosmetic development is so-called "natural" cosmetics. Naturally derived ingredients in cosmetics have been used for decades. While nature has some wonderful chemicals to contribute to the cosmetics industry, they are not sufficient by themselves, nor are they always superior to synthetic chemicals.

The fact is that in one form or another everything comes from the earth! Think about it. Even the ingredients used to make plastic come from Mother Nature!

Natural products can also cause allergic reactions. For more on this, see the chapter on allergies. Do not choose a cosmetic solely on the basis of its "naturalness."

Organic Cosmetics

This is probably also supposed to mean that the cosmetic ingredients used are derived from "natural" sources. The term *organic* actually means that the chemistry of a substance involves the element carbon.

Puffing

Puffing is a term used to describe the way some companies make their products sound better. This is actually an insulting term, because it is usually used to mean that the cosmetic company is making the product sound better than it actually is.

Most companies want their products to sound good. Companies that use outrageous claims to promote their products, like "face lift in-a-jar," make the entire industry suffer. Companies that promote their cosmetics for their real benefits are fortunately in the majority. However, there is always one unscrupulous company that will make outrageous claims in order to make money. Fortunately, consumers soon find that their claims aren't true.

Animal Testing

Some companies claim that they do not perform testing on animals. While many companies do not believe in excessive animal testing, certain tests must be performed to insure a safe product.

Formulas sometimes are not tested on animals, but almost all ingredients used in cosmetics have, at one time or another, been tested on animals. This is the only way to make sure that the individual ingredients are safe for human use.

In general, cosmetics companies have made a legitimate effort to reduce animal testing, eliminating excessive and unnecessary testing. However, some important tests cannot be performed without using animals.

Some estheticians are single-mindedly against animal testing. Many of these estheticians do not understand that it is vital to insure ingredient safety. Some of these safety tests cannot be run without the use of animals.

In the future, technology will be developed so laboratory tests should substitute for most animal tests. Progress is being made, but until testing is developed, some tests will still have to be run on animals to insure that products are completely safe to be used by the American consumer.

International Companies

Some products are imported from other countries where the laws regarding cosmetics may be different than those of the United States. Because of this, some companies make claims that are legitimate by their country's standards, but are illegal or misleading by U. S. standards. Importers of these products should be aware of these differences and change claims that are not permitted in the United States. While many companies are extremely conscientious about this, a few companies, out of ignorance, do not make the proper changes.

Today's consumer is generally better informed than consumers of years past and know better than to believe unrealistic claims. Unfortunately, enough "bad guy" companies have "cried wolf" often enough that the consumer is often wary when buying cosmetics.

Discussing Claims with Clients

Always try to be honest with clients about a product's true benefits. Hard-selling only offends clients. Estheticians should educate their clients about proper products for their skin. The client is only interested in making the skin look the best it can look. Do not make promises you can't keep. Each client has unique problems and conditions, and clients will not always react to products in the same way. There is no way an esthetician can absolutely be sure any product will work. All an esthetician can do is give the best advice possible.

Buying Products for Your Salon

You will, no doubt, attend many trade shows throughout your career where cosmetics companies display their products for you to purchase. You should do your homework before you purchase products from any company.

You should ask many questions before buying a product line. Some of these questions are:

1. Are the theories used by the company's products rational?

2. Do they make legitimate claims? If the product sounds too good to be true, it probably is too good to be true!

3. How much care do they take in developing cosmetics?

4. Are their products formulated with allergies and comedogenicity in mind?

5. If they make claims about hypoallergenic or noncomedogenic products, do they test their products?

6. Are these tests run by the company or by an independent testing company? (It is better if they are performed by an outside company—they are less likely to be biased.)

7. Are they willing to let you see the test results?

8. Are their prices competitive with similar products?

9. Do they use ingredients that you have never heard of? If you are current on your skin-care journal reading, you should be aware of new and innovative ingredients that are legitimate.

10. What is the company's history? Who is their founder, and what are the founder's credentials?

The more education you have, the better you will be at selecting the best, reputable companies. Be careful not to be pressured. Good solid companies don't mind if you think about a purchase before making it.

Many more questions should be asked of companies before you choose a line. You should investigate their reputation with colleagues you respect. You should look into their marketing programs and find out if they are accessible if you have questions, and how fast their service is.

The bottom line is are they honest, and do they have a quality, legitimate product?

1. What does the FDA regulate?

2. Why is the FDA called a "disapproving" agency?

3. Discuss the Food and Drug Act's definitions of cosmetics and drugs. How do these definitions differ?

4. What is the reason for listing ingredients on a cosmetic label?

5. What are the labelling laws for drug products?

6. Discuss the terms *noncomedogenic* and *nonacnegenic*. What tests should be run to legitimately make these claims?

CHAPTER

12

Acne and the Esthetician

OBJECTIVES

In this chapter you will learn about factors that influence the development of different types of acne. You will learn to identify the different types of acne lesions and will learn about several acne-like medical conditions. You will learn how dermatologists treat acne and when you should refer a client to a dermatologist. A variety of treatments, ingredients, drugs, and products will also be studied.

Acne is a skin condition that results in inflammatory and non-inflammatory lesions. Commonly associated with teenage and adolescent skin, it actually affects many age groups at different stages of life. There are many forms of acne and acne-related conditions that the esthetician sees every day. While many forms of acne require the care of a dermatologist, many clients can benefit from esthetic treatments for problem skin.

Common Acne

The most common form of acne is called **acne vulgaris**. This is the type of acne so often associated with teenagers. It usually begins at the onset of puberty, at which time teenagers begin producing larger amounts of sex hormones. (See the chapter on hormones.) These hormones cause stimulation of the sebaceous gland, which produces an over-abundance of sebum.

This extra oil adds to a condition called **retention hyperkeratosis**. As we learned earlier, the epidermal cells, particularly the corneum, is constantly shedding and being replaced by younger cells. Retention hyperkeratosis is a condition in which these cells are retained, stick to the surface of the skin, and begin lining the inside walls of the follicles. We will, for simplicity, refer to retention hyperkeratosis as "cell buildup." The cells build up inside the follicles much like wax has a tendency to build up on the surface of furniture.

This process of buildup is complicated by the fact that the cells continue to push to the surface of the epidermis at a faster rate. *Hyper* means more than normal, so hyperkeratosis means the process of keratinization (turnover of cells) occurs at a rate much faster than normal.

Retention hyperkeratosis is a hereditary condition. If a child's parents both had acne, there is a very good chance that the child, also, will have a strong tendency to develop acne.

Some researchers believe that retention hyperkeratosis is caused by an inability of the body to produce intercellular structures called lamellar granules. These granules are theorized to release an enzyme that causes dead cells to break away from the corneum in the normal manner. It has been determined that chronic acne patients do not have as many of these active structures present in their follicular cells.

As cells build up on the inside of the follicle wall they form a small impaction called a **microcomedo**. Microcomedones (plural) are actually a mixture of dead cells, bacteria, fatty acids from sebum, and other cellular debris. Microcomedones are invisible. They cannot be seen without a microscope. They continue to retain more and more of the mixture of dead cells, sebum, and bacteria, until they become a visible lesion on the surface of the skin (Figure 12-1).

Noninflammatory and Inflammatory Acne Lesions

There is a point in the development of the impaction where the microcomedo either becomes an inflammatory or noninflammatory lesion. **Noninflammatory** means that the impaction is not red or inflamed. Examples of noninflammatory acne lesions are **open comedones** (blackheads) and **closed comedones** (whiteheads) (Figure 12-2).

Open comedones occur when the follicle is large enough to hold all of the debris retained by the follicle. The **osteum**, or opening, in these follicles is dilated by the mass of the impaction, allowing the comedo to push towards the surface opening.

Cornybacterium acnes is the scientific name of the bacteria that causes acne vulgaris. These bacteria are **anaerobic**, which means that they do not need oxygen to grow and survive. These bacteria are present in the follicles in small numbers. They are kept from reproducing to large numbers by the oxygen that is constantly aerating the open follicle. However, when the follicle gets blocked from oxygen circulation, these bacteria multiply in great numbers, feeding off the sebum produced by overactive sebaceous glands (Figure 12-3). Open comedones do not encourage development of this bacterial growth because the follicle opening is large enough to expose the follicle to oxygen. The oxygen is also what causes the "blackhead" to form at the

FIGURE 12–1 The progression of acne

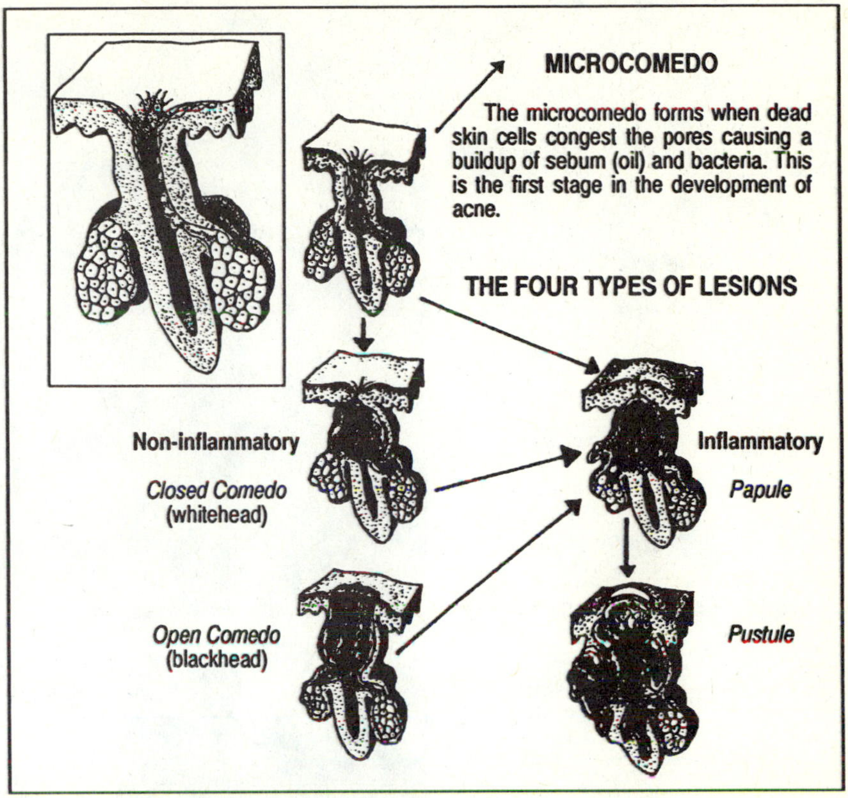

MICROCOMEDO

The microcomedo forms when dead skin cells congest the pores causing a buildup of sebum (oil) and bacteria. This is the first stage in the development of acne.

THE FOUR TYPES OF LESIONS

Non-inflammatory

Closed Comedo (whitehead)

Open Comedo (blackhead)

Inflammatory

Papule

Pustule

exposed part of the impaction. This darkening is caused by the exposure of the top of the comedo to the oxygen in the air outside the follicle. The sebum turns a brown color, similar to the way mayonnaise will turn yellow if left out on a picnic table for a period of time. The darkness is also caused by clumps of **melanin** (skin pigment) present in the dead cells in the comedo. This theory is easily demonstrated by observing an extracted open comedo. It is a solid cylindrical plug, topped by a dark area that gets lighter as the deeper parts of the impaction are extracted.

Open comedones, therefore, rarely develop into inflammatory lesions. Unfortunately the same cannot be said for closed comedones. Closed comedones have very small pore openings, which prevents oxygen from readily penetrating the follicle. The walls of the follicle stretch to hold the contents of the impaction, but the follicle opening does not. Because of this lack of oxygen, the lesions can easily become inflamed due to the increasing number of bacteria multiplying in the anaerobic environment.

FIGURE 12–2 Open and closed comedones. *Courtesy Michael J. Bond, M.D.*

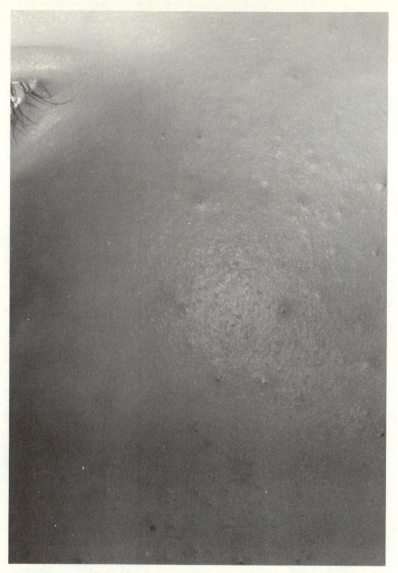

Closed comedones are easily recognizable. They are frequently seen in adult women, often in the blush line of makeup users. They are small "underground" bumps and are not easily extracted. They are frequently associated with the use of comedogenic cosmetics (see the chapter on comedogenicity), as indicated in the blush line of some women.

When enough bacteria form inside the closed comedone and the impaction becomes large enough, a small tear occurs in the

FIGURE 12–3 The development of acne in a young girl

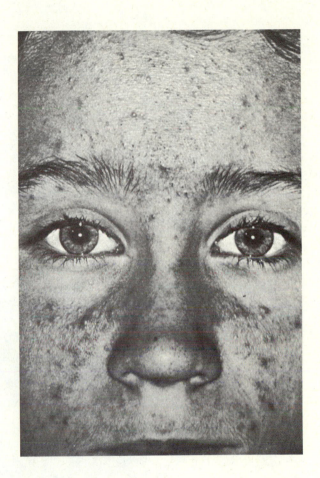

follicle wall, which stimulates the immune system to investigate (see the chapter on the immune system), releasing white blood cells into the area. This begins the inflammatory process.

A **papule** is a red, sore bump without a "whitehead" (no pus) (Figure 12-4). This is the beginning of the "rescue" by the white blood cells. When enough white blood cells arrive, they may form a "clump" and rise to the surface, creating what is known as a **pustule** (Figure 12-5). *Pus* is the common name for this

FIGURE 12–4 The papule

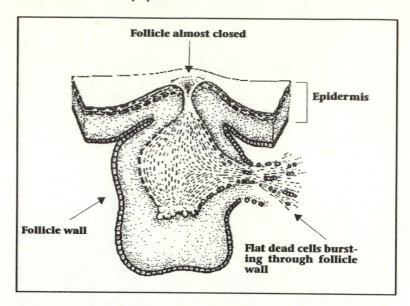

FIGURE 12–5 The pustule

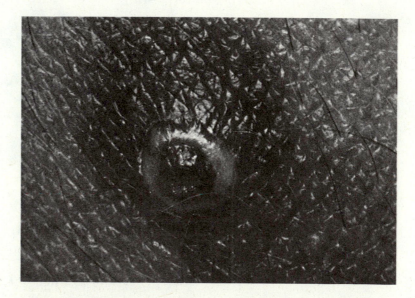

"clump" of white blood cells. For practical purposes, a papule is often described by the client as a large, red, sore bump that never "comes to a head." Papules seem sometimes to "magically disappear." This is because the immune system has "won the battle" and disposed of the impaction through enzymes and absorption, and the body has disposed of the remains through normal blood excretion. Papules affect the nerve endings more than pustules because they are deeper in the skin. This explains the soreness. Pustules have "migrated" the impaction toward the skin surface, dilating the follicle opening and relieving the pressure on the nerve endings, resulting in less pain.

A **nodule** is similar to a papule, but is deeper in the skin and feels very solid and sore. **Cysts** are deep infections caused by a deep, massive invasion of white blood cells. They are very pustular and very large (Figure 12-6).

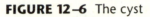

FIGURE 12–6 The cyst

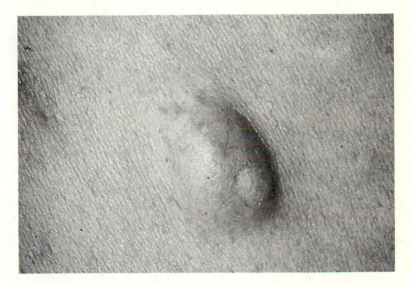

The Grades of Acne

Acne is "graded" by dermatologists on a four-point scale. (See Figure 12-7.)

- **Grade 1 acne**—mostly open and closed comedones with an occasional pimple. Grade 1 acne is typical of a teenager just beginning puberty.

- **Grade 2 acne**—very large number of closed comedones, with occasional pustules or papules.

- **Grade 3 acne** is thought of by most people as "typical teenage acne." It involves large numbers of open and closed comedones and many papules and pustules as well. It is very inflamed and red.

- **Grade 4 acne** is commonly referred to as cystic acne, with many deep cysts and scar formation.

FIGURE 12–7a Grade 1 acne. *Courtesy Melvin L. Elson, M.D.*

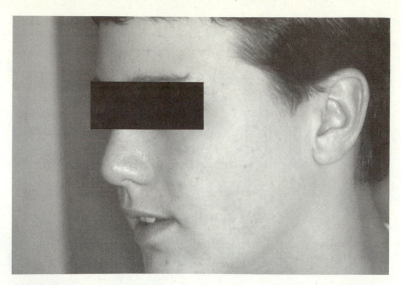

FIGURE 12–7b Grade 2 acne. *Courtesy Rube J. Pardo, M.D., Ph.D.*

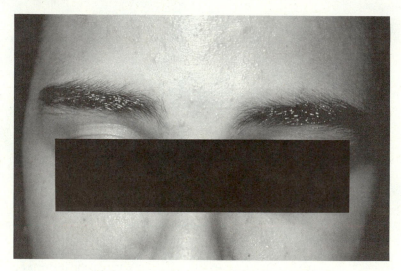

Why Scars Form

Scars form when the skin, in a desperate attempt to heal itself, produces lots of collagen to try to compensate for the lack of normal skin functioning. This type of scar will usually be raised. Acne "pit" scarring occurs from actual destruction of the tissue during the inflammatory process. Cystic acne is almost always associated with scarring (Figure 12-8).

Hormones

Hormones are often associated with acne because they have the ability to stimulate the sebaceous glands, causing the manufacture of more sebum, which is the food for the acne bacteria.

FIGURE 12–7c Grade 3 acne. *Courtesy Melvin L. Elson, M.D.*

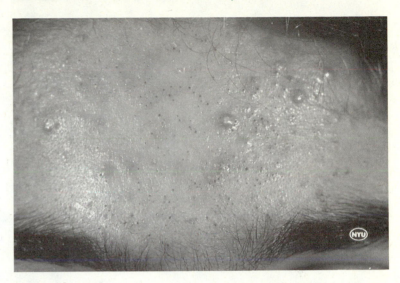

FIGURE 12–7d Grade 4 acne. *Courtesy Melvin L. Elson, M.D.*

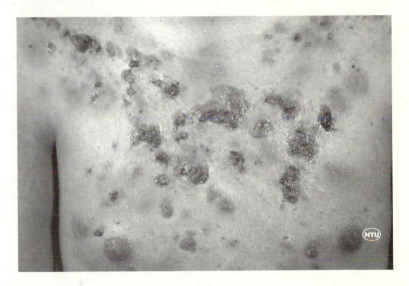

As discussed in the earlier chapter on hormones, both males and females produce both male and female hormones. The male hormones, the androgens, may stimulate the overproduction of sebum in acne sufferers.

The predominence of androgens over estrogens during certain times of life, such as during the premenstrual and menopausal, periods can cause acne flareups in adult women. Premenstrual breakouts are theorized to be caused by a predominance of male hormones during premensus. This abundance of andro-

FIGURE 12–8 Facial scarring

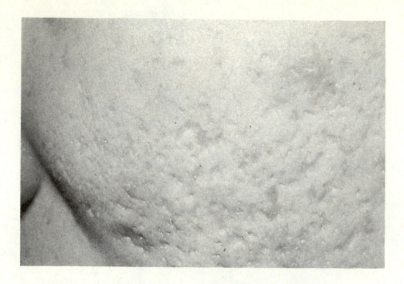

gens causes the egg to be lost during mensus and also causes the overabundance of sebum that can easily cause an acne flareup during premensus.

Chin Acne

Many women notice that during premensus they develop papules and pustules in the chin area. Some researchers believe this may be caused by the fact that while the sebaceous glands in the chin area are fairly large, the actual follicle openings in these adult women are not large. When a large amount of sebum production is stimulated by the androgens, these follicles in the chin area fill up quickly with sebum and cannot handle the large amount. They therefore become inflamed and become papules.

Many women notice that these papules do not linger for long periods of time and do not turn into pustules. This may be because once the hormones restabilize, the oil production returns to normal, and the follicles return to normal.

During menopause, however, this androgenic stimulation may not slow down, and the woman may develop a full-blown acne condition.

Stress

Stress is what causes "pimples on prom night." Many acne sufferers, as well as dermatologists and estheticians, have noticed acne flareups when a patient is under stress. A final exam at school, dating problems, financial problems, or difficulties at work seem to frequently accompany breakouts.

There is a fairly simple explanation for this relationship. Stress causes the brain to manufacture a hormone that, in turn, causes the adrenal gland to make more hormones, which causes an abundance of oil to be produced. The reaction is very similar to the premenstrual reaction.

Birth Control Pills

Birth control pills can cause an androgenic flareup that can contribute to acne. When starting birth control pills the skin may get better or worse. The same may be true when discontinuing birth control pills. Women using birth control pills may find that their monthly premenstrual breakouts occur at a different time in the cycle.

The reasoning here is simple. Birth control pills affect hormone levels and may affect different women in different ways. (See the hormone chapter for more information).

Pregnancy

Pregnancy may also produce unpredictable flareups or clearing of acne. The usual course is that acne gets worse during the first three months of pregnancy, then gets dramatically better. The acne may flare up again after childbirth or after breastfeeding is discontinued. Theoretically this is due to obvious hormone changes, but stress levels may be partially responsible.

Acne in the 20- to 30-Year-Old

Some women never have acne until their early 20s or 30s. This may be due to many factors. We have already mentioned premenstrual hormonal flares, birth control, pregnancy, and stress, all of which can certainly affect this age group. Cosmetics are very popular with this age group also, and comedogenic factors may certainly play a part. The esthetician often hears the complaint of sudden breakout in this age bracket. Treat these cases as you would any acne case.

The Beginning of Teenage Acne

The beginning of teenage acne is characterized by minor breakouts in the nose area. Small blackheads and clogged follicles, small papules, and small milia are found. The esthetician will only notice the beginning of visible pores in the nose and chin and sometimes the forehead. This is the beginning of adolescent pore structure, and usually, puberty and adolescence. Usually within six months more pimples will develop. Boys may notice small pimples in the lower cheeks. This may be caused by the beginning of beard hair growth. The hair is beginning to grow, but the follicle is not large enough to accommodate the hair.

Young teenagers should be treated every two to three months until breakouts become persistent. At that time regular treatments are recommended. Recommend a gentle, nonmedicated, foaming cleanser, a toner for oily/combination skin, and a mild gel of salicylic acid or 2 1/2 percent benzoyl peroxide. Used regularly, these products will help prepubescent teens through this period. Teenagers usually do not need a moisturizer except in cold weather.

Lack of Care

Young teenagers may not be disciplined when it comes to a regular facial care routine. Sit them down and gently explain the need for consistent care. They usually will take advice from you before they will from Mom at this age.

Teenagers are not the only age group that suffers from lack of skin hygiene. Even though acne is not caused by dirt, many adults neglect their skin. Sleeping in makeup is not only unhygenic, it also means that the night treatment is not applied. Explain to the client that she may come to have a treatment at the salon twice a month, but she is responsible for the other 60 times a month that the skin is cleansed and conditioned! Help her find simple routines that she enjoys doing. Teach her to clean her face as soon as she gets home for the evening. This is also a good time to floss her teeth, right after dinner. When she gets sleepy later in the evening, she can walk past the bathroom guilt-free!

Environmental Factors that Influence Acne

Heat and Humidity

There is no question that acne is more likely to flare up in the summer months when heat and humidity are high. Heat causes the skin to swell slightly, and humidity causes tremendous swelling of the outer epidermis. It is reasonable to assume that this could possibly exert enough pressure on the follicles to further complicate an already existing condition.

It has been observed over the years that people who live in tropical, warm climates with high humidity experience a fairly predictable seasonal pattern of flareups. Estheticians should bring this to the attention of their clients and encourage them to come to the salon more often for treatments during this type of weather if the client notices a consistent relationship.

Sun Exposure

While sun exposure may have an immediate drying effect on acne lesions, sun damages skin and is documented to cause more "cell buildup," which can add to or increase the chances of acne flareup.

Many acne patients claim their acne improves with sun exposure. Tanning masks the redness, and as the buildup of tan cells occurs on the surface of the skin, acne may appear better. As soon as beach season is over, however, these same patients notice reoccurrence of their acne. What actually happens is that the tan fades and the cell buildup subsides, suddenly exposing a tremendous number of clogged follicles and closed comedones.

The most unfortunate part of this situation is that these clients have a strong tendency to neglect treating their acne during beach season, making it more complicated when the tan fades. It is up to the esthetician to educate the client before sun season to avoid this problem.

Greasy Workplaces

Acne patients who work in environments where their skin is constantly exposed to large amounts of occlusive grease or airborne grease, such as that present in fast-food restaurants, may notice a strong flareup in their conditions. Occupations such as car mechanics and short-order cooks are good examples of such situations. It is best for these individuals to avoid working for prolonged periods of time under these conditions. Advise clients who must work in these types of jobs to cleanse their skin at regular intervals (about twice during an eight-hour period) with a mild cleanser that will remove the environmental oil without drying the skin too much.

Overcleaning

Clients are constantly under the impression that acne is directly caused by lack of cleansing. While keeping skin as clean as possible is certainly important, acne is not caused by dirt. In fact, acne can be aggravated by too much cleaning. Repeated exposure to detergents in facial cleansers, for example, can aggravate acne if the client is using the cleansers too often. Estheticians often find that their clients are cleaning the face numerous times daily (eight to ten times). This causes enough irritation to precipitate not only an acne aggravation, but other sensitivities. Instruct these clients to cleanse two or three times a day only.

Self-Trauma Excoriations

This essentially means that the client is scratching or picking at the skin until the raised portion of the acne lesion is literally scraped off the face (usually with the fingernails). Most clients pick at their lesions subconsciously. These lesions will appear red, flat, and raw on the surface of the skin, similar to a freshly scraped knee or brush burn (Figure 12-9).

These clients usually pick at the skin as a habit. It must be pointed out to these clients that the lesions will never heal properly as long as they continue to pull off the scabs, and that the fingernails carry many germs that can cause other types of infections besides acne. Encourage these clients to use a mask treatment at home routinely (but not too often). Suggest that

FIGURE 12–9 Self-trauma excoriation

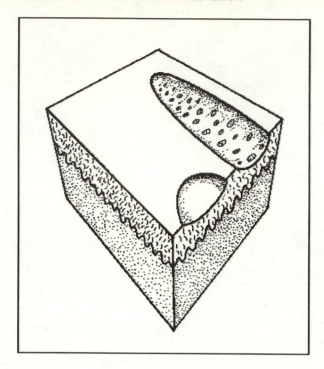

they wear loosely fitting gloves while reading or watching television. The touch of the glove material will signal them and make them aware when they are scraping at their skin.

It should be pointed out here that, while a number of clients pick absentmindedly, many "self traumatizers" are troubled mentally or are under a tremendous amount of stress. Handle these clients gently. They need lots of understanding as well as good skin care.

Nutrition and Diet

There are numerous falsehoods regarding the effects of food on acne. Chocolate, nuts, seafood, greasy "teenage" foods such as burgers and french fries, milk, and milk products have all been falsely accused at one time of causing or worsening acne. While some of these foods are not healthy in large quantities because they may be high in sugar, cholesterol, or triglycerides, they do not directly or indirectly cause acne. Many acne patients and, unfortunately, estheticians are still under the mistaken impression that these foods cause acne.

It is important to have a properly balanced diet to have good skin and good health. The only food group that has consistently been implicated in aggravating acne conditions is iodides. Foods that are high in iodides include some types of shellfish, kelp, squid, asparagus, and iodized salt in salty foods. Iodine causes a follicular irritancy when ingested in large quantities. Consumed in reasonable quantities occasionally, these foods probably do not cause serious problems. It stands to reason, though, that excessive consumption of foods high in iodides can cause acne to flare up.

Zinc supplements are furnished to some acne patients by dermatologists. Prescribed in inflamed acne to reduce redness and inflammation, the usual dosage is 100 mg per day. It is best to check with a dermatologist before suggesting zinc supplements to your clients, as estheticians are not registered dieticians and therefore are not authorities on nutritional science. It is best to leave advice to the specialists in this area.

Acne and Cosmetics

Probably the best service an esthetician can render to an acne patient is helping the patient choose cosmetics and skin-care products that are noncomedogenic. (See Chapter 13.)

So many factors cause or contribute to acne, but the esthetician has control over only a few. Heredity and hormones are not part of the practice of esthetics. Even though we may know a lot about these subjects, there is little the esthetician can do to control or affect these factors. Estheticians can temporarily reduce stress by administering soothing treatments, but the stress reducing effects of these therapies are not long lasting when the client gets in an argument with the boss or forgets when a term paper is due.

The point here is that the only real factors over which estheticians have control is how the client cleanses the skin and what cosmetics and skin-care products the client uses routinely.

It is imperative that the esthetician fully understand comedogenicity for acne and problem skin clients. It is the best service we can offer them. The client may come in for treatment only once a month but she exposes herself to cosmetics and skin care up to 60 times a month.

The esthetician must eliminate all possible comedogenic factors from the home care and cosmetic regime of the acne patient.

Cosmetics, skin care, and topical drugs are the only things that are in constant, direct contact with the skin.

Acne-Related Conditions

Seborrhea (Seborrheic Dermatitis)

Seborrhea is an irritation associated with oily skin and oily areas. Dandruff is a type of seborrhea. Seborrhea is characterized by dry looking, flaky, crusty patches. Redness is often apparent under these crusty patches. Seborrhea is normally seen in the scalp, around the hairline, along the sides of the nose, and in the ears (Figure 12-10).

FIGURE 12–10 Seborrheic dermatitis. *Courtesy Rube J. Pardo, M.D., Ph.D.*

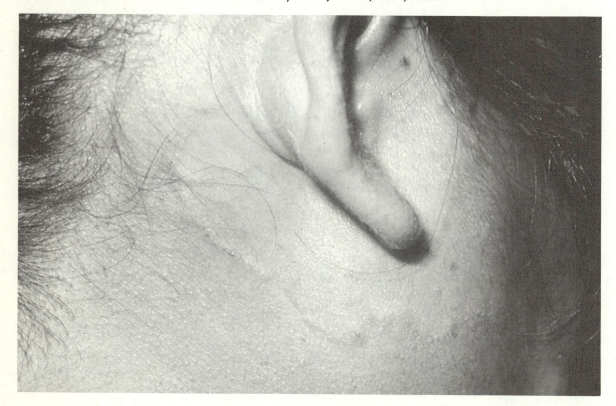

Seborrhea is often misdiagnosed by the client or an inexperienced esthetician as "dry skin," when it is actually associated with oily skin. Seborrhea is best treated by a dermatologist, but the esthetician should be involved in choosing the correct skin-care program. Again, it is important to avoid comedogenic products. Suggest a gentle but thorough cleanser, toner, and very light, noncomedogenic moisturizer. Overmoisturizing can be a contributing factor to seborrhea.

Low humidity and poor or lack of cleansing both contribute to this irritating condition. This is one situation that small amounts of sun exposure actually seems to help. If the client does not improve immediately, the client should be referred to a dermatologist, as this condition can be chronic and volatile. Typical dermatological treatment includes the use of hydrocortisone, coal tar shampoos, salicylic acid, selenium sulfide, and zinc pyrithione medications. In the salon, avoid excessive massage and stimulating treatments. Use soothing, nonirritating treatments. Mild extraction of the areas often helps to reduce follicle inflammation by removing impactions.

Acne Rosacea

Acne rosacea is a condition of the skin, referred to as adult acne by many doctors, that causes large red papules and pustules to form in the nose and cheek areas. These lesions are very large and painful, accompanied by diffuse redness, telangectasias (broken and enlarged capillaries), and general redness (Figure 12-11).

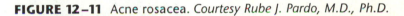

FIGURE 12–11 Acne rosacea. *Courtesy Rube J. Pardo, M.D., Ph.D.*

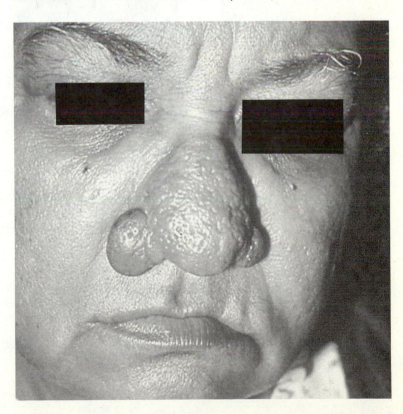

In its severe form, it may result in a condition called **rhino-phyma**, an enlargening of the nose. The famous comedian W.C. Fields suffered from rosacea and rhinophyma, which is why he had the "famous" large, red nose (Figure 12-12).

FIGURE 12–12 Rhinophyma. *Courtesy Rube J. Pardo, M.D., Ph.D.*

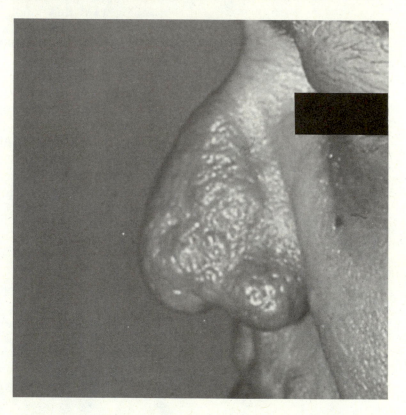

The exact cause of rosacea is unknown. Thought by many research-ers to be hereditary, it is also thought that constant blushing and enlargening of the blood vessels may be the cause of rosacea.

Rosacea should be treated by a dermatologist, who will use oral antibiotics such as tetracycline, topical medications such as anti-fungals, and sulfur preparations to combat the flareups, which are typical of the conditions. Flareups have been associated with ingestion of alcohol, tobacco, spicy foods, citrus, and hot bever-ages. External heat and sun exposure are also implicated. Advise clients with rosacea to avoid these irritating factors.

Recently a new drug has been developed for rosacea. Metrogel® is a topical cream, available only by prescription, that has proven to be helpful in controlling rosaceal flareups.

Rosacea is sometimes hard to recognize in its mild forms. It almost always affects the nose area, the distinct large red pustules among large red patches of underlying skin. Oily skin often accompanies rosacea, but not always. Sometimes rosacea will flare up during menopause, or when hormone therapy is discontinued.

Sometimes skin that the esthetician has treated for some time will suddenly flare up with rosacea. This is not the fault of the esthetician. The esthetician should always refer the client with rosacea to a dermatologist. Rosacea almost always requires drug therapy at some point. Unless the dermatologist directs otherwise, there is no reason to discontinue esthetic treatment. Treat the rosacea skin with gentle products for oily or combination skin. Noncomedogenic cosmetics and skin care are, again, helpful. Do not attempt to extract the pustules. They are much larger and more complicated than those of acne vulgaris. Avoid harsh treatments, large amounts of alcohol, essential oils, and spicy or highly fragranced products. Excessive steam is not beneficial. Massage should also be avoided on the nose, cheeks, and surrounding areas. Suggest a gentle, foaming cleanser (nonfragranced), mild toner, very light noncomedogenic moisturizers, sunscreens, and hydrating products. Avoid all oil-based products, heavy creams, and super-tightening masks.

The use of concealing color toners, such as green underbase, is recommended. Make sure that all makeup products are also water-based and noncomedogenic. Rosacea clients can generally wear makeup. Occasionally the dermatologist will ask that the client avoid makeup altogether, usually during severe flareups

Perioral Dermatitis

Perioral dermatitis, which is dermatitis around the mouth, is also considered an acne-related disorder. Red papules and pustules in the mouth, nose, and chin area, usually small in size and in clusters of several lesions, are apparent. Almost always found in women, perioral dermatitis often occurs during the childbearing years, 20 to 35 years (Figure 12-13).

The condition is sometimes accompanied by scaliness and stinging dehydration. Moisturizers may complicate the condition. If a moisturizer is used, it should be water-based, noncomedogenic, and used sparingly. Perioral dermatitis is, again, in the domain of the dermatologist. Mild cortisone creams, antibiotics, and acne medications are often prescribed.

Avoid massage and instruct the client not to touch or rub the area, as this can worsen the condition. Mild sulfur acne preparations may be helpful.

FIGURE 12–13 Typical pattern of perioral dermatitis on the chin. Perioral dermatitis can also appear on the cheeks or anywhere around the mouth area. *Courtesy George Fisher, M.D.*

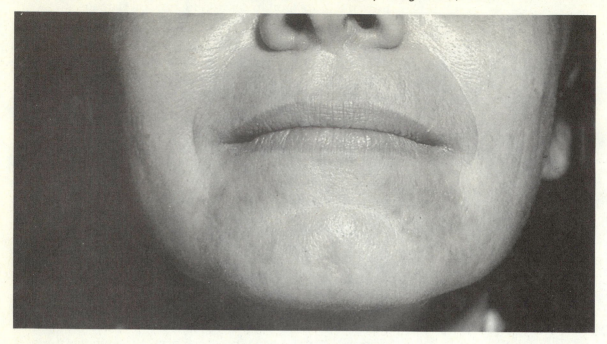

In the salon, avoid massage or overstimulation of the area. Esthetic treatments can help the client's other problems, but you must refer the client to a dermatologist for treatment of the perioral dermatitis. Mild foaming cleansers and toners for oily and combination skin are recommended. Concealing color toner, such as green underbase, is recommended.

Treatment Products and Ingredients for Acne

Benzoyl Peroxide

Benzoyl peroxide works well on most forms of acne vulgaris and occasional pimples. Benzoyl peroxide works by peeling off excess cell buildup, temporarily dilating the follicles, and breaking up follicle impactions and debris. Benzoyl peroxide also releases oxygen in the follicle, helping to kill bacteria. Benzoyl peroxide is available in a variety of bases, from drying clay bases to masks, creams, gels, and lotions. The lotions and gels are most frequently used by estheticians.

Benzoyl peroxide normally is made in three strengths:

- $2\,^1\!/_2$ percent for mild acne and thin, sensitive skin.

- 5 percent for moderate acne.
- 10 percent for more severe acne.

Additional strengths are available by physician's prescription. Scrubs and foaming washes containing benzoyl peroxide are also widely used. Unfortunately, many people are or become allergic to benzoyl peroxide (see the chapter on allergies). Benzoyl peroxide is also a bleach and may bleach fabric and hair if contact is made. Benzoyl peroxide may also be used in the treatment room as a treatment after extraction.

Recommended Usage of Benzoyl Peroxide

1. First and most important, check to see if the client has ever experienced an allergy to benzoyl peroxide. Many clients will overuse a benzoyl peroxide product, resulting in peeling and irritation, which the client may assume is an allergy. But, when in doubt, don't.

2. Benzoyl peroxide may be used as a keratolytic (see the chemistry chapter) to loosen impactions (open and closed comedones), or as a treatment for papules and pustules. Therefore, benzoyl peroxide can be used on present pimples or used as a preventative for development of future lesions.

3. Benzoyl peroxide can be a very aggressive drying agent. Visible peeling of skin will often occur. Some clients, especially older women, will confuse this peeling with "aging." Tightness of the peeling skin may accentuate lines and wrinkles for a short period of time. As the dead skin buildup is removed, the visible peeling lessens or subsides with continual use of benzoyl peroxide. Unfortunately, these clients will often stop using the benzoyl peroxide just as it is beginning to work. It is best to explain this peeling procedure to the client at the first consultation, before it actually begins. Explain that the peeling will be temporary and is not the same type of drying that occurs with aging. Many older clients find that, with continued use of a peeling agent, their aging skin looks better, and their acne is controlled. With many clients, especially older ones, it is good to recommend a light, noncomedogenic moisturizer that they can use to combat the visible flaking and peeling from drying agents, which will make the skin more comfortable as well as making the drying areas look smoother.

4. Occasionally a client will call complaining of severe itching, burning, urticaria (hives), and rash. This is most likely an allergic reaction. Tell the client to discontinue treatment immediately. Severe allergic reactions should be

seen by a dermatologist. Overuse of benzoyl peroxide products, as previously discussed, can cause an irritation reaction similar in appearance. The client should wait until the irritation completely subsides before retrying benzoyl peroxide. The client should then try applying the benzoyl peroxide to a small area for the first day or two of application. If the irritation returns to the small test area, she should completely discontinue use.

5. Benzoyl peroxide should be used with extreme caution on black skins. It is recommended not to exceed 5 percent benzoyl peroxide in these clients. The area around the mouth should be treated very lightly, as occasionally black clients will experience darkening (hyperpigmentation) of this area.

Sulfur and Resorcinol

Sulfur and resorcinol are often combined in an acne-drying product. These products are usually available in gels, creams, masks, and clay-based "spot" treatment products. They are ideal for use when a client is allergic to benzoyl peroxide products. These products are also irritants and can cause irritations or allergic reactions. They can be used in the same way as benzoyl peroxide products. They help to peel away excessive cell accumulations and loosen follicle impactions. They do not, however, release oxygen as benzoyl peroxide does. As a general rule, they are not quite as aggressive as benzoyl peroxide. While benzoyl peroxide is usually the more effective treatment, sulfur-resorcinol products are very helpful in drying acne lesions. If an allergy occurs, follow the same procedures as recommended for benzoyl peroxide.

Salicylic Acid

Probably the mildest of the drying agents, this chemical is ideal for use on older, dryer skin types. It usually comes in lotion form and can be incorporated in a moisturizing base. It is available in various strengths. Many companies will automatically include salicylic acid in their moisturizers for problem skin. In thin or sensitive skin, it is often used as a day treatment, while benzoyl peroxide or sulfur-resorcinol is used as a night treatment.

Some people are very allergic to salicylates, the family of salicylic acid-type products. Salicylic acid, in its oral form, is aspirin. If your client is allergic to aspirin, avoid using salicylic acid.

Glycolic Acid

One of the newest treatments, glycolic acid is used to help break up follicular impactions. It is available in over-the-counter and prescription strengths. It does not produce quite as much visible peeling as benzoyl peroxide. Glycolic acid burns slightly when applied and burns more if applied to already-irritated skin. Research on the use of this product is still in progress at the time of this writing; however, it shows promise in helping impactions and may be very effective when combined with other prescription drugs.

Products for Home Care for Acne Clients

Scrubs and washes are very popular treatment cleansers for the acne patient. There are several types of these rinseable cleansers available.

The base of most of these washes is water and a mild to aggressive detergent. These detergents (see the chapter on cosmetic chemistry) are surfactants that help remove excess oil from the skin's surface, which helps keep the oil from further clogging follicles. Examples of detergents are sodium lauryl (or laureth) sulfate (moderate strength), ammonium lauryl sulfate (strong—for very oily and acne skin), and disodium lauryl sulfosuccinate (a milder detergent used for more sensitive skin and less drying).

Acne medications such as benzoyl peroxide, sulfur-resorcinol, and salicylic acid are sometimes added to these detergent bases. These are referred to as **medicated cleansers**. They can be considerably more active than regular cosmetic detergent cleansers. For extremely oily, problem skin, these medicated cleansers sometimes contain small, bead-like granules made of polyethylene or ground nuts, seeds, or hulls. These **exfoliating cleansers** help to mechanically remove surface cell buildup, helping the detergents or medication penetrate the surface better. However, they can be very abrasive on red, sensitive, thin skin, and are not recommended for Retin-A or Accutane patients. They should only be used on the thickest, oiliest skin types.

Cleansing milks for acne are generally only recommended for makeup removal. Their use should be followed by a mild to moderate detergent cleanser to remove any traces of the cleansing milk. These cleansing milks are generally used at night only and should be made of noncomedogenic ingredients.

Astringents and Toners

Astringents and toners are usually recommended for acne clients to use after cleansing. These toners are helpful in controlling surface oils and in lowering the pH after cleansing. They are always water-based, with astringent chemicals such as witch hazel, isopropyl or S.D. alcohol, lemon extract, or citric acid. Some toners are made with antiseptics such as benzalkonium chloride. Some astringents use salicylic acid to help exfoliate the skin.

Toners containing more aggressive drying agents such as alcohol and salicylic acid should be avoided on sensitive skin or the skin of someone using Retin-A.

Day Treatments and Protective Lotions

Two basic types of day treatments are used for acne-prone skin. The first is a light keratolytic cream containing a mild drying agent like salicylic acid in a noncomedogenic base. The second is an alcohol and water lotion that may contain other keratolytic agents.

Clients with mild acne and older clients usually prefer the creams, while alcohol lotions may be helpful to teenagers and people with thicker, oilier skins.

Occasionally the acne client may need a light moisturizer during the day to combat the esthetic effects of peeling agents. Noncomedogenic moisturizers for acne-prone skin are made without the use of fats and oils, so they are often referred to as "lipid-free" moisturizers. If a moisturizer is needed, they must be noncomedogenic and light enough in weight to be comfortable for oily skin. Retin-A patients and clients who spend a lot of time outdoors should be given a moisturizer with a sunscreen.

Night Treatments

Medicated gels have already been briefly discussed. These gels or creams contain peeling agents to help remove cell buildup and are extremely beneficial to acne clients. They contain benzoyl peroxide, salicylic acid, sulfur, resorcinol, or glycolic acid.

Hydrating fluids are sometimes needed by acne clients to combat flaking caused by the medicated gels. Adult acne patients frequently require the use of these hydrating fluids. A good hydrating fluid for problem skin will be extremely light in texture, made without comedogenic ingredients. They are often alternated with peeling treatments, used on skin with acne tendencies and during colder seasons.

Masks for Acne

Masks for acne clients are almost always in a clay-type drying base. The clay most frequently used is **bentonite**, which has excellent oil-absorbing qualities. Masks for acne are frequently also medicated, containing benzoyl peroxide, sulfur, or sulfurated lime. They are available in a variety of strengths. Camphor is a popular ingredient for more sensitive and adult skins, because it is less drying than the keratolytic agents. Some clay masks also contain a mechanical granule such as pumice or polyethylene to help exfoliate during application and rinsing.

Masks should be applied for 15 to 20 minutes after night cleansing. After drying, they should be removed by wetting the mask, then gently wiping off with a very soft cloth or sponge. Toner and night treatment should then be applied.

Masks are used two or three times a week, depending on the client's condition and oiliness. Weather and climate may also influence use frequency.

Home Care Treatment for Beginning Teenage Acne

1. Wash the face thoroughly with rinseable foaming cleanser. Use a sponge or soft cloth to help exfoliate surface cells. Rinse thoroughly.

2. Apply mild antiseptic toner with damp cotton ball or gauze to entire face.

3. Moisturizer is seldom needed for very young skin. If weather or climate overdries the skin's surface, use a light noncomedogenic day cream sparingly.

Night Treatment

1. Remove any makeup thoroughly with noncomedogenic cleansing milk.

2. Wash face thoroughly with rinseable cleanser as shown above. Apply toner.

3. Apply a small amount of $2\frac{1}{2}$ or 5 percent benzoyl peroxide gel to clogged areas. Gently massage until the gel penetrates. Apply additional dabs of gel to individual raised lesions (papules and pustules). The only medication seen should be on the lesions. Excessive peeling may result, particularly in young, sensitive skin if too much medication gel is used.

Salon Treatment

Salon treatment should be administered whenever clogs and comedones are present. Sometimes treatment is necessary only every month or two during the very beginning stages of the teenage years. Treatment should be more frequent when apparent blemishes are more frequent. (Parents should be consulted and advised when treating very young skin, so that they may advise children at home. It is often best to consult with the young client without the parent present, and then discreetly talk to the parent afterwards. Teenagers will often perform home care better if they do not feel "supervised." It is important to advise parents to bring the young client in as soon as pimples start to develop. Unfortunately many parents will neglect a child's acne, thinking they will "outgrow it," until the teenager has a more serious condition. "An ounce of prevention is worth a pound of cure!")

Home Care Treatment for Grade 1 Acne

Morning

1. Wash face with granular (nongranular if sensitive or thin skin) medicated cleanser, with wet fingertips, then with wet sponge or very soft cloth. Rinse thoroughly with room temperature water.

2. Apply moderate strength toner to entire face (except eyes). Allow to dry briefly.

3. Apply salicylic acid cream or alcohol lotion. Apply non-comedogenic makeup only (if desired).

Afternoon

It is sometimes advisable in very oily skins to repeat the morning procedure in the mid-afternoon, or after school for teenagers. Cleansing should be repeated in the afternoon if working in a greasy environment or after exercising.

Evening

1. Remove makeup thoroughly with noncomedogenic cleansing milk.

2. Wash face again with medicated cleanser. Nonmedicated foaming cleanser can be substituted if the skin is irritated, sensitive, or peeling.

3. Apply toner as in the morning.

4. Apply 5 percent benzoyl peroxide, sulfur-resorcinol, or salicylic gel or lotion to all clogged and oily areas lightly. This treatment should penetrate almost immediately. Apply additional dabs to pimples and raised lesions. It is important that the client understand that they are not only to treat raised lesions. Treating unaffected but oily areas routinely with light applications will help break up "cell buildup" and help prevent future lesions.

Frequency of Salon Treatments

Treatments are advised weekly or biweekly until the acne clears substantially This normally takes between three to six months. After clearing, the client should be treated every three to four weeks in the salon and should use masks two to three times a week at home. The client should be reminded that acne is a controllable, not curable, condition, and that upkeep is very important.

Home Care for Grade 2 Acne

The home care routine is the same as for grade 1 acne; however, avoid very strong toners. Remember, there are usually many closed comedones in grade 2 acne. These lesions have smaller pore openings, and astringents may prevent these follicle openings from loosening with home care therapy.

Grade 2 acne is one of the hardest types to clear. It requires diligent attention from both client and esthetician. Treatments in the salon should be weekly or biweekly. Extensive extraction is necessary. After the first consultation, allow the client to use products two weeks before the second salon treatment. The closed comedones usually will be much easier to extract after two weeks of proper home care. It is especially important that these clients avoid comedogenic products. The esthetician should check every product carefully for comedogenic ingredients.

Home Care for Grade 3 Acne

Most grade 3 acne cases should be seen by both the dermatologist and the esthetician. The esthetician must pay careful attention to the dermatologist's instructions and prescriptions. Benzoyl peroxide granular washes, stronger astringents, and 10 percent benzoyl peroxide gel may be used, if not contraindicated by the dermatologist. Oral medication is often required for these clients. They will also need help choosing noncomedogenic products and makeup.

Treatment is advised weekly, unless otherwise directed by the dermatologist. Once clear, the client should be seen for salon treatment every three to four weeks.

Home Care for Grade 4 (Cystic) Acne

Grade 4 acne always requires a dermatologist. This is the oiliest and worst acne condition. Home care should be the same as for grade 3 acne, again following any specific instructions from the dermatologist. Salon treatment should be frequent to help prevent lesions by removing clogs and open and closed comedones. Be very careful if cysts or nodules are present during treatment. Refer the client to the dermatologist immediately for treatment of any cysts, nodules, or deep papules. Again, avoidance of comedogenic ingredients is a must for these clients.

Drugs Often Prescribed by the Dermatologist for Acne Treatment

Retin-A

Tretinoin, better known as Retin-A, is a vitamin A acid that was developed in the late 1960s at the University of Pennsylvania by a team of researchers headed by Dr. Albert Kligman. Retin-A works by helping "flush out" follicular debris, helping to clear the follicles of comedones. It also is an excellent drying agent for oily skin and pimples. It is used extensively as a prescription in all grades of acne and is often used for other skin problems. (See the chapter on photoaging and sun damage). Retin-A requires a physician's prescription, as it is a potent topical acid. It is available in cream, gel, and liquid forms.

Because it is a powerful keratolytic, it is usually not used with other keratolytics such as benzoyl peroxide, sulfur-resorcinol, or salicylic acid, except by dermatologist recommendation. Occasional cases do well with benzoyl peroxide and Retin-A. This is a dermatological decision. Do not add keratolytics to a Retin-A user's regime without consulting the dermatologist.

Retinoic acid does not have a substantial direct effect on bacteria within the follicle, however. It is often used with a topical antibiotic called *clindamycin* (trade name Cleocin-T™), which is a powerful antibiotic. It is in an alcohol base, and by itself can be quite drying. The theory here is to use a powerful "follicle flusher" along with an antibiotic to kill bacteria and remove comedones and impactions. Because Retin-A is such a powerful keratolytic, it is also an irritant. It is not unusual for clients beginning Retin-A to experience flaking, dry skin, redness, irritation, and slight discomfort. The prescribed dosage varies with the client and the dermatologist, but many dermatologists start patients on Retin-A every third night, slowly increasing the frequency to nightly applications.

Because of the irritating side effects of this drug, clients often find that their present skin-care program and cosmetics may be irritating or over-drying. It is up to the esthetician to work with the client or dermatologist to find products that work with retinoic acid therapy.

Products for Retinoic Acid Users

1. First, eliminate any other keratolytics from the client's home-care program. As discussed previously, avoid benzoyl peroxide, sulfur, resorcinol, salicylic, and glycolic acid. Use these products with Retin-A clients only with the approval of the dermatologist.

2. Eliminate high alcohol products, particularly those containing isopropyl alcohol.

3. Avoid fragranced products.

4. Avoid spicy, stimulating products.

5. Avoid large amounts of citric acid.

6. Eliminate essential oils from the regime. Large amounts of many plant extracts may cause further irritation.

7. Sometimes it is necessary to totally eliminate the use of astringents or fresheners, particularly during the first six to eight weeks of Retin-A therapy.

8. Encourage the use of sunscreens, as Retin-A also makes the skin photosensitive.

9. Eliminate the use of granular scrub cleansers or tight drying masks, particularly during the first part of the Retin-A therapy. Later in the therapy (six to eight weeks), a gentle granular exfoliant, diluted with cleansing milk, may be beneficial in helping to remove dry, dead cells.

10. Highly stripping cleansers, soaps, and abrasives must be discontinued.

Basic Home Care for Acne Clients Using Retin-A

Morning

1. Cleanse the face with a gentle foaming cleanser for oily or combination skin.

2. Apply a gentle, nonalcoholic toner if not too irritated from beginning treatment.

3. Apply a noncomedogenic moisturizer with sunscreen. If using clindamycin, apply sunscreen after clindamycin application, or follow dermatologist's specific instructions.

Evening

1. Remove makeup with a gentle cleansing milk. Extremely oily skin may need to be washed gently with a foaming cleanser. Apply toner if not too sensitive.

2. Wait 20 minutes.

3. Apply Retin-A as directed by a physician.

If the skin is very dehydrated, 20 minutes later a light, nonfragranced, noncomedogenic, hydrating fluid may be applied. Check to make sure that this is approved by the physician. If Retin-A is used on alternate nights, the client may choose to use the same noncomedogenic hydrating fluid on alternate nights to combat dehydration.

Salon Treatment Changes for Retin-A Patients

1. Do not use wax on Retin-A patients. Waxing is extremely irritating to retinized skin. Electrolysis is usually acceptable to continue.

2. Avoid enzyme treatment, particularly when starting Retin-A. After eight weeks or so, these may be acceptable.

3. No mechanical abrasion, brushing, or "rub off" type masks.

4. Avoid all keratolytics previously discussed during treatment.

5. Camphor masks can usually be tolerated if the skin is not red and irritated.

6. Avoid excessive massage.

7. Electrical therapy should be shortened in duration and performed at a lower intensity.

8. Avoid heavy, thick creams, as with all acne clients.

Tetracyline is an oral antibiotic often prescribed for patients with chronic and persistent acne. Minocycline (Minocin™) is another oral antibiotic often used for chronic acne sufferers. Erythromycin is prescribed in both oral and topical medications. It is also an antibiotic.

Accutane

Accutane is a cousin of retinoic acid. It is an oral medication prescribed for patients with severe, chronic, grades 3 and 4 acne with multiple cysts. It is very useful when treating this type of patient.

Accutane has numerous side effects, including severe drying of the skin and mucous membranes, nosebleeds, and severely dry, cracked lips. More severe side effects include birth defects in children of women who take Accutane during their childbearing years. Many doctors insist on a pregnancy test for women planning to undergo Accutane therapy. Other side effects include muscle aches. Periodic blood, kidney, and liver function tests are administered during Accutane therapy. These side effects may sound frightening, but Accutane can be the most effective acne drug for hard-to-treat cases. Every precaution is taken by dermatologists. Under these circumstances it can be a safe, effective treatment.

Skin Care for the Accutane Patient

Follow the same precautions as recommended for Retin-A patients. No waxing **on any part of the body** should be done during or for several months after Accutane is discontinued. You may need to administer soothing hydrating treatments to the Accutane patient, using light, noncomedogenic, hydrating fluids and gentle gel or cream masks.

Again, avoid all keratolytics, excessive massage, and any stimulating treatments. Extractions on Accutane patients should be extremely gentle, as the skin becomes extremely thin and fragile and reddens and bruises easily.

Help the Accutane patient with light hydrating fluids and gentle cleanser. This may be the first time this type of client has ever used a moisturizer. Take some time to re-instruct the client in the uses of the new products.

After Accutane therapy, the skin usually returns to being somewhat oily—rarely is it as oily as it was before treatment. Within two or three months after Accutane is discontinued, re-evaluate the skin and recommend the correct home-care regime.

Dermatological Treatment of Cysts

The dermatologist will treat cysts by a number of different methods. Extraction is used, using a small incision to drain the cyst. This technique is known as acne surgery.

Sometimes the dermatologist will inject the cyst with a steroid. The steroid usually clears the lesion in between one and three days of injection. It is an extremely effective treatment for cysts. The doctor will usually also prescribe an oral antibiotic for these patients. Avoid pressure or extraction around a freshly treated cyst. Sometimes the dermatologist will suggest avoiding facial treatment until the cyst is completely healed.

Analysis Technique for Acne or Problem Skin

Before treating problem skin, the esthetician should take a thorough health history of the client. This is best accomplished by having the client fill out a health form. On your form you should include:

1. Client name, address, and phone numbers.

2. The client's occupation. This tells you if the client is in a high-stress job, or if the client is employed in a situation where there is constant exposure to "greasy air," such as a fast-food restaurant.

3. Is the client already seeing a dermatologist? If so, was medication prescribed? Is the client using the medication as instructed by the dermatologist? (Often a client is not using the medication correctly, or has discontinued it because of excessive drying or irritation. Do not interfere with a doctor's prescription or attempt to instruct about medication! Refer your client back to the dermatologist for further instruction. Never instruct a client to discontinue prescribed medication!) If questions arise, call and consult with the dermatologist.

4. How long has the client experienced problem skin? (This may tell you if it is a long-term hereditary problem or if it is caused by short-term factors such as comedogenic cosmetics, hormones, drugs, stress, etc.)

5. When does the client have flareups? Shortly before her period? During stressful times?

6. Is the client under a lot of stress?

7. What cosmetics and skin-care products does the client use presently? Request that the client bring in products presently used during the first visit. This will allow you to check for comedogenic products and to see what steps the client is taking to help.

8. Is the client using birth control pills, and what type?

9. Has the client had any history of hormone problems? Is she experiencing menopause? Is she taking prescribed hormones?

10. Is she pregnant?

11. Does the client have allergies to any cosmetics, foods, or drugs?

12. Does the client have any other health problems or use any other form of medication?

13. Does the client eat a balanced diet?

14. Does the client take vitamin supplements?

15. Does the client have a history of acne in the family?

16. How often does the client clean the skin and with what product?

17. Does the client pick at acne lesions?

18. The client's age. Sometimes this will indicate the nature of the problem.

These standard questions should also be asked on the preliminary form completed on the first visit. It is generally recommended that any client who has not visited in six months fill out a new health evaluation form. Make sure you check for any other health problems or contraindications for home-care or salon treatments (such as electrical therapy, heart problems, etc.) just as you would on any client.

Hands-On Analysis

Remove the client's makeup and cleanse the skin's surface thoroughly. Analyze the client's skin through a magnifying lamp. It is a good idea at some point in the beginning of analysis to look at the skin with the client in a magnifying mirror. The best way to accomplish this is to use one of the two-way mirror devices available through equipment manufacturers. This interaction will allow the client to see what you are describing. Explain each type of problem to the client as thoroughly and simply as possible. Remember, the client is a consumer, not a professional. The bottom line of interest for the client is how you can help with beauty problems and problem skin.

Ask the client lots of questions about any skin problems:

- How often are you having break-outs?
- Where do they occur?
- Do they seem to come at certain times of the month?
- What do the blemishes look like when they occur?
- Do you normally have more or less breakout than this?
- Explain what you are doing now at home.

Even though the client may have written some of these answers down on the health form, it's a good idea to discuss them. Clients sometimes forget to write something down, or the esthetician may discover that the client is doing something incorrectly.

This is also a good opportunity to review any experiences that the client has had with previous esthetic or dermatological treatment.

While observing the skin under the magnifying lamp, make detailed, written notes of any problems and any discussion you have with the client. You should particularly note the following:

1. Number of lesions.

2. What type of lesions? Open comedones? Closed comedones? Papules? Pustules? Nodules? Cysts?

3. Chin breakouts, particularly if isolated to that area.

4. Breakout around the mouth, isolated to that area. (This could possibly be perioral dermatitis.)

5. Flaking in the hairline, sides of nose, eyebrows, and ear areas. (Possibly seborrhea.)

6. What is the thickness of the skin? Is it sensitive? Does it turn red easily?

7. Are the unaffected follicles clogged and enlarged? (An indication of generally oily skin.)

8. Large red pustules and surrounding redness in the nose area. (Possibly rosacea.)

9. Flat red lesions that look like scraped skin, sometimes with scabs. (Client is probably scraping with the fingernails.)

10. Scarring—make special notes of any existing scarring, icepick scars, raised (hypertrophic) scars, and any scars from cyst removal.

11. Macules, which are lesions that have healed but are still red or tan in color. They are flat and are most often found in the fleshy areas of the face, such as the cheeks.

12. Is there any surface flaking or dehydration? Is the skin tight or pliable?

13. What grade of acne exists?

The esthetician must check to see if any client with rosacea, seborrhea, perioral dermatitis, or cysts is seeing a dermatologist. These conditions are dermatological, not esthetic. It is not the esthetician's place to diagnose or suggest these conditions to the client. Simply suggest that the client see a dermatologist. After the client sees the doctor, call the doctor and discuss esthetic concerns or arrange for the client to obtain a letter from the doctor.

Salon Treatments

Before discussing salon treatments, a few important procedures and precautions should be discussed:

1. Do not use any product or ingredient to which the client is allergic.

2. Extraction should never last more than 10 or 15 minutes in one session. If you are uncomfortable with extraction procedures, omit this step completely. Extraction is probably the most important part of esthetic salon treatment, but can also be the most harmful if done improperly. Never extract a lesion you are not sure about. Open and closed comedones and pustules are the only lesions that the esthetician should extract. Leave papules, nodules, and cysts alone!

3. The esthetician should wear disposable latex gloves during the entire acne treatment.

4. If lancets are used they must be sterile and disposable.

5. Active acne should never be massaged. After the acne is completely cleared, then consider a light massage.

6. Clients should be told not to wear makeup for at least two hours after treatment.

7. Skin that has been exposed to Retin-A should not be exfoliated. Eliminate the use of all keratolytics, including beonzoyl peroxide, salicylic acid, sulfur, resorcinol, glycolic acid, for clients using Retin-A.

8. Be careful how much you extract on the first visit. As the client begins home care, the impactions will be much softer and easier to extract and a lot more comfortable for the client. Explain this so the client will understand that you will do more extraction on the second visit, when the client has been using the correct products for a week or two.

Basic Salon Acne Treatment

1. Thoroughly cleanse and analyze.

2. Re-cleanse with a foaming cleanser.

3. Apply a desincrusting pre-mask (see the chapter on products). Begin the steam treatment during the pre-mask. Allow to sit for 8 minutes.

4. Remove the pre-mask. Proceed with galvanic desincrustation as normal, about 5 minutes in duration.

5. Begin extraction in the chin area first, moving up the face, finishing at the forehead. This will avoid contact with any minor blood or fluids. As previously mentioned, the esthetician should wear latex disposable gloves during extraction and throughout the remainder of treatment.

6. After extraction, apply a generous amount of antibacterial toner to the entire area extracted.

7. Unfold a 12-ply piece of gauze and place across the client's entire face. Avoiding the eye area, apply high-frequency current to the client's face (through the gauze) for about 1 to 2 minutes. Remove the gauze.

8. Apply a small amount of 5 percent benzoyl peroxide to the extracted areas.

9. Apply a drying mask with camphor. (For more severe conditions, you may use a sulfur drying mask or benzoyl peroxide mask.) Avoid the eye areas.

10. Allow the mask to sit for about 15 minutes. Wet the mask well with a cold spray solution of toner to loosen before removal. Remove with wet sponges or a soft cloth. Spray the face again with toner mixture to remove any excess mask.

11. Apply a small amount of salicylic cream to finish the treatment.

Alternative Treatment #1 for Acne

This treatment is effective for thicker skin types with grades 2 and 3 acne.

1. Thoroughly cleanse and analyze.

2. Re-cleanse with an alkaline pre-mask or an alkaline rinseable cleanser.

3. Apply a soft-setting enzyme treatment to help dissolve surface cell buildup and dilate follicles. Begin the steam treatment during the enzyme treatment. Allow to sit for 8 minutes.

4. Remove the enzyme treatment. Proceed with galvanic desincrustation as normal, about 5 minutes in duration.

5. If you are using a lancet, begin dilating the follicle openings of the closed comedones in the chin area, moving up the face to the cheeks and finishing on the forehead. Proceed with extraction. Gently dilate the top of any follicles with pustules with separate lancets. Extract pustules.

6. After extraction, apply a generous amount of antibacterial toner to the entire area extracted.

7. Unfold a 12-ply piece of gauze and place across the clients entire face. Avoiding the eye area, apply high-frequency current to the client's face (through the gauze) for about 1 to 2 minutes. Remove gauze.

8. Apply a small amount of 5 percent benzoyl peroxide to extracted areas.

9. Apply a drying sulfur or benzoyl peroxide mask, avoiding the eye area. For more sensitive skins, apply a drying mask with camphor.

10. Allow the mask to sit for about 15 minutes. Wet the mask well with a cold spray solution of toner to loosen before removal. Remove with wet sponges or a soft cloth. Spray the face again with toner mixture to remove any excess mask.

11. Apply a small amount of salicylic cream to finish the treatment.

1. Thoroughly cleanse and analyze, paying particular attention to any red or sensitive areas.

2. If the skin is red or sensitive, apply a light, noncomedogenic hydrating fluid. Proceed with steam for 5 to 8 minutes. Be very careful not to get the skin hot from the steam. For skin that appears noninflamed, apply a disincrustant pre-mask instead of the hydrating fluid.

3. Remove the pre-mask or hydrating fluid. Galvanic is best avoided on clients just beginning Retin-A treatment.

4. Begin extraction gently in the same chin to forehead pattern.

5. Apply a generous amount of antibacterial non-alcoholic toner on a cool, wet, cotton pad or soft cloth. Apply to all extracted areas. If you prefer, you may use a diluted cold spray toner solution.

6. Apply a noncomedogenic hydrating fluid. Cover with gauze and proceed with high frequency (mushroom attachment) for 1 to 2 minutes.

7. Apply a cool, soothing treatment with aloe, azulene, bisabolol, or chamomile. Gel masks are very beneficial and gentle, as long as they are free of alcohol and fragrance. For thicker skins, you may try a light application of light-setting, clay-based camphor mask.

8. Do not allow to sit for more than 5 to 7 minutes. Remove the mask by thoroughly wetting it with cold spray, then gently wiping with cool, wet, cotton or soft cloths.

9. Apply a light, noncomedogenic moisturizer with sunscreen.

TOPICS FOR DISCUSSION

1. What is acne?

2. Trace the development of the comedo.

3. Name some environmental factors influencing acne development.

4. Explain various cleansers, toners, and treatment creams and lotions available for acne, and their action on the skin.

5. Discuss some acne-related conditions that should be referred to the dermatologist.

6. What are some questions that should be asked of the client during the first consultation?

CHAPTER

13

Comedogenicity

OBJECTIVES

Many ingredients used in cosmetics can make acne worse and can contribute to the development of comedones of all types. In the 1980s, comedogenicity became a very important subject for estheticians and is one of the most important areas of esthetics practice.

In this chapter you will learn about these ingredients and how they affect the skin. You will learn how to check ingredient lists for possible comedogenic ingredients. You will also learn about the many products that are helpful for clog-prone, oily skin.

Background

For many years, dermatologists often told women who had acne or problem skin to avoid using makeup. Many doctors said this as a blanket statement and encouraged women with acne to avoid all cosmetics.

These doctors noticed that women often did not respond to traditional acne therapy. They also noticed that many of the women continued to use makeup and cosmetics on a regular basis.

These dermatologists did not know at the time specifically why the cosmetics caused acne to become worse or not to improve during treatment. Many thought that the cosmetics sat on the skin and occluded aeration of the follicles, not allowing oxygen to penetrate the follicles. Others were aware that many of the cosmetics had a high fat or oil content. It seemed to make sense that oily skin that developed acne lesions easily did not need additional oil from the outside.

These theories made sense, and some studies touched on the subject of cosmetics and hair products aggravating acne, but it wasn't until the early 1970s that doctors published studies that showed increased retention hyperkeratosis or a buildup of cells within the follicle in patients using some types of cosmetics.

217

It was discovered that the use of certain ingredients within cosmetics was more likely to cause a pronounced buildup of cells within the follicle. This buildup lined the follicle walls, and when enough accumulated it began forming a microcomedo. The microcomedo eventually evolved into an open or closed comedone and then possibly into an inflammatory acne lesion, such as a papule or pustule.

The acne-prone women who used the cosmetics in question already had a predisposition to clog development. In other words, they already had a tendency to develop clogged pores from hereditary retention hyperkeratosis.

The doctors coined a term for this condition, *acne cosmetica*, meaning "cosmetic acne." They were able to correlate excessive buildup of dead cells within the follicles of patients using certain cosmetics. These cosmetics were said to be **comedogenic**. *Comedogenic* means the tendency of a topical ingredient or product to increase the buildup of dead cells within the follicle, eventually causing comedone formation. *Noncomedogenic* means that the ingredient or product does not cause excessive follicular hyperkeratosis, and therefore is unlikely to cause comedone development (Figure 13-1).

Testing for Comedogenicity

Researchers developed a test for comedogenicity using the inside of a rabbit's ear. Cosmetic or drug topical products were applied to the inside of the ear. The follicles inside the rabbit ear develop comedones much faster than human skin. Within three weeks most cosmetics can be tested using the rabbit ear method.

The procedure for rabbit ear assays, as they are called by the scientific community, is really quite simple. A product is applied to the inside of one ear of a male albino rabbit at least 12 weeks old. The reason for the specifics of sex and age of the rabbit are due to the size of these particular animals' follicles, which are better for evaluation of comedo development.

The other ear of the rabbit is left alone, as a control. A *control* is an experimental factor that remains the same throughout the experiment. Scientists can compare the two ears at the end of the three-week period to determine the difference seen in the follicles of the skin of the two different ears of the rabbit model.

The product is applied to the test area daily for three weeks. Each day the ear is observed for obvious changes to the skin and checked carefully for comedo formation.

FIGURE 13 –1a Grade 2 acne due to cosmetics.

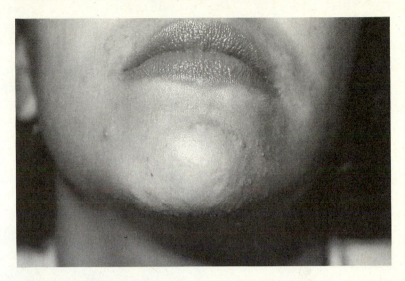

FIGURE 13 –1b Pomade acne due to hair conditioners.
Courtesy Rube J. Pardo, M.D., Ph.D.

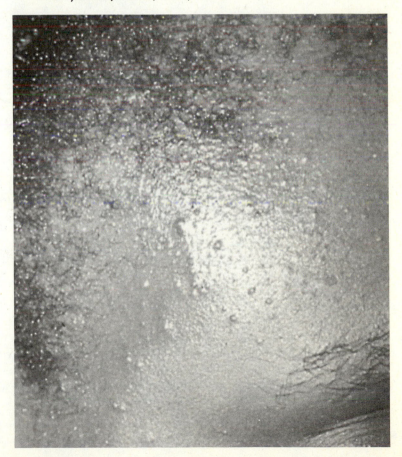

If after three weeks there are no comedones, the product testing is finished. However, to be absolutely sure there is no excessive follicular hyperkeratosis, small tissue samples are taken surgically from the skin of the ear and examined under the microscope. Any hyperkeratosis will be obvious as it lines the follicle walls. At the same time the follicle is examined for irritation that might cause immediate acne reactions due to follicle irritation. The test is not fully complete if this microscopic test is not run. This test is called a histopathological study (Figure 13-2).

FIGURE 13–2 The microscopic view of retention hyperkeratosis shows excessive cell buildup and swelling. This slide represents a positive test for comedogenicity.

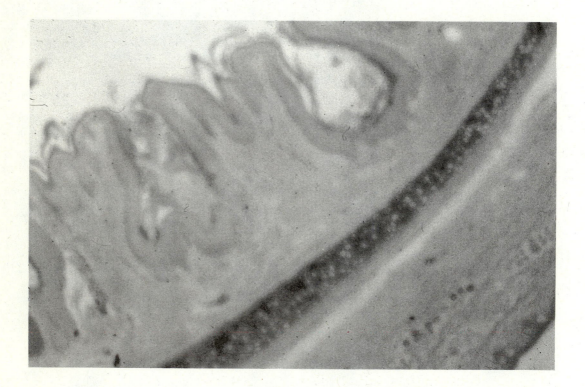

If comedone formation is detected, it is rated on a scale of 0 to 3. A score of 0 means that no comedones formed. A score of 3 means that the product or ingredient is comedogenic. Only products with overall scores of 0 on all rabbits tested are claimed to be noncomedogenic.

The hyperkeratosis within the follicle found during the histopathological examination is also rated on the same scale. While most follicles will develop a small amount of irritation and keratosis while being tested, large amounts of keratosis may indicate a delayed comedogenic reaction. In other words, a high test score in the histopathogy report may indicate that longer exposure time to the product or ingredient may cause comedone development or that the test material causes sufficient irritation within the follicle to possibly promote sudden acne flares.

Materials that are both found to be noncomedogenic and show no significant irritancy or retention hyperkeratosis within the histopathological examination are said to be nonacnegenic.

A few scientists and physicians use a five-point scale. Both tests are run using scores of 0 to 5, rather than 0 to 3. If you look at various studies, you will notice that both scales are used, but the three-point scale is more often used and is widely accepted as standard by the cosmetic industry. If you look at comedogenicity studies or charts, you will notice that one rating number is followed by a slash mark and then a 3 or a 5. As an example you may see a rating of 2/3. This means that out of 3 possible points, the product or ingredient tested had a rating of 2, making it significantly comedogenic. Scores of 3/3, 4/5, or 5/5 indicate highly comedogenic materials or products.

A score of 1/3, 1/5, or 2/5 means that the product or material showed comedogenic results in the rabbit ear, but not as strong as material with a higher score.

Remember, clients who are subject to easy development of clogged pores, comedones, and other acne lesions must first hereditarily develop retention hyperkeratosis. A client who does not develop clogged pores easily and has fairly oil-dry skin may show no reaction when treated with a product that has a low score of comedogenicity of approximately 1/3 or 2/5. Clients who easily develop acne flareups may be much more sensitive to even a mildly comedogenic material.

Other Tests

Some companies conduct tests for comedogenicity on humans instead of on rabbit ears. In the human studies, the product or material is applied routinely to the skin on an individual's back. The skin is observed for comedo development. In the opinion of this author and many other scientists, the rabbit ear assay is a much more accurate test for determining comedogenicity. There are several reasons for this opinion. First, the rabbit ear forms comedones much faster than humans, making the testing procedure much faster and therefore more economical. Second, rabbit ear skin is very sensitive to comedone development. Human skin develops clogged pores much more slowly. The skin of the back of a human may not necessarily develop retention hyperkeratosis hereditarily. Third, and probably most important, a rabbit can be easily controlled, and there are very few variables involved with testing. The rabbit is in a controlled environment, with a controlled diet and climate. Humans, on the other hand, are not confined, and you must consider literally hundreds of variables when you interpret test results. As examples, human models may have different diets, different environments, and different activities.

Because of these variables, many scientists believe that human studies are not as reliable or as accurate as rabbit ear studies.

At this point in time, there is no non-animal test available to measure comedogenicity or retention hyperkeratosis. Some day we hope to have better non-animal testing measures. In the meantime, some tests must still be performed on animals.

Types of Ingredients that Are Often Comedogenic

Often the vehicle ingredient, rather than the active agent, is comedogenic in a product. Emollients, fats, waxes, esters, and oils used in cosmetics are the most common comedogenic ingredients.

These oils and other substances are used in cosmetics to smooth the surface of the skin, help spread the cosmetic, and help replace the sebum in an alipidic skin type. However, the type of skin that develops clogged pores easily is not alipidic; in fact, it is usually oily, already producing too much sebum. These ingredients are similar to sebum in texture and chemical makeup. Is it any wonder that these ingredients, simulating human sebum, add to the problem of cell buildup and comedone development?

Think of the dead corneum cells constantly shedding from the walls of the follicles as flakes of oatmeal lining a drinking glass. Because of the hereditary tendency to retain cells and because of this type of skin's oiliness, the flakes of dead cells naturally stick to the follicle walls.

Now imagine pouring oil down the sides of this glass filled with oatmeal. Imagine how oil would make the oatmeal sticky and clump together.

This may be a very rough metaphor, but it does illustrate the point. Many of the fats, oils, esters, and emollient ingredients used in cosmetics do penetrate the follicles of already clog-prone individuals, adding fatty substances to the follicles of skin that is already burdened with too much sebum and cell buildup.

These ingredients are considered comedogenic. Their purpose in cosmetics is to lubricate or serve as a spreading agent. While this may be helpful to truly dry skins that do not produce enough oil, it is bad for clog-prone skin.

Emollients and Oils

Emollients that often clog the pores are derived from fats or waxes of animal or vegetable origin. We will divide these substances into several categories.

Oils

Many vegetable and animal oils are comedogenic. Coconut oil, cocoa butter, peach kernel oil, linseed oil, grape seed oil, and sesame oil are comedogenic oils. Less comedogenic oils include avocado oil, safflower oil, castor oil, jojoba oil, and sunflower oil. Mineral oil is also noncomedogenic.

Other Waxes and Fats

Beeswax is noncomedogenic, particularly in small quantities of concentration, as it is often used. Emulsifying wax, carnuba wax, and candelilla wax, often used in lipstick, are noncomedogenic. Petrolatum is also noncomedogenic. However, because petrolatum is relatively greasy, it is not often used in cosmetics for oily and clog-prone skin, especially in large concentrations.

Fatty Acids

Probably the most comedogenic group of cosmetic chemicals are the fatty acids. Fatty acids, which are used to give cosmetics a creamy consistency, are often comedogenic. These substances are derived from animal and plant oils and include oleic acid, lauric acid, isostearic acid, palmitic acid, and myristic acid. Capric acid, caprylic acid, and behenic acid are less comedogenic, but still should not be used in large concentrations for oily, problem skin.

Esters

The fatty esters obtained from combining alcohols with fatty acids are also often comedogenic. As we learned in the cosmetic chemistry chapter, these esters are often used in cosmetics because they feel less oily than raw fatty acids. However, their chemical alteration to an ester often renders them comedogenic. The esters that are comedogenic include isopropyl myristate, very well known as a highly comedogenic ingredient. Other comedogenic esters are isopropyl palmitate, octyl palmitate, isopropyl isostearate, decyl oleate, sorbitan oleate, isopropyl lanolate, isopropyl linoleate, butyl stearate, and myristyl myristate.

Fatty Alcohols

Fatty alcohols are used in cosmetics as emollients. They are generally less comedogenic than their parent acids or esters. The comedogenic fatty alcohols include oleyl alcohol, isostearyl alcohol, and octyldodecanol.

Lanolin

Lanolin is derived from sheep sebum. It is an excellent emollient, and in its purest form, in a small quantity, does not cause many problems for clog-prone skin. However, chemically altered lanolins, such as lanolic acid, isopropyl lanolate, and acetylated lanolin alcohol, are comedogenic.

Active Agents

It is interesting that most extracts, pigments, humectants, and other active agents are noncomedogenic ingredients. Emollients and fatty-type ingredients create the most problems. The other ingredient type that creates problems is inorganic pigments, specifically the red dyes.

The Red Dyes

Almost every red dye is comedogenic. This explains why you may often notice closed comedones on women's cheekbones. Red dyes are frequently used in blushes.

These dyes are derivatives of coal tar. Coal tar is extremely comedogenic. Red dyes are used in blush, lipsticks, powders, foundations, and skin-care products. They are not permitted to be used in eyeshadows. Coal tar is known to be a major eye irritant and is not safe for use in the eye area.

Unfortunately, many of the beautiful shades of blush or lipstick cannot be made without D & C red dyes. There is a red color in an organic pigment called carmine and in certain colors of iron oxide. Carmine is more expensive to use than D & C red dyes and does not produce as vivid red colors.

Because of these facts, you may correctly assume that, in general, the more red a product is, the more likely it is to contain D & C red dyes and the more likely it is to be comedogenic. Again, these dyes produce no problems for many clients who are not acne-prone. However, they should be avoided in oily and acne-prone clients. Some cosmetic companies do manufacture blushes that are free of coal tar dyes.

Chemistry Behind Comedogenicity

The chemical reasons why certain cosmetic ingredients are comedogenic is not fully understood. It is certainly logical that the fats that simulate human sebum could potentially cause problems for oily, problem skin. It is believed that the size of the molecule has a great deal to do with comedogenic potential. The larger the molecule, the less likely it is to be comedogenic. This explains why some fatty acids become more or less comedogenic when they are altered chemically. When a large molecular structure is added to a fatty acid, it tends to become less comedogenic. When a fat is broken down to a smaller molecule, it is more comedogenic. This is theorized to be linked to the size of the molecule and its ability to penetrate the follicle. It makes sense that smaller fatty molecules penetrate more easily into the follicle and therefore they may cause more problems.

Concentration of Comedogenic Ingredients

The amount of comedogenic ingredients used within a particular cosmetic formulation may also have an effect on the overall comedogenicity of the product. Moisturizers with large amounts of known comedogenic ingredients are more likely to be comedogenic than products with less concentration of comedogenic ingredients.

Controversy continues over the amount of comedogenic ingredients that should be used in cosmetics. Some scientists believe that as long as comedogenic ingredients make up less than 5 percent of the product, there will be no effect on the comedogenicity. The flaw in this idea is that neither the consumer nor the esthetician knows exactly how much comedogenic chemical is used in any particular product, since no cosmetic company publishes its percentages on the label. This makes this theory impossible to use practically.

The other argument against this theory is that known comedogenic ingredients should simply not be used in products that are designed for clog-prone, oily, or acne-prone skin. Many estheticians agree with this statement.

Pressing Agents

Besides the problem with D & C red dyes, the other problem with blushes, as well as pressed powders, is the pressing agent. Emollients are added to talc and other products to create cake-type blush and powder. Pressed powder is an example. By mixing the powder with a sticky emollient, a pressed cake forms, which is usually marketed as a compact or powder blush.

If a comedogenic emollient is used to press the powder or blush, the product may indeed cause or increase comedone development. If a blush with D & C red dyes is pressed with a comedogenic agent, you get a "double-whammy" as far as comedogenicity is concerned!

Zinc stearate and mineral oil are safe ingredients to use in pressing powders. They do not cause clogging and make good pressing agents.

The other problem with pressing agents is that they involve mixing a fat, which is liquid or semi-liquid, with a nonsoluble powder. This means that, unlike moisturizers, which are usually water based and always liquid, there are no liquid ingredients to "water down" the comedogenic effects of the emollient pressing agent.

Because of this, comedogenic powders tend to be very comedogenic because the skin is more directly exposed to the concentrated emollient.

Loose Powders

Loose powders are not immune from comedogenicity just because they are not in a cake form. Emollients are also added to loose powders to give them a silky texture and to help them adhere to the skin. Check powders carefully to make sure they are free of both comedogenic emollients and coal tar-derived D & C red dyes.

Skin-Care Products

Skin-care products are often comedogenic, particularly many types of moisturizers, lotions, fluids, and creams. They may be made with comedogenic emollients or other fatty ingredients. If you are treating a clog-prone client, check ingredients carefully (Figure 13-3).

The Controversy Over Ingredient Lists

Some scientists have objected to comedogenic ingredient lists (like the one included here). Their objection is based on the theory that mixtures of ingredients may not be as harmful as the individual ingredient's test score indicates.

While it is true that the bottom line is to have the final product tested, many companies do not test their products or publish the results of testing.

Testing for comedogenicity can be expensive and time-consuming. This is an additional expense for the company. Theoretically, claims testing should always be performed by an independent testing firm. By having testing performed outside the cosmetic company, the test results will be more likely to be accurate, reliable, and nonbiased. The reason lists like this one exist is so that estheticians and consumers can check the labels of their skin-care products and cosmetics for comedogenic ingredients. Even though this may not always be the most scientific or accurate method of determining potential comedogenicity, it is certainly the most practical for helping clients choose the right products.

Comedogenic Product Analysis

When you consult with a client who has acne or develops clogged pores easily, ask the client to bring in the products being used currently, so that you may check them for comedogenic ingredients.

Consumers today have heard the word *noncomedogenic*, but they generally are not aware of the variety of cosmetic ingredients that are comedogenic. One of the most important duties of the esthetician is to educate consumers about cosmetic chemistry. While your clients do not need to know everything in this chapter, they will appreciate your knowledge about comedogenic ingredients and products, as well as the advice you can

FIGURE 13–3 Chart of common comedogenic ingredients

Common Comedogenic Ingredients

Highly Comedogenic (4-5/5 or 5/3)

Linseed oil
Olive oil
Cocoa butter
Oleic Acid
Coal Tar
Isopropyl Isostearate
Squalene
Isopropyl Myristate
Myristyl Myristate
Acetylated Lanolin
Isopropyl Palmitate
Isopropyl Linoleate
Oleyl Alcohol
Octyl Palmitate
Isostearic Acid
Myreth 3 Myristate
Butyl Stearate
Lanolic Acid

Moderately Comedogenic (3-4/5 or 2/3)

Decyl Oleate
Sorbitan Oleate
Myristyl Lactate
Coconut Oil
Grape Seed Oil
Sesame Oil
Hexylene Glycol
Tocopherol
Isostearyl Neopentanoate
Most D & C Red Pigments
Octyldodecanol
Peanut Oil
Lauric Acid
Mink Oil

Mildly Comedogenic (2-3/5 or 1/3)

Corn Oil
Safflower Oil
Lauryl Alcohol
Lanolin Alcohol
Glyceryl Stearate
Lanolin
Sunflower Oil
Avocado Oil
Mineral Oil
(Please note mildly comedogenic ingredients are generally not a problem when used in diluted concentrations. Check to see their ranking of concentration on the ingredient label.)

Non-Comedogenic

Glycerin
Squalane
Sorbitol
Sodium PCA
Zinc Stearate
Octyldodecyl Stearate
SD Alcohol
Propylene Glycol
Allantoin
Panthenol
Water
Iron Oxides
Dimethicone
Cyclomethicone
Polysorbates
Cetyl Palmitate
Propylene Glycol Dicaprate/Dicaprylate
Jojoba Oil
Isopropyl Alcohol
Sodium Hyaluronate
Octylmethoxycinnimate
Oxybenzone
Petrolatum

give about eliminating comedogenic products from home skin care and cosmetic routines.

While you cannot run a rabbit ear assay on every product that your client might bring in, you can check the products for containing comedogenic ingredients. Check each ingredient against charts like the one here. Companies that produce noncomedogenic cosmetics often have charts available that list ingredients and their comedogenic levels. On request, many of these same companies will be glad to share their comedogenic studies on their own products with you.

Returning to your product analysis, check with your clients to see what products they are routinely using. Clients will often bring in products that they are not actually using. It is important that your client is honest with you regarding daily habits.

Begin by checking your client's moisturizers and treatment preparations. The most important products to observe are products that remain on clog-prone areas of the face for prolonged periods of time. This will include day creams, night treatment creams, moisturizers, hydrators, sunscreens, foundations, powders, blushes, and any other specialty products that the client uses that stay on the face for long periods of time.

Cleansers and toners should also be noncomedogenic, but these products do not stay on the face for eight hours at a time. Cleansers should be very easily rinseable and should not leave residues on the face. Superfatted soaps, for example, tend to leave a film on the face. Often the fat added to these soaps is comedogenic. Toner can also be made with fats, particularly if they are designed for extra dry, alipidic skin.

A good noncomedogenic cleanser should be made with noncomedogenic emulsifiers. Many contain a detergent. They may vary in strength, but many will be on the stronger side, because most skin types that develop clogs easily are also predominantly oily, making thorough cleansing a necessity. These detergent cleansers will do a good job of cleansing surface oil and debris. The cleansers may be too strong for very dry skin, but most alipidic skins do not clog easily.

A foaming cleanser is often used. These cleansers are extremely rinseable and leave the skin feeling very clean, a feeling clients often describe as "squeaky." There is nothing wrong with this feeling, as long as the cleanser does not have a high pH, stripping off too much oil. Most oily clients like to feel super-clean. They enjoy and will use a foaming type cleanser, particularly if they use soap on a regular basis. In short, foaming cleansers give the client the feeling of using soap without the undesirable effects of some soaps. Foaming cleansers are also convenient and can be used in the shower or bath easily.

Toners should be, as previously discussed, free of fats. They should have moderately strong astringent action, helping to remove excess oils and cell buildup. Some may contain an anti-bacterial, and some of the stronger ones for oily skin may contain a mild peeling agent like salicylic acid. Cleansing milk can be used for makeup removal, but should be easily removed and should not leave a residue on the skin. For oilier skin, clients may want to use a foaming cleanser after removal of makeup with a cleansing milk. Cold-cream type cleansers should not be used for clog-prone skin because they leave too much of a residue and do not remove enough oil from the surface.

Day Creams

Day creams should certainly be noncomedogenic, because they are worn in direct contact with the skin for eight hours or more. There are several types of day creams for clog-prone skin. Some may contain a mild peeling agent like salicylic acid, and some will be a hydrating protectant with a sunscreen ingredient and some sort of protectant ingredient like dimethicone, a silicone derivative. Day creams should be extremely light. The heavier they are, the more likely they are to occlude the follicle openings, and the more likely they are, as a general rule, to be comedogenic.

Night Treatments

There are two basic types of night treatments for clogged and problem skin, hydrators and peeling creams.

Hydrating creams or fluids are made for skin that is clogged or acne-prone, but still dehydrated—in other words, skin that really needs hydration, but also breaks out easily. These fluids will be water-based, very light in texture, noncomedogenic, free of the offending ingredients we have discussed, and contain hydrating agents that will not clog such as sodium PCA, glycerin, sorbitol, or hyaluronic acid. These agents hydrate without causing clog development and may be used in products without high levels of fatty emollients. Peeling treatment creams and fluids are designed to help exfoliate oily, clogged, and acne-prone skin, helping to eliminate excess dead cell buildup to break loose impactions. These products will contain peeling agents such as benzoyl peroxide, salicylic acid, glycolic acid, resorcinol, sulfur, or a combination of these. They should be used in a lightweight vehicle base that is noncomedogenic. For more information on how to use these acne treatments, please see the chapter on acne.

Foundations for Clog-Prone Skin

Foundation makeup for clogged and acne-prone skin must be noncomedogenic, preferably in a "fat-free," water-based liquid. As a general rule, liquid foundations are the only appropriate type of foundation for clogged and acne-prone skin. The foundation should be completely free of comedogenic ingredients and should be very lightweight. Coverage can still be attained if you look for foundations that contain a lot of talc and pigment. Many of these foundations will contain some sort of evaporating agent, like witch hazel, to help control surface oiliness. These foundations often dry to a matte finish, a good characteristic for oily skin. Some of the newer foundations contain silicones like cyclomethicone as a spreading agent. These foundations are good for older clients with acne problems, because they do not dry as matte.

Other Products that May Be Comedogenic

Hair products and many kinds of face creams may contain comedogenic agents. The purposes of these creams, or claims, may vary greatly. They may not fall into the categories just mentioned. Check all products that come in contact with clog-prone areas.

Some items such as lipstick, eyeshadows, eye creams, and other products need not be noncomedogenic, because they are not being used in clog- or acne-prone areas. The only reason you may want to check these is if the client has an isolated clogged area, such as the lipline (you should check her lipstick or lip conditioner), or if the client is using the product in an area for which it was not intended (i.e., using a hair conditioner on the face). Hair conditioners and styling products often contain fats, oils, and other comedogenic ingredients. They were not designed to be used on the face.

Comedogenic ingredients are also sometimes used in ointments and prescription topical drugs. While you should never tell a client to discontinue the use of a prescribed drug, you should be aware that some topical medications can be comedogenic.

Dehydrated, Clogged Skin

Many women, particularly mature women, suffer from dehydrated skin that is also clogged. This is caused by the client mistaking dehydrated skin for dry skin. In other words, the client actually has dehydrated (water-dry) skin, but mistakenly uses products designed for dry (oil-dry) skin. These products designed for mature alipidic skin are often full of fatty acids, esters, waxes, oils, and fats. In the attempt to treat their dehydrated skin or wrinkles, they expose oily areas to the excessive fats and oils present in these emollient products.

Unfortunately these clients have often been misdiagnosed by a cosmetic salesperson, or more unfortunately, a poorly educated esthetician. Many women have a fear of "dry skin," because they fear aging and associate "dry skin" with aging. They do not understand that aging is not only caused by "dryness," but by hereditary factors and sun damage. They attempt to treat aging with oils.

It is very important to educate this client about dehydration versus oil dryness. Explain to clients that dehydration makes the skin look dry and flaky, but this does not mean that they need oil; they need water!

Hydration can be achieved in one of two ways. Hydrating active agents can be used to increase the water level of the surface cells, easing dehydration and flaking, and making the skin look smoother, softer, and feel better.

Adding oily products to this type of skin keeps the skin from further dehydration, but it does not necessarily add significant water to the surface cells. Fatty, oily products often contain comedogenic ingredients. While these clients attempt to "moisturize," they actually cause clogged pores to form, possibly developing into acne, and are not best treating their dehydrated skin.

Almost all hydrating active agents are noncomedogenic. Many emollient-active agents for oil-dry skin are comedogenic. Retrain clients to use noncomedogenic products with noncomedogenic emollient ingredients, and use good noncomedogenic hydrating agents such as sorbitol, sodium PCA, glycerin, or hyaluronic acid. Make sure you check the vehicle ingredients for comedogenic ingredients. Most often the spreading agents are comedogenic.

Avoid using over-drying peeling agents on these clients. Psychologically they will feel that their skin is even more dry, particularly in the first few days of treatment. It is important to make sure that the client is comfortable to ensure compliance with the new program.

Heavy Creams

Many heavy creams can make acne-prone or oily clog-prone skin worse. Some of these creams are not actually comedogenic, but they contain large amounts of oils or petrolatum. They are simply too heavy for these oily skinned clients. While neither petrolatum or mineral oil is particularly comedogenic, they are not appropriate in large concentrations for oily, clogged, or acne-prone skin.

Oil-Free and Water-Based

These two claims are often made for products supposedly designed for oily skin. Neither of these two terms mean the same thing as *noncomedogenic*. *Oil-free* means, technically, that there are no oils in the product. That doesn't mean that there are no fatty esters, fatty acids, or other comedogenic ingredients.

Water-based simply means that the main ingredient is water, which might be mixed with comedogenic ingredients. The bottom line is, check the product carefully for comedogenic ingredients.

Clinical Comedogenics

Some clients will have a sudden acne flareup when introduced to certain new products. While there can be many reasons for this reaction, occasionally even a noncomedogenic product can cause an acne flareup due to irritation of the follicles. If your client reports such a flareup, advise your client to try the cream again after a short time. If the reaction continues, the client should discontinue use of the product.

Checklist of Products

The following products should be checked during a comedogenic analysis:

- Cleansers, washes, and soaps.

- Toners, fresheners, and astringents.

- Day creams, moisturizers, and sunscreens.

- Night fluids, creams, specialty products, and ampoules.

- Foundation makeup.

- Powder—both loose and pressed.

- Blush.

- Any other product that is being used over a clog-prone area of the face for a prolonged period of time.

Checklist of Analysis Procedures

1. Analyze the skin and the areas that have comedones, clogged pores, sebaceous filaments, or other acne lesions.

2. Check the client's current products for comedogenic ingredients.

3. Are the products the client is using really correct for the skin type, or is the client using products for oil-dry skin when the skin is actually dehydrated?

4. Is the client using fluids and lotions or creams?

5. Are the products the client is using simply too heavy for the skin?

6. Is the client skipping steps that should be done?

7. If the products the client uses contain comedogenic ingredients, are they high or low on the ingredient list? If the client has a minimal number of clogged pores, it may not be caused by the products. Remember, in order to have a comedogenic reaction, you must have comedogenic products and a skin type that tends to clog due to hereditary oiliness and hyperkeratosis.

Client Product Analysis

As we have previously discussed, you should ask a client who is clog-prone to bring in all products for analysis on the first visit. First check the products with the checklist for analysis.

After checking the products for correct skin type, etc., then begin checking the products for comedogenic ingredients. Let's look at a typical label. You have already established that the client is definitely clog-prone. Here are the products the client is using:

Product: Cleansing Cream. Ingredients: Mineral oil, purified water, beeswax, sodium borate, isopropyl palmitate, petrolatum, stearyl alcohol, lanolin alcohol, ceteareth-20, magnesium aluminum silicate, sodium dehydroacetate, methyl paraben, propyl paraben, D & C red #6.

Analysis: More than comedogenic, this cleansing cream is simply much too greasy and heavy for oily, clog-prone skin. It contains isopropyl palmitate, a known comedogenic ingredient. However, the ingredient is fairly low on the ingredient list. It also contains D & C red #6, which is not very comedogenic compared to other D & C red dyes and is present in a fairly small quantity. The biggest problem with this cleanser is that it is oil based, very heavy, and is probably not being rinsed off well, which can be a real problem for oily, clog-prone skin. This cleanser is a good cleanser for dryer skin types or for those who wear heavy or theatrical makeup and need a thorough oil-based cleanser. It should be replaced for your client with a rinseable foaming cleanser and/or a nongreasy cleansing milk.

Product: Day Protectant. Ingredients: Water, isopropyl palmitate, isopropyl myristate, mineral oil, propylene glycol, propylene glycol stearate, stearic acid, magnesium aluminum silicate, oleic acid, cellulose gum, methyl paraben, propyl paraben, fragrance.

Analysis: This day cream is loaded with potentially comedogenic ingredients. Isopropyl myristate, isopropyl palmitate, and oleic acid are all comedogenic chemicals. Isopropyl myristate and isopropyl palmitate are extremely high on the ingredient list, indicating a fairly large concentration of these problem agents. This cream is left on the face all day, creating a true exposure time. This day cream should only be used on skin types that are not clog prone. Your client should discontinue this product.

Product: Liquid makeup. Ingredients: Water, propylene glycol, SD alcohol 40, titanium dioxide, talc, witch hazel extract, zinc oxide, magnesium aluminum silicate, methyl paraben, propyl paraben; may contain: iron oxides, ultramarine blue.

Analysis: This is an excellent example of a noncomedogenic product. It contains no comedogenic ingredients and no real emollient fats. It contains witch hazel and S.D. alcohol as mild drying agents—a plus for oily skins. This makeup is safe enough to be used on acne. Your client made a good choice here and should continue to use this product.

Product: Loose powder. Ingredients: talc, myristyl myristate, zinc stearate, fragrance, methyl paraben, propyl paraben, iron oxides, fragrance.

Analysis: This product would be acceptable if it did not have myristyl myristate as a pressing agent. It should not be used on oily, acne, or clogged skin.

These are only a few examples of how to do a comedogenic analysis. Use your head and the facts you have been taught. The bottom line of all of this testing and analysis is: Is your client's skin developing clogged pores? If it is, something is not working correctly!

You should of course have available to your clients an entire range of noncomedogenic products. When purchasing products for your salon, remember to check carefully for the ingredients and testing procedures we have discussed throughout this chapter.

TOPICS FOR DISCUSSION

1. Discuss testing for comedogenicity.
2. Discuss the difference between noncomedogenic and non-acnegenic products.
3. Discuss the concentration of possible comedogenic ingredients in a product and how this may affect comedogenicity.
4. Why are comedogenic ingredient lists controversial?
5. Discuss the various types of products for clog-prone skin. What should you look for in a day cream? Night treatment? Foundation?
6. Discuss treatment of adult, mature, clogged, and dehydrated skin.

14

Extraction

Extraction is an extremely important part of the esthetician's skills, and it is a difficult process to master.

With proper hands-on supervision, this chapter will help the esthetician learn about extraction procedures for many different types of follicle impactions. Different methods of extraction will be discussed as well as specific unusual problems that may be encountered during extraction.

One of the most important parts of an esthetics practice is extraction. It is also one of the most difficult to learn and master.

Extraction refers to the removal of dead cells, sebum, bacteria, and other debris from the skin's follicles. This expulsion technique is probably the most important function of a facial treatment. The solid mass of sebum, dead cells, and other matter stuck in the follicles are both an esthetic and a physiological problem. Besides being unsightly, failure to treat these lesions may lead to more serious acne and health problems, not to mention permanent scarring.

Extraction techniques cannot be learned simply by studying a book. You must have hands-on training in all areas of extraction, taught by a well-qualified instructor. Do not attempt any of the procedures outlined in this chapter without the supervision and hands-on demonstration of a qualified, licensed instructor.

Extraction is a very important part of the esthetics profession and is possibly the most important service that estheticians perform. It can also be an uncomfortable and unsafe procedure if performed incorrectly.

Some states do not allow the use of lancets for extraction. Check with your esthetics instructor or school for laws governing the use of lancets by estheticians in your state.

Analysis of the Need for Extraction

Almost every skin that you will see under the magnifying lamp will need at least some extraction. Even dry, older skin will be likely to have some clogged follicles in the nose area. Observe your client's skin closely under a magnifying lamp. Check all areas of the face well, including behind and in front of the ears, the neck, and the jawline.

On combination skin you will likely see small clogged pores through the T-zone area and scattered larger clogged pores or blackheads. In any area you may see small white bumps or closed comedones, milia (whiteheads), pustules, and papules associated with acne. The width of the T-zone will determine the oiliness of the area and therefore the number of clogged pores. Clogged pores are always a sign of an oily area (Figure 14-1).

FIGURE 14–1   T-zone of clogged pores

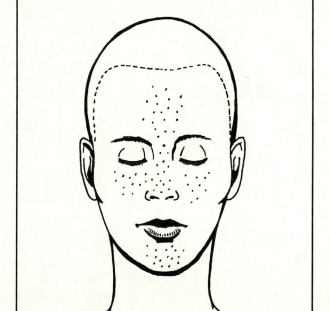

The perimeter of the face is an ideal place for clogged pores and acne lesions to form. These are areas your clients often miss while cleansing. You can think of these areas as "cobwebs" in the corner of a room! (See Figure 14-2.)

FIGURE 14–2   Examination procedures

Exam Procedures for Extraction

1. Cleanse the skin well.
2. Using a magnifying lamp, examine the skin observing areas with enlarged pores, noting areas with smaller and larger pores.
3. Combination skin—Note enlarged pores through the T-zone indicating oilier skin, smaller pores around the edges of the face, indicating less oil production. The width of the oily T-zone determines whether the skin is oily-combination or dry-combination. The wider the visible enlarged pore structure, the oilier the skin is.
4. Clogged pores, comedones, closed comedones, papules and pustules are more likely to be seen in the oilier areas.
5. The small clogged pores in the nose are usually sebaceous filaments, not open comedones; they are simply follicles filled with oxidized sebum.
6. IN THE OILY AREAS ... Pull the skin taut with the thumb and forefinger and observe any small white bumps under the skin. These are closed comedones.
7. Check the perimeter of the face well, including under the chin, jawline, the neck, and in front and behind the ears.

Think about your client doing at-home cleaning. The client is not a skin-care specialist and probably does not take the time or care cleaning as you would cleaning your own face. The client applies the cleanser and massages it but does not notice the remnants of cleanser or makeup left in front of the ears, in the hairline, and under the jawline. The client may also omit toner as a followup in these areas.

Failure to remove makeup and cleanser in these areas means that dead cells buildup here. Clogs will inevitably form.

The first thing you should do when you encounter "perimeter acne" is to gently make the client aware of it and why it is probably there. Instruct your client to pay extra attention to cleaning these areas and to use toner after cleansing. You may also suggest that a foaming cleanser be used as a second cleanser after makeup removal. This not only helps to remove any emollients left from a cleansing milk, but the foam itself is very obvious when it is still on the face or in one of those hidden corners! Your client will see the foam and rinse off the area.

Continuing the Analysis...

Gently spread the skin with your thumb and forefinger. Move the fingers across the face, constantly spreading the skin gently. Observe if there are any small white bumps that are only visible when the skin is pulled taut. These are often closed comedones and can be seen on any area of the face, but especially can be hidden in the chin area, just under the lower lip, and under the chin and jawline.

Check the skin for sebaceous filaments, which are not really open comedones. They are what most clients refer to as "clogged pores." These are follicles that have filled with sebum, sometimes over a very short period of time. They are most noticeable on the nose, but can appear in any area. On very oily skin, they can literally seem to be in every single area.

Sebaceous filaments indicate an oily area. They are not nearly as large or dilated as an open comedone, but they are basically the same type of lesion. The only real difference is that a sebaceous filament is mostly sebum, whereas a real open comedone will be dilated, much larger, and filled with many dead cells. An open comedone may take weeks to form, but sebaceous filaments may form in just a few days. The debris extracted from a sebaceous filament will be much smaller than that of an open comedone, and you will also notice that the plug is not as deep or as solid.

Open Comedones

Open comedones may appear anywhere on the face. They are most noticeable in acne conditions and in clients who have neglected their skin for a long time. They are also frequently observed in young adolescents who have a budding adolescent acne problem, but may not be cleaning well and have not taken a true interest in their personal appearance yet.

Open comedones can certainly appear in any skin type, but they are more prevalent in the above-mentioned situations. Clients who are very conscientious will be aware of these lesions and will either have them extracted or attempt to do so themselves. Open comedones are often about the size of a pinhead. They have a large black top, hence the term *blackhead*. Open comedones are the easiest lesions to extract.

Presoftening Before Extraction

The procedure you follow before extraction will significantly help loosen follicle impactions, making extractions less difficult for the esthetician and less uncomfortable for the client. The skin must be pretreated before extraction. This pretreatment will help soften the accumulations in the follicles, as well as the surface of the skin, making the skin more soft and flexible during the extraction procedure.

Desincrustation

Desincrustation refers to the process of softening the skin and sebaceous impaction by applying a chemical that helps to liquify the sebum, reducing hard, solid plugs to a softer consistency. This technique softens clogs significantly. The chemical used for this procedure is usually an anionic surfactant. Thus, desincrustation solutions usually have a higher, or more alkaline, pH.

Desincrustation solutions are usually either liquids or a soft gel-cream consistency, often referred to as a pre-mask.

The liquid is applied to the affected areas of the face after preliminary cleansing or is sometimes poured onto cotton compresses and then applied to the face.

The "pre-masks" can be applied to the face either with a brush or your hands. Pre-masks have a thicker consistency than liquid solutions. They can be seen on the skin, whereas liquids cannot. Being careful to follow manufacturer's instructions, allow the solution or pre-mask to sit on the face for 5 to 10 minutes. Steam treatment is frequently used at the same time. The water from the steam helps to provide additional softening effects. Galvanic desincrustation may be applied over the pre-mask or liquid, depending on the manufacturer's instructions. Galvanic treatment with a desincrustant chemical provides for better penetration of the product and better reduction of the plug due to chemical reactions produced by the electricity within the follicle. (See *Milady's Standard Textbook of Cosmetology* for further explanation and instructions for use of galvanic current.)

The oilier and more impacted the skin, the better it is to use galvanic treatment. Some clients who have a minimal number of clogged follicles and more dehydrated skin may find galvanic treatment to be too drying. It is a good idea to use galvanic treatment routinely on acne conditions, provided that there are no medical contraindications for use.

After the "soak" period with desincrustation solution or pre-mask, or galvanic treatment is completed, remove the desincrustant product well and proceed with extraction.

Desincrustant chemicals are often slippery and must be removed thoroughly before extraction. Otherwise the skin will be too slippery for extraction procedures.

Other Pre-Extraction Procedures

The use of a brushing machine may help loosen dead cells, particularly on skin that is both dehydrated and clogged.

The electric rotating brush should be gently applied after steaming. The brush should be used over a layer of emulsion-type cleanser to prevent too much scratching of the face during the brushing procedure. Do not use the brush on acne, couperosed, or sensitive skin. (For further instruction on brushing, see *Milady's Standard Textbook of Cosmetology.*)

Suction, or vacuuming, may be performed with a skin suction machine after desincrustation or steaming. Suction may help to further loosen impactions that have already been loosened with desincrustation. Suction removes very little debris from the follicle, but the procedure feels good to the client and has a nice psychological effect. Again, suction should not be used on sensitive or couperose skin or acne. See *Milady's Standard Textbook of Cosmetology* for instruction on suction machines.

Enzyme Treatments and Peels

Light peeling treatments performed with enzymes can help to loosen clogged pores and impaction significantly. The light exfoliating effects help to remove dead cells from the skin's surface and helps to loosen and slightly dilate the follicle openings. This makes extraction easier. Clients who are both dehydrated and clogged may particularly benefit from an enzyme pore-treatment.

Enzymes are normally applied during the steam treatment for an 8 to 12 minute period of time. For further information on how to use enzymes, see the chapter on chemical peeling.

Hygiene and Extraction

It is very important to always wear gloves during extraction. It is generally good practice to wear gloves throughout the treatment, especially if there are any acne lesions present. Please review the sterilization and hygiene chapter before beginning extraction.

Extraction of Open Comedones

After presoftening the accumulations, remove all products from the skin, leaving the face moist but not wet. Wet skin or skin that still has product on it is impossible to extract. Take two cotton swabs. Hold them as you would hold two pencils. It is best to use the type of swab that has a soft, flexible plastic stick. These plastic cotton swabs are much easier to work with and will snap if too much pressure is applied, a built-in safety feature.

Place a swab on each side of the open comedone. Gently press down on the swabs and then gently move the swabs closer together, with the tips touching the skin. This will have a lifting effect on the solid plug. Keep applying gentle pressure until you see the plug come out of the follicle. If the plug does not come out easily, move the swabs to another angle around the sides of the comedone and repeat the procedure. Once the plug is out, continue to press gently on the sides of the follicle to make sure all of the debris has been removed.

Finger Technique

Wrap your gloved forefingers in damp cotton. Using the same gentle downward and inward pressure technique, attempt to extract the comedone. Work your fingers all around the comedone with the same pressure technique.

Cotton swabs are easier for many people because they are smaller than fingers. It is the consensus of clients that the cotton swab technique is more comfortable and more efficient.

Extractor Technique

Comedone extractors are best to use on non-fleshy parts of the face, such as the forehead or cheekbones, or on clients whose skin does not have a fleshy thickness that can be physically manipulated. Comedone extractors should never be used on thin, fragile, sensitive, or couperose skin.

Place the extractor over the open comedone, with the hole in the extractor directly over the comedone. It is very important that the lesion be smaller than the hole in the metal extractor. If the lesion is wider than the hole in the extractor, do not use the extractor. Either try a larger extractor or try the cotton swab method.

Assuming that the comedone can easily fit into the hole in the extractor, gently press straight down on the extractor, using the leverage of the handle end to exert pressure. The plug should come out of the follicle and be noticeable inside the hole of the extractor. It is a good idea to follow this extraction procedure with another gentle expression of the follicle with the cotton swabs to check for any further debris that might be trapped in the follicle.

Remember when using a metal extractor that the extractor is metal and is not flexible. The use of a comedone extractor can be very painful for the client, particularly if used over the entire face. They should be reserved for use on boney areas or non-fleshy skin.

Comedone extractors are available in a variety of sizes. Some are made with a slight bend for better leverage. Some are made with a round hole, and some with an oval or rectangular hole. You should have some of each type available, and you will, over time, develop a feel for which is appropriate to use. Comedone extractors must be sterilized after each client. They are not disposable. See the chapter on sterile and aseptic procedure for sterilizing techniques.

Closed Comedones

Closed comedones appear as small bumps just underneath the surface of the skin. They can be found on any area of the face, but are frequently found on the cheeks, jawline, and chin. Often you will see a large number of closed comedones on the cheekbones of female clients. These are often caused by a comdogenic reaction to a blush. (See the chapter on comedogenicity.) The closed comedone is just beneath the skin and normally has a very small follicle opening. If you look carefully through a magnifying lamp, you may detect a very small opening in the top of the closed comedone. Often, these follicles must be dilated with a lancet before extraction.

Extraction of Closed Comedones

Closed comedones are the most difficult of any lesion to extract, because they are just beneath the surface of the skin, have a very small pore opening, and may vary greatly in size. If you can see the opening of the follicle well, and the white area surrounding the opening does not appear to be very large, you may attempt to extract the area by using the cotton swab technique. Place the tip of the cotton swabs on either side of the closed comedone, being careful to make sure you are clear about the border of the lesion. In other words, make sure you have the entire comedone within the placement of your swabs. Failure to do so may result in extracting only part of the comedone. Gently press down on the swabs and then gently turn them inward while pulling the skin taut with the outside fingers. A solid white stream of sebaceous material will emerge from the comedone. Continue to gently press the area until no more material emerges.

In many closed comedones, follicle dilation is necessary. This procedure is performed for three reasons. Dilation of the follicle allows more room for the sebaceous material to emerge. Secondly, dilation of the closed comedone relieves pressure on the follicle walls, helping to avoid follicle wall rupture during extraction. Finally, relieving the pressure on the lesion by lancet dilation makes the extraction procedure much more comfortable for the client.

To dilate the follicle find the small opening in the top of the closed comedone. Using a sterile, disposable lancet, gently dilate this follicle opening by gently pressing the tip of the lancet through the follicle opening. DO NOT attempt to force the lancet into the follicle (Figure 14-3).

FIGURE 14–3   Dilation using a lancet

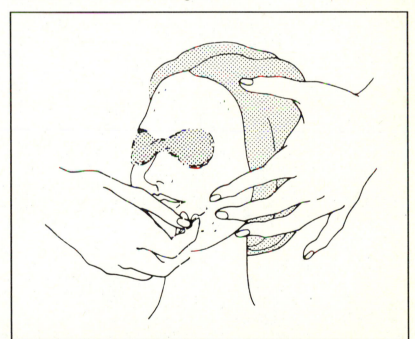

After the follicle is dilated, extract the comedone using the cotton swab technique. Waiting a few seconds after lancet dilation sometimes helps to expel the debris. Relief of the pressure accomplished by dilation will often cause some "self-expelling" action. This will help make the extraction process easier. It is not advisable to use comedone extractors on closed comedones. Closed comedones are often found in fleshy areas of the face, making use of an extractor cumbersome and difficult. Second, closed comedones often have a larger diameter than that of the opening in a comedone extractor, making the use of the extractor unsafe and inappropriate.

Extraction of Pustules

Pustules are raised, inflammatory acne lesions. They have a "head" that is filled with pus. Most of the pustule and its contents are above the surface of the skin (Figure 14-4).

FIGURE 14–4   The lancet lifts the top of the pustule

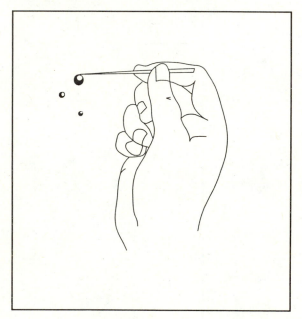

To extract a pustule, gently place the tip of a sterile disposable lancet against the side of the pustule. Bracing the outside of your hand against the face, gently "lift" the very top of the pustule away with the lancet. This procedure is similar to removing a splinter from your finger, except that the lesion is above the skin. Because you are strictly removing dead cells from the top of the pustule, this procedure should not be very uncomfortable to the client.

When the top of this dead cell layer has been removed, the pus will begin to emerge from the follicle opening. Placing two cotton swabs on the sides of the lesion, gently press downward and inward on the swabs, being careful to hold the area taut with the outside fingers. The rest of the impaction should emerge from the follicle. Following the pus will be the emergence of the actual comedone, often referred to as the "core." This part of the extracted material will look much like the debris extracted from an open or closed comedone, except that these impactions will be slightly harder and more dense.

It is not unusual for a small amount of bleeding to occur while extracting pustules. Remember, the follicle wall has ruptured in a pustule, allowing blood to come into the follicle. A slight amount of red blood appearing after extracting a pustule indicates that there is no more debris or sebum present in the follicle. Papules, nodules, and cysts are deep inflammatory lesions and are the domain of the dermatologist. Do not attempt to extract these lesions. While papules will often develop into pustules or dissipate without treatment, cysts and nodules should be referred to the dermatologist for treatment.

Facial Treatment Before and After Extraction

We have discussed the actual extraction procedures used in removing debris from the follicles. Treatment before and after extraction is very important, to help ease the extraction process by softening the follicle accumulations, to treat the area after extraction to prevent infection, and help further dry the lesions. The following is a suggested treatment in which extraction takes place. This treatment is known in the esthetics industry as "deep-pore cleansing."

1. Completely remove all the makeup from the face with a liquid cleanser.

2. Analyze the skin under the magnifying lamp. Check all areas of the face for clogged pores (sebaceous filaments), open and closed comedones, milia, and pustules. At the same time, of course, check for other disorders of the skin.

3. Apply steam treatment to the face with a vapor machine in the usual manner. Apply a desincrustant pre-mask, desincrustation lotion compresses, or enzyme treatment to the skin.

4. Remove the desincrustant treatment or enzyme treatment after allowing the treatment to sit on the face for about 8 to 10 minutes, or the time prescribed by the product manufacturer.

5. Galvanic desincrustation treatment may be used to further loosen the debris in the follicle, especially in cases of multiple impactions or acne.

6. Suction may be used, providing that there are no contraindications, as previously discussed.

7. Begin extraction in the chin and jawline area first, working upward on the face. This order of extraction helps the esthetician avoid contaminating the hands or other areas of the face from debris extracted from the lower part of the face. It is the most hygienic and aseptic pattern of treatment.

8. After extraction is completed, apply an antiseptic toner to the face with damp sponges or cotton pads. This will help kill any bacteria on the surface of the skin. It will also lower the pH from the use of the alkaline desincrustant treatment.

9. Apply the appropriate treatment for the particular skin type. An ampoule or antiseptic lotion may be appropriate. Benzoyl peroxide or salicylic acid can be used on oilier and acne-prone skin.

10. Apply high frequency over the face. This also further helps to kill surface bacteria. Using a piece of gauze over the face while extracting helps intensify the frequency treatment and helps the electrode move easily across the skin.

11. Apply a drying clay-based mask to the area that was extracted. A mask containing sulfur, salicylic acid, or benzoyl peroxide may be used for acne. A bentonite based mask with camphor may be more appropriate for oily or more sensitive clogged areas. The mask should be allowed to dry completely, usually for about 15 to 20 minutes.

12. Remove the mask with damp, soft cloths, sponges, or cotton pads. Apply more toner after mask removal.

13. Apply a noncomedogenic hydrating protectant or a treatment fluid for problem skin.

It is strongly advised that clients not wear makeup for about two hours after extraction. Extraction can be slightly irritating, and application of makeup to freshly extracted areas may be more irritating.

Extraction of Milia

Milia are small deposits of sebum between the follicle and the corneum. A milium is not the same as a comedone. The sebaceous material is trapped above the skin's surface, covered with a layer of dead cells. Milia may occur for several reasons. For more information on milia, see the chapter on comdogenicity. Milia will frequently be seen on older, mature skin. This may be associated with the use of heavy creams loaded with emollients for treating dry, dehydrated skin. Injuries to the skin sometimes also cause milia to develop. Dermabrasion by a plastic surgeon is often followed by a large number of milia forming. This will be discussed more in detail in the chapter on plastic surgery (Figure 14-5).

FIGURE 14–5   Milia

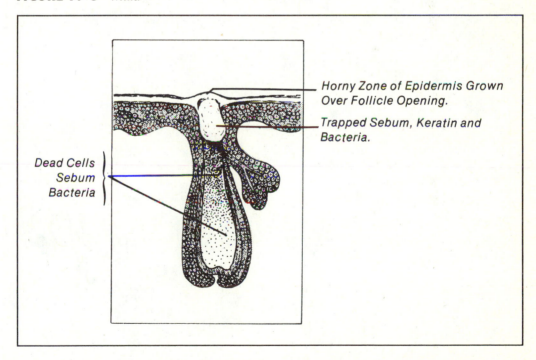

Horny Zone of Epidermis Grown Over Follicle Opening.

Trapped Sebum, Keratin and Bacteria.

Dead Cells
Sebum
Bacteria

To extract a milium, make sure that it is large enough to be extracted. Milia are almost always perfectly round in shape and are found on any area of the face, but especially the cheeks and the forehead. A milium must be large enough to easily lift off the top with a lancet. This is about the size of the heads of two pins. Make sure that you are absolutely positive that the lesion is a milium. Other types of skin lesions look like milia, including some types of skin growths. Check the shape carefully. The milium should not have any capillaries running through it. If the lesion has a capillary associated with it, leave it alone. Also, if the milium seems to give you any resistance while using the lancet, leave it alone. The dead cell layer on the top of a milium is very thin. Milia are easily treated with a lancet and should not give any resistance to pressure from the lancet

Gently spread the skin taut around the milium with your fingertips. Using a sterile disposable lancet gently lift off the top cell layers from the milium. Gently place the lancet against the side of the top of the milium. The lancet should slide easily into the top. These are all dead cells in the elevated part of the milium, so the client should barely feel the lancet at all (Figure 14-6).

FIGURE 14–6 Lancing milia

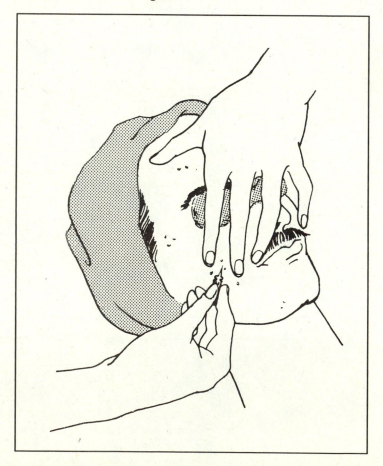

You should barely see the opening you have created in the top of the milium. Sometimes a very small amount of sebaceous material will emerge from the side of the milium where you have lifted the dead skin. After the lancet procedure is complete, place a cotton swab on both sides of the milium and gently press and lift on the milium. You may find it helpful to put slightly more pressure on the "unopened" side of the milium. This pressure will help the sebaceous material exit the milium easier.

If the milium does not extract easily, you may try lifting more dead cells with the lancet. Sometimes when the milium is small enough, it is easier to use a comedone extractor, particularly on non-fleshy areas of the face such as the forehead. Place the comedone extractor over the milium. Gently press down on the unopened side of the milium, moving the extractor very slowly towards the open side of the milium. You should see the emerging sebaceous material.

If the milium does not respond to treatment, do not continue attempting to extract it! You must have lots of experience to extract milia! Do not extract milia until you have been given hands-on instruction by a qualified licensed instructor.

Lesions Around the Eyes

Many clients will complain of small milia-like lesions around the eye area. Some of these lesions are milia. Some are other types of skin growth or lesions called xanthalasmas. **Xanthalasmas** are much flatter than milia, have a yellowish appearance, are below the skin's surface, and may have irregular shape. They are rarely round like a milium. These lesions should be referred to a dermatologist—they are not in the domain of the esthetician. Xanthalasmas can sometimes be indicative of other diseases or disorders, such as high cholesterol. Refer the client to a dermatologist for treatment and followup (Figure 14-7).

Other small milia in the eye area are often associated with the use of heavy eye creams, concealers, and other eye cosmetics that are thick, heavy, and loaded with fatty emollients. This can cause a buildup of dead cells in the area. Advise the client to switch to a lighter eye cream or a gel-type treatment. These have fewer or lesser concentrations of emollients.

Improper cleansing has also been associated with milia development around the eyes. Clients who do not remove their eye makeup well on a nightly basis have a tendency to develop milia. They leave traces of makeup or do not remove the eye makeup at all. Instruct the client in the correct procedure for

FIGURE 14–7 Xanthalasma. *Courtesy Timothy G. Berger, M.D.*

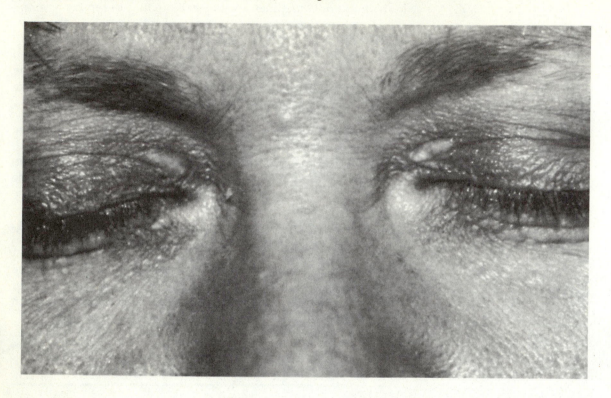

removing eye makeup and make sure she is using a proper eye makeup remover.

Clients who are very rough in removing their eye makeup may also suffer from milia development around the eyes. Injuries and excessive manipulation of the eyelid tissue have been associated with milia development.

Do not attempt to remove milia found on the eyelids. This tissue is extremely difficult to handle properly and is extremely fragile. Refer this client to an opthalmologist or dermatologist and give proper home care advice. Sometimes milia will disappear after the adjustment of proper home care.

Treating Clogged and Dehydrated Skin

Skin that is both clogged and dehydrated is extremely difficult to treat. The client's skin will feel dry, but is actually oily and dehydrated. The follicle will become "crimped shut" from the tightness of the surface dehydration, making extraction difficult if not impossible.

You should avoid heavily drying products. Products that are made with high levels of humectants and low levels of emollients are appropriate for this skin problem. The hydrating agents will help to hydrate the skin's surface, making it less dry feeling and more pliable so that extraction is more easily accomplished.

To treat this type of skin apply a hydrating fluid during salon steam treatment. Allow to steam with the humectant-based hydrating fluid for 8 to 10 minutes. This water from the steam and the humectant will help to soften the skin, hydrate the surface, and reduce the "crimped" effect on the follicles.

After this procedure, proceed with extraction. Follow extraction with a toner and then apply hydrating fluid to the skin before applying a gentle, clay-based drying mask. Applying a drying clay-based mask without applying a hydration fluid can be over-drying to this type of skin problem. Clients should be instructed to use the hydrating treatment with the mask at home too. Twice a week application will help to clear the clogged pores.

The client with both dehydrated skin and clogged pores will often be middle aged, trying desperately to "fight aging" through the use of heavy moisturizing, and believing that he or she is "drying up" with age. These heavier, and often come-dogenic, cosmetics (see the chapter on comedogenicity) clog the skin while the client attempts to treat the wrinkles and lines associated with aging, dehydrating, and sun damage.

This client needs lots of education about the aging process, sun damage, and comedogenic cosmetics. It is up to the esthetician to provide this education and help the client find a product program that helps dehydration but will not be clogging to this clog-prone skin condition.

Solar Blackheads

In older clients, often men, you will find a concentration of large open comedones round the eye area. While the development of these huge blackheads is similar to acne-related blackheads, these lesions are caused by excessive long-term sun exposure. This condition is called Favre-Racouchot Syndrome. More on this condition will be discussed in the chapter on sun and sun damage (Figure 14-8).

FIGURE 14—8 Favre Racouchot (senile solar comedones) in a typical pattern on a sun-damaged individual. *Courtesy Rube J. Pardo, M.D., Ph.D.*

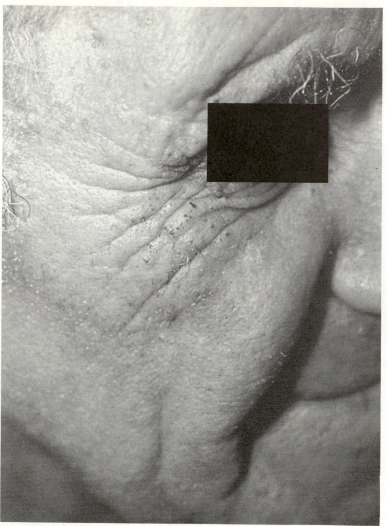

Extraction of solar comedones must be very gentle. This type of skin often has extremely fragile capillaries, also associated with excessive sun exposure and damage. This sun-damaged skin bruises easily, and it is easy to cause redness that lasts for days after treatment. You must be extremely gentle while treating this fragile skin.

Begin by cleansing or steaming the skin. Applying a fluid hydrating agent while steaming will help to loosen the impactions and make the skin more pliable. Very gently extract the lesions with the cotton swab technique. Do not attempt to remove every single clog in one session. Advise the client to have weekly treatments in the salon until the problem is clear, and then regular monthly treatments to prevent or control their return. Favre-Racouchot is a chronic problem, and this client will often have other sun-related skin problems. There are medical treatments for Favre-Racouchot Syndrome and other sun damage conditions.

Duration of Extraction

Extraction should not be performed for more than 10 to 15 minutes on any client during one treatment visit. Extraction that is longer than this can be painful and traumatic to both the client and the skin. You will, of course, have to access the needs and the duration for each client as an individual.

Clogged skin should never be massaged, at least not for prolonged periods of time. Avoid massage on excessively clogged skin, until such time that the skin is almost completely clear of clogged pores and any other type of acne lesion. As a general rule, if you take 10 minutes or more for extraction on a client, that client should not be massaged. Massaging of the clogged skin will simply stimulate more oil production and apply pressure to clogs, forcing them to become more impacted in the skin.

TOPICS FOR DISCUSSION

1. Discuss extraction—can any skin type need extractions?

2. Why is it important to presoften the skin before extraction? What are some techniques used to presoften the skin for extraction?

3. Describe the extraction process for closed comedones. When is follicle dilation necessary? Describe the extraction procedure for pustules.

4. Describe the order of facial treatment procedures involved in a deep cleansing treatment.

5. Discuss problem impactions around the eyes. Which should be referred to the dermatologist?

6. What are some special procedures used for treating clogged skin that is also dehydrated?

15

The Aging Process

Aging is a process that almost every person fears. Changes in the skin inevitably happen as years pass. In this chapter we will discuss the way the skin changes as it becomes older, and some of the ways we can manipulate these changes to make the skin look better.

It is the natural order of life that matter changes as it ages. Skin is not immune to this natural law.

A human baby has beautiful, supple, smooth skin that is all one color. As skin is exposed to the environment, defends itself against disease, and is affected by nutrition, health habits, exposure, and time, it begins to change.

Scrapes and accidents we receive as children inevitably leave scar tissue, which develops from injuries. At puberty, the hormonal system begins functioning in a new way. Suddenly pores begin to enlarge, skin becomes oilier, apocrine glands start functioning differently, and the skin's appearance changes. Pimples form from impacted follicles and sometimes leave scars, particularly from the more severe forms of acne. Body hair begins growing, and skin texture changes as well.

Most teenagers are more concerned with the zit on their cheek than with how they will look at age 35 or 55. Many take their good skin for granted.

During the early twenties is when most people notice the beginnings of changes associated with aging skin. They begin to notice small lines and wrinkles around the eyes and sometimes other areas.

If you look closely and carefully at a square inch of skin on a baby's face and compare it with a square inch of skin on the face of someone in their twenties, you will notice many differences. The skin will look rougher; the texture will be coarser to the touch. The skin will no longer be all one color, but multicolored due to melanin deposits.

If you again compare this square inch of skin with that of someone in their 40s or 50s, you will notice even more dramatic changes. Many of these changes are due to sun exposure, which we will discuss much more completely in the next chapter.

However, some of these changes happen naturally as years go by. The natural aging process of the skin is called intrinsic aging. In other words, these changes happen within the body and are not directly associated with external factors such as sun or weather (Figure 15-1).

Heredity

Much of the intrinsic aging factors are hereditary. Family history and ethnic background will largely govern skin aging. For example, red-headed, thin-skinned, and fair-skinned individuals develop the skin characteristics of aging much more rapidly than thicker, darker skin, such as black or hispanic skin. While it is true that darker skins produce more melanin and therefore ward off more solar damage, the skin itself is very different between different ethnic groups.

In general, the darker the skin, the less visible aging will take place, depending on the amount of sun exposure an individual experiences. Thicker skin does not show signs of aging as fast as thinner, fragile skin types.

This is certainly not to say that dark skin types cannot or do not age. It is just that they are less likely to look aged as fast. A lot of this depends on how the skin is cared for.

What Causes Aging?

We will discuss several factors that influence aging. Gravity is certainly a strong factor. The gravity of the earth constantly pulls on our bodies, including the facial skin. This gravity is what causes skin and muscle to sag. Even an individual who takes immaculate care of both skin and body will have some sagging of the face over a period of years. Even persons who have never exposed their faces to the sun will have some sagging. This sagging is referred to clinically as **elastosis**, which means loss of elasticity. While facial treatments and good products can help the surface appearance temporarily, the appearance of sagging skin can only be corrected on a long-term basis by plastic surgery.

FIGURE 15–1   Samples of skin tissue from the buttocks and faces of people in different age groups. a and b are photographs of a 2-year-old girl; c and d are of a 49-year-old woman; e and f are of a 77-year-old woman; and g and h are of an 80-year-old woman. *Photographs reprinted courtesy of J. Bedford Shelmire, Jr., M.D., author of* The Art of Looking Younger, *St. Martin's Press, New York.*

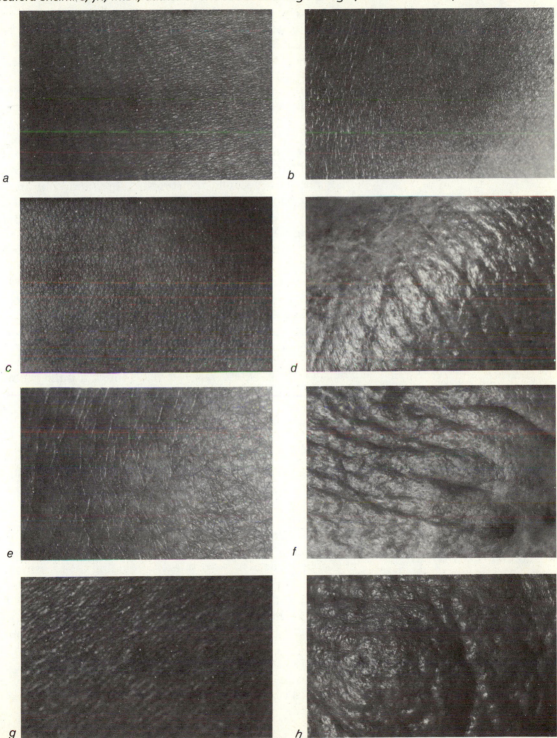

Let's look at an example of elastosis. If you purchase a new pair of underwear, it has an elastic waistband. If you wear these underwear many, many times, the elastic will begin to wear out. At some point the elastic waistband will no longer "snap back" the way it did when the underwear were brand new. Skin is the same way—aging causes a wearing down of the elastin fibrils in the dermis that give skin its elasticity. If you pinch the skin of a 50-year-old's cheek, it will not "snap back" as fast as that of a 20-year-old.

Gravity also causes the nose to droop downwards and the ears to become larger over a period of years.

Expression Lines

Expression lines are another symptom of intrinsic aging. Individuals will develop lines from consistent and repetitive facial movements. "Smile" lines occur in the nasolabial area. "Frown" lines may also occur in the forehead, eye, and chin area. Any repetitive movement of a facial expression such as raising the eyebrows, frowning, smiling, scowling, or any other facial movement will eventually cause a crease to occur, just as pants will wrinkle more the more you wear them. "Eye smilers" smile and squint at the same time, creating additional eyelines. Squint lines also occur around the eyes from squinting due to sun exposure, light exposure, or facial expression. It is important to wear ultraviolet protective sunglasses while outside to provide protection against both ultraviolet light exposure and the tendency to squint when exposed to light.

Smokers will inevitably get "smoker's lines" around the mouth and eyes from continually moving these areas during smoking activities.

Sleep habits, such as sleeping on one side or directly on the face, will eventually create lines and elasticity problems. Advise clients to sleep on their backs as much as possible, helping to avoid "sleep creases," which when they happen repetitively have a strong effect on the aging symptoms of the face.

The "Wearing-Out" of the Foundation

As time progresses, the muscles, fat, and skin on our faces undergo structural changes. The amount of fat in the subcutaneous layer decreases with age, providing less cushion and plumpness to the skin, resulting in less support. People who are overweight often do not have as many noticeable wrinkles on the face as thin people or people of normal weight. This does not mean that the skin has not aged; it simply means that there is more fat to "plump out" the skin, creating a smoother looking appearance. The skin is stretched back and forth over a lifetime, causing an "enlargening" of the skin, and gravity pulls down on the skin. The muscles have partially receded, causing the effect of more elastosis.

Prevention of Aging Skin

While there is really very little anyone can do to prevent inevitable intrinsic aging of the skin, one can develop certain health habits that will help delay the onset and possibly lessen the severity of intrinsic aging symptoms. Prevention of sun exposure is the biggest preventable factor. Sun exposure is, of course, an example of extrinsic aging, which will be covered in great detail in the next chapter.

Diet and Exercise

Again, this will not prevent intrinsic aging, but good health habits will help the body to nourish the skin better and therefore help to fight aging. Avoiding alcohol will also help the body function better. A regular aerobic exercise program and a well-balanced, healthy diet can certainly help an individual live longer and better, as well as helping the skin function in a more healthy manner.

We learn more and more each day about nutrition and its relation to health. While we will not focus on nutrition in this book, many estheticians find it helpful to receive a good nutrition education. While it is not the role of the esthetician to give nutritional advice and counseling (this is the role of the physician and registered dietician), the esthetician should have a working knowledge of the elements of nutrition in order to better understand skin function and health and be able to refer clients with nutritional or eating disorders to the proper qualified professionals. Investigate taking courses in nutrition through the departments of health or home economics at your local community college or university.

Good Skin Care

Using good skin-care products and developing a routine facial skin-care program will obviously help the skin look better. As the skin ages, production of intercellular cement decreases, which decreases the skin's ability to hold water. This is **dehydration**, and it results in a rough-textured appearance. Many theories support the use of hydrating agents in lessening the signs of aging. While many researchers believe that good skin care with proper conditioners, free-radicals scavengers, stimulating chemicals, hydrating agents, and sunscreens may help lessen the physical aging of the skin, these theories are all new and controversial. Nevertheless, it is obvious that many of these conditioning treatment agents help the skin look better, regardless of any long-term positive effects. Research continues in the use of these many agents to help lessen the symptoms of skin aging.

Plenty of Sleep

This is another good health habit, giving the body time to regenerate its tissues and repair damaged cells. Lack of sleep can cause eye circles, puffiness, and contribute to stress that can have a debilitating effect on both the mind and the body.

Stress

Each day medical researchers are learning more and more about stress and its effect on health, nutrition, and aging. Avoiding high amounts of stress certainly will help avoid premature aging signs of not only the skin, but of the other organs of the body.

You can help your clients reduce stress through massage and other services that help to ease daily tension. Again, while estheticians cannot permanently change their clients' lifestyles, they should be abreast of the newest research regarding stress and health in order to help give their clients the best esthetic care possible and be aware of referral services to qualified professionals who handle stress, such as psychologists.

The Beginning of Aging

Many clients will notice signs of aging and occasionally "freak out" at the first wrinkle. Be understanding and give them the best advice you can, teaching them realistic preventative techniques. The word *realistic* should be emphasized, as ethical estheticians do not endorse "miracle" treatments, but rather advise clients about the best proper realistic skin-care program.

The use of hydrators should begin early in life, but, realistically, many clients do not start using proper care or develop good skin-care habits until they notice the first signs of aging. Designing programs for home care should always first take into account the skin type, and second the aging process. The vehicle of the products is most crucial in treating the skin type, while active agents such as hydrators and conditioners benefit the aging symptoms.

Good hydrating ingredients include sorbitol sodium PCA, glycerin, hyaluronic acid, collagen, elastin, lecithin, liposomes, and glycosaminoglycans. These will all help to "plump" the surface with water, helping to reduce the appearance of fine lines and smooth the surface.

Other conditioning agents such as tocopherol acetate, retinyl palmitate, beta glucans, panthenol, and others will help to lessen visible signs of aging.

Certainly, using sunscreens is a must both on a daily basis and more intensively if the skin is directly exposed to the sun.

The use of keratolytic agents and exfoliants is often recommended for aging skin symptoms. As the skin ages the cells "turn over" more slowly, resulting in rough texture as well as dehydration, which occurs more and more the older the skin gets. This dehydration is theoretically related to the slowdown of the cells' turnover, resulting in a decrease of production of intercellular cement between the epidermal cells, which is a vitally important factor in natural hydration. Substituting cosmetic hydrators can help the skin hold more water in the surface epidermis.

Exfoliants and mild keratolytics remove dried-out, dead, crusty cells, helping the surface appear smoother, but also helping to stimulate the skin. Many researchers feel that the key to combating skin aging is routine mild exfoliation, which seems to help "re-layer" the surface cells and improve hydration and the functioning of the epidermis. This is still somewhat controversial and may border on a product "drug" claim. Nevertheless it is obvious that, in many instances, routine mild exfoliation helps smooth the surface, improve the hydration level, and minimize the appearance of lines and wrinkles.

Exfoliation can take place with the use of mild abrasants such as polyethylene granules, corn meal, ground almonds, or with the use of an implement such as an exfoliating cloth or brushing machine. When exfoliating aging skin, be careful not to apply too much pressure, as aging skin can sometimes be very thin and can redden or become easily irritated due to the closeness of small capillaries to the surface.

Keratolytics help to dissolve the dead cells to facilitate removal. Keratolytics for aging skin include proteolytic enzymes such as papain, retinoic acid (Retin-A), glycolic acid, and lactic acid. For more information on these materials and their use, please see the chapters on retinoids and chemical peeling.

Dermal and Epidermal Structural Changes

Several histological changes take place as the skin ages within the dermis and the epidermis. These changes are often associated with sun damage and chronic sun exposure, but some of this occurs through the natural intrinsic aging process.

The epidermis slowly becomes thinner with age, and the dermis increases in thickness. Breakdown of the network of collagen and elastin fibrils within the dermis also occurs. Blood vessels tend to fragment, causing redness—telangectasias, known to many estheticians as couperose. Because of this fragmented blood vessel formation the blood supply is also fragmented, resulting in poorer blood distribution than in younger skin.

Older skin, as we previously discussed, tends to be thinner than younger skin. Clients must be careful not to over-exfoliate, use harsh abrasives or use too much pressure. Hot water and extremely cold water should be avoided on skin with couperose or capillary fragility. Avoid using hot masks or steaming the face too closely. Clients who have extreme redness should be told to avoid alcoholic beverages, tobacco, and spicy foods, as all of these are **vasodilators**, which means they cause dilation of the blood vessels and sudden surges of blood flow in the already fragile vessels.

"Age Spots"

Also known as "liver spots," these dark brown patches on the face and hands are areas with large amounts of melanin present. Skin discoloration begins in the late teens and early twenties and gets continuously worse. The main difference between teenage skin and skin in the early 20s may be the discoloration caused by deposits of melanin. If you look carefully at make-over pictures, one of the biggest differences between the "before" and "after" photographs is the even coloring of the individual. Hormones can also play a significant role in the formation of hyperpigmented areas.

Sun is one of the worst causes of hyperpigmentation on the face and hands. You may notice that many clients do not exhibit hyperpigmentation on the body as they do on the face and hands. While there are exceptions to this rule, these are areas that have been chronically exposed to the sun for a long period of time. Hence the splotches are much worse in these areas.

Hyperpigmentation is treated by having the client apply a solution containing hydroquinone, a bleaching agent derived from the quinine plant. This bleaching agents breaks up melanin deposits in the skin.

Have the client apply the hydroquinone product to the hyperpigmented area twice a day. Some peeling may occur in especially thin-skinned clients. Occasionally a client will be allergic to hydroquinone. The strongest over-the-counter hydroquinone solution available to estheticians is 2 percent. Stronger solutions are available by prescription through the dermatologist. Use of retinoic acid and glycolic acid along with hydroquinone seems to help penetrate the hydroquinone better, showing a better and more rapid bleaching effect. Retinoic acid is, of course, only available by prescription. Glycolic acid can be used in a cosmetic preparation by the esthetician.

Bleaching hyperpigmented areas can be very difficult. The more chronic the sun damage, the longer it take's for results from bleaching solutions. Some clients may have to use a bleaching product for months and months before seeing results. Others may see results in weeks.

It is imperative that the client use a sunscreen and completely avoid sunbathing. Explain to clients that wherever they show a hyperpigmented area, there is a concentration of active melanocytes in the lower epidermis and upper dermis of these areas. While hydroquinone has a bleaching effect on the hyperpigmentation, it has no effect per se on the melanocytes themselves. Explain that the hyperpigmentation is the "product" of the melanocytes, the "factory." Bleaching solutions affect the "product", but cannot stop the "factory." As long as the client continues to sunbathe and not use sunscreens routinely, melanin production will continue. You must explain this well to the client, as this type of client has a tendency to be quite a sun worshipper, which is how the hyperpigmentation occurred in the first place. It is essential that clients change their sunny lifestyles to achieve any appreciable results.

Psychological Effects of Aging

Clients may experience psychological effects when they realize that the aging process has begun. They may seek "immediate result" treatments, which do not exist. Work with these clients to establish a good, solid home-care program, coupled with good salon treatments. The more often the client comes into the salon, the better the program will be, because this client needs lots of encouragement and "coaching."

Try to steer the client away from unrealistic "nonsurgical face lift" approaches to skin care. Stress using sunscreens, avoiding sun exposure, using good hydrators designed for the client's skin type, and using specialty products, such as conditioners containing glycolic acid.

This type of client will also sometimes have a tendency to "drown" in heavy moisturizers, often causing comedogenic or acnegenic results. Explain to the client that aging is not a lack of oil. Only clients who are truly alipidic (oil dry) need to be using heavy oily products, and then they need to contain the right kind of emollient.

Home Care for the Aging Client

Home care should be adapted to help the client's aging signs, whatever their severity. Begin by thoroughly analyzing the skin. Always adapt the entire program to the skin type. Treatment conditioners for aging skin will not be useful if they are for the wrong skin type. Aging clients will still be predominantly dry or oily. For oily clients, stick to noncomedogenic fluids, lotions, or gels. For more oil-dry skin, you can use heavier emollients.

Stick to very gentle cleansers with little or no detergents. Remember, the aging skin already has fewer intercellular lipids. You do not want to strip these essential lipids by using too aggressive a cleanser. Low-foaming washes and cleansing milks are best to use for the aging skin.

Toners should be alcohol-free and should contain a humectant such as propylene glycol or glycerin. Toners should not have a strong astringent action.

Day creams should contain a sunscreen and a sealant agent such as dimethicone, mineral oil, or cyclomethicone. These agents will help the skin retain water better in the surface layers. The consistency of the day cream will vary depending on the oiliness or dryness of the skin. "Poreless" skin with poor sebum production will need more emollients, and the cream should generally be heavier. Oily skin should be treated with a noncomedogenic day cream containing less emollient and more hydration agents.

Night treatment will vary, again depending on the skin type. Hydrators such as lecithin (liposomes), sorbitol, sodium PCA, glycerin, and hyaluronic acid are appropriate.

Special treatment products for the eye and neck areas are very helpful to the aging skin. The skin of the eyes and the neck is much thinner than the rest of the facial skin, and is therefore very likely to show signs of aging. Heavier emollients are often used for these areas, with the exception of some of the newer liposome gels. The client should use eye and neck care products 24 hours a day for best results.

Many estheticians vary the night treatment for clients, alternating different types of night treatments. The theory here is that the change in night treatment will help to stimulate sluggish skin.

Facial Treatments for Aging Skin

Salon facial treatments for aging skin must be administered frequently. You should begin by treating the skin weekly or biweekly for 6 to 12 treatments, slowly decreasing to once every four weeks. Treatment should vary so that the skin is slightly stimulated.

You should always design the facial based on skin type and conditions. Aging skin often will be thin, so be careful with harsh exfoliants, brushing, and suction machines. As skin gets older, it tends to become more oil-dry, particularly after age 50. Keep this in mind when treating the skin. Occasionally you will see an oily or, more often, a combination aging skin. Because many treatment products designed for aging skin contain larger percentages of emollients and fats, be careful not to use creams that are too oily or heavy for combination and oily skin types.

Exfoliation

Mild exfoliation is good for aging skin. It gently stimulates the skin and removes dead, dry cells on the surface, helping the skin look and feel smoother and softer, and also helping to minimize the appearance of rough textures and wrinkles. Mild enzyme peeling treatments are effective for helping to remove this dead cell buildup. For more information on peeling treatments, see Chapter 18.

Massage helps to sooth and hydrate aging skin, stimulating blood flow. Be careful not to over-massage or use rough massage techniques on fragile, thin, aging skin with distended capillaries.

Treatment for Aging Skin

1. Remove makeup by gently massaging a cleansing milk into the skin and then removing the makeup and cleanser with damp, soft, facial cloths, sponges, or cotton pads. Follow with gentle toner on cool wet pads or a soft cloth.

2. After cleansing and toning, carefully examine the skin for elasticity, dryness, dehydration, couperose, or distended capillaries, hyperpigmentation, and sun damage symptoms (see Chapter 16).

3. Apply a very lightweight hydrating fluid during steam treatment. Steam the skin at a distance of 14 to 20 inches with the hydrating fluid on the skin. This will help to soften the skin and attract the steam. Do not use oil-based fluid or heavier creams. This will repel water instead of attracting it. As an alternative treatment a gentle enzyme mask may be applied during steam instead of a hydrating fluid.

4. If the skin is not too fragile, you may use the brushing machine over a thick coat of hydrating fluid. (Do not use the brushing machine after enzyme treatment). Avoid brushing if the skin is thin, red, or couperose.

5. Gently extract any clogged pores or comedones.

6. Use cold spray with a mild toner solution after extraction.

7. Apply a hydrating fluid, ampoule, or cream to the skin, designed for both the aging skin and the individual skin type. Gently massage the skin. Massage should last about 10 minutes. If using an ampoule, you may want to use electrical treatment before continuing massage.

8. Apply high frequency at a low setting or ionization rollers over the ampoule, hydrating fluid, or specialty cream. Make sure to check all health precautions and contraindications before using electrical therapy.

9. Apply masks appropriate for the particular skin types. Most masks for aging skin are creamy and soft-setting, or are the gel variety. Clay masks may be used on oily or clogged areas.

10. Allow the mask to sit for 15 to 20 minutes. For extra dry skin, you may apply extra hydrating fluid or cream in lieu of a mask.

11. After 15 to 20 minutes, spray the mask with an atomized cold spray of diluted toner or conditioning water. This will help to soften and loosen the mask. Apply strips of cool, wet cotton or soft facial cloths in a compress technique, gently molding the compresses to the face. Remove the strips one at a time, wiping the mask off the skin as you remove the compress.

12. Finish by applying an appropriate day cream with sunscreen.

Aging skin can be stimulated, cleansed, softened, firmed, and hydrated. With careful management, aging skin can be made to look much softer and smoother. However, no one can actually turn back the clock. Avoid using "miraculous" "anti-aging" treatments. Explain sensible care to your client, emphasizing the importance of careful, consistent, diligent care both in the salon and at home.

TOPICS FOR DISCUSSION

1. What changes occur in the skin from birth, to the twenties, to the forties and fifties?

2. Discuss hereditary characteristics and aging.

3. What is the difference between intrinsic and extrinsic aging?

4. Discuss other factors related to aging.

5. Discuss home care procedures for aging skin.

6. Discuss salon treatment for aging skin.

16

Sun and Sun Damage

The sun is a phenomenal structure that helps plants convert carbon dioxide to pure oxygen. We cannot live without oxygen, and we cannot live without the sun. Yet the sun is, by far, the worst enemy of the skin. Repetitive exposure to the sun causes severe skin damage, premature aging, and skin cancer. In this chapter we will learn all about the way the sun affects the skin, in both the long and short term. We will learn about the best ways to prevent sun damage and skin cancer, as well as how to detect skin cancer.

Over 93 million miles away, the sun is a source of energy for the earth and our ecosystems. It is a vitally important part of human life.

It is also the worst enemy of the skin. It is the number one cause of premature aging and skin cancer. Yet many people continue to bask in the sun's rays, achieving a golden tan, but also accumulating terrible irreversible damage to skin.

The sun projects three basic kinds of **ultraviolet rays**, or UV rays (Figure 16-1). UVC rays are short rays that are blocked by the ozone layer. They have germicidal properties, and in large doses are deadly to live creatures.

FIGURE 16–1 Dispersion of light rays by a prism

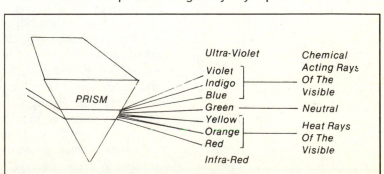

PRISM

Ultra-Violet

Violet
Indigo
Blue
Green
Yellow
Orange
Red

Infra-Red

Chemical
Acting Rays
Of The
Visible

Neutral

Heat Rays
Of The
Visible

Ultraviolet B rays (UVB) are the next longest ultraviolet ray. UVB rays cause most skin cancers and are responsible for sunburns. They penetrate the epidermis to the basal layer. Some UVB rays penetrate the dermis, but most stop at the basal layer. UVB are much stronger than UVA rays, even though UVA rays are longer rays and penetrate the dermis.

Within the basal layer and upper dermis are the **melanocytes**, the pigment-producing cells. These cells are stimulated by exposure to ultraviolet rays and manufacture **melanin**, the skin pigment that is the body's natural sunscreen. While many people think a tan is healthy, a tan is actual a chemical reaction of the body defending itself from the damaging rays of the sun! A tan is actually the body and the skin saying "don't do this to me"—just like a warrior picking up a shield to ward off an enemy!

Again, UVA rays are longer rays, penetrating the dermis and the precious collagen and elastin fibrils. UVA only burns in large doses and is therefore the type of UV ray used in most tanning beds and booths. While the tanning bed is unlikely to burn the skin, the damaging UVA rays penetrate the dermis, affecting the supportive structure of the collagen and elastin fibrils and causing other detrimental changes to the skin.

Short-Term Sun Problems

Most of us know that long-term sun exposure causes skin aging and skin cancer, but very few people are aware of the short-term damaging effects of ultraviolet and sun exposure. Sun exposure causes a variety of short-term skin and esthetic problems. These may affect both beauty and health.

Sunburns happen very frequently, especially in the summer months. They can be mild to severe. The skin becomes very red, sore, and sensitive to the touch, caused by dilation of blood vessels and stimulation of nerve endings in the skin. The skin will eventually peel due to the extreme dryness associated with the sunburn. The skin literally bakes to a very dehydrated condition, just as cookies will burn and become dry if cooked too long in the oven. Many of these sunburns happen because people are ignorant about sun protection. While Floridians and Californians are very familiar with sun protection, tourists from areas where sunbathing is not popular due to the climate are especially vulnerable to sunburn. It is important that estheticians be very familiar with sun protection methods to help their clients protect themselves from sunburn as well as from long- and short-term sun damage.

A variety of remedies can ease the pain of a minor sunburn. These include cool baths with vinegar added to the cool water, applying cool packs, applying plain yogurt to the area, and using local spray anesthetics. The latter must be used with caution, although the spray anesthetics can provide temporary pain relief to the sunburned area, many people have allergies to localized skin anesthetics. Advise clients to be very careful if using these products. Sunburn is actually a medical condition and therefore is in the domain of the physician, not the esthetician. Severe sunburns can cause shock, fever, nausea, and even death. Any "bubbling" of the skin or severe blistering should always be referred to a medical doctor.

After the initial burn is relieved, your client may ask you for help with the remaining esthetic skin problems associated with a sunburn. The skin may be extremely dehydrated, flaking, and peeling. You may also notice discolorations caused by peeling skin. Occasionally, these discolorations may be long term. First and most important, strongly advise the client not to expose him- or herself to any more sun until all the symptoms of the sunburn are completely gone, especially peeling of the skin. Further sun exposure during the peeling process following a sunburn often results in further long-term skin damage and permanent solar lentigenes (freckles induced by the sun) and other skin discolorations.

You should not attempt to treat sunburned skin that is still red or sensitive. If the skin is no longer red or sensitive, you may use very gentle techniques to hydrate the skin. Use cool steam, fragrance-free hydrating fluids and lotions, non-hardening, non-stimulating masks, and other products designed for super-sensitive skin. Avoid exfoliating or stimulating treatments including brushing, galvanic desincrustation, or heavy massage. Advise the client to use similar procedures at home until all symptoms subside. Give the client good instruction about the proper use of sunscreens to avoid a reoccurrence of the situation.

Other Short-Term Sun-Related Problems

Hyperpigmentation is both a long- and short-term cosmetic problem caused by the sun. Skin that has been repeatedly burned or has not healed from the sun before additional sun exposure is especially vulnerable. If you look at the skin of a 15-year-old and compare it to that of a 25-year-old, the biggest difference you will notice is in the skin pigmentation. Hyperpigmentation occurs in many patterns and is also associated with hormone fluctuations and pregnancy. (See the chapter on hormones.) Hyperpigmentation can usually be treated, as we will learn in the chapter on therapy for photoaging skin.

The best treatment, of course, is preventing the hyperpigmentation by avoiding the sun and using proper sunscreens. The reaction of the skin to the sun is **hyperpigmentation**. The melanocytes make melanin react when exposed to the sun. It is the skin's natural method of producing its own sunscreen. The skin is saying, "I don't like this — don't do this to me!"

Tinea versicolor is what many refer to as sun "spots" or sun "fungus." These white splotches, which usually appear on the chest and back of avid sunbathers, are actually a fungal condition. If you have a client with this condition, refer the client to a dermatologist for treatment (Figure 16-2.).

FIGURE 16–2 Tinea versicolor. *Courtesy Rube J. Pardo, M.D., Ph.D.*

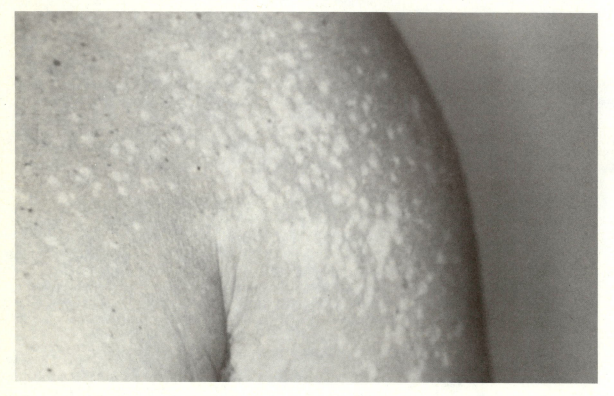

What You Don't Know About Short-Term Sun Exposure

There is growing evidence that sun exposure may actually suppress the immune functions of the skin. Exposure to sunlight "chases off" your protective macrophage "guard cells," allowing substances and organisms to enter the skin, increasing the chance of infection. Sun exposure has also been shown to increase the formation of **free radicals**, which can affect normal cell reproduction. Sun "freckles" found on the faces of teenagers may represent problem areas in the future. It is so important to protect children from sun. The truth is that we receive about 80 percent of the sun's damage to the skin before the age of 18. Most of this sun exposure is not from sunbathing, but from day-to-day exposure. Think about how many children play outdoors. Everytime they go outside, they expose themselves to harmful ultraviolet rays. That's why every time they go outdoors, they should be protected with a good sunscreen! We tend to think about sunscreens during the summer months, but it should be a year-round consideration.

Long-Term Photo Damage

Dermatoheliosis is the medical term coined to describe long-term damage to the skin caused by sun exposure. The skin is severely affected by long-term exposure.

Collagen and elastin fibrils in the dermis begin a process called **cross-linking**. In essence, collagen and elastin fibrils collapse, causing the support system for the skin also to collapse. Esthetically, this results in deep wrinkling of the skin, sagging, and elastosis.

Sun-damaged skin appears much more severely aged than skin that has aged solely from intrinsic factors. The wrinkling does not only appear in expression lines. Many, many lines develop, in all areas and in all directions. Wrinkles may be both horizontal and vertical. Normal expression lines are much deeper in sun-damaged skin.

The abnormal structure of the dermis and the epidermis gives the skin a "leathery" appearance and feel. This type of skin is also severely discolored due to melanin deposits and hyperpigmentation.

The skin of a sun-damaged person is very rough to the touch, and the surface is actually uneven. This is caused by damage to the cells, which causes the corneum and other epidermal cells not to shed in a normal, even manner. This is due to the altering of the DNA from chronic sun exposure. The cells become "confused," divide unevenly, and no longer retain their normal shape. If you look at a cross section of normal skin, you will notice that the cells in the epidermis form layers that look like layers of brick in a brick wall. In sun-damaged skin, this same structure looks like a brick wall that is collapsing, made with uneven bricks that are poorly made!

The epidermis of sun-damaged skin becomes progressively thinner, and the dermis slowly begins to atrophy, or collapse, and fall apart. This is how the sun eventually "zaps" the skin and destroys it!

Your sun-damaged client will have multiple wrinkles, not just around the eyes and neck, but all over the face. There will be many more pronounced wrinkles than in other clients. Their skin is literally a multitude of uneven colors, very freckled. This skin will have a leathery feel and look. There may be patches of dryness frequently, and clients may frequently complain about how "dry" their skin is. The truth is that as the skin cells become disfigured, they also fail to produce sufficient amounts of intercellular cement, making proper hydration of the skin practically impossible. Strong hydrators such as hyaluronic acid, lactic acid, sodium PCA, and sorbitol may help to moisten this skin, but will not repair these dysfunctional cells to any degree.

Sun-damaged skin may also have many telangectasias or couperose areas. Sun damage also causes collapse of some of the blood vessels and decreased blood flow. The small capillaries look like tributaries of a river. These vessels may be very fragile, and bruises may appear easily. You may notice how easily some of your older clients bruise. While this may be due to many medical factors, sun-damaged skin bruises much more easily than normal, healthy, non-damaged skin. You will also notice that these clients who bruise easily have very thin-looking, dry, hyperpigmented skin. This is because the skin is almost always severely sun-damaged.

Skin Cancers and Other Sun-Related Skin Growths

Skin cancer is caused by the damage to the DNA that we have been discussing. The cells begin dividing unevenly and rapidly, but the genetic material in the DNA is damaged from the sun. This rapid dividing of the cells may take the form of small tumors, which we know as skin cancer.

There are three major kinds of skin cancer. **Basal cell carcinomas** are the most common. They are almost always found on sun-exposed areas, typically on the face, hands, legs, back, and chest. They look like small pearls. Sometimes they have a small blood vessel running through them. They are not usually perfectly round like a milium. On older hyperpigmented skin, they may be hard to differentiate from milia. You must look carefully to tell the difference (Figure 16-3).

Estheticians are not in the business of diagnosing skin cancer. However, you should know the signs of the major forms of skin cancer and be able to refer suspicious looking lesions and areas to a dermatologist.

FIGURE 16–3 Basal cell carcinoma. *Courtesy Rube J. Pardo, M.D., Ph.D.*

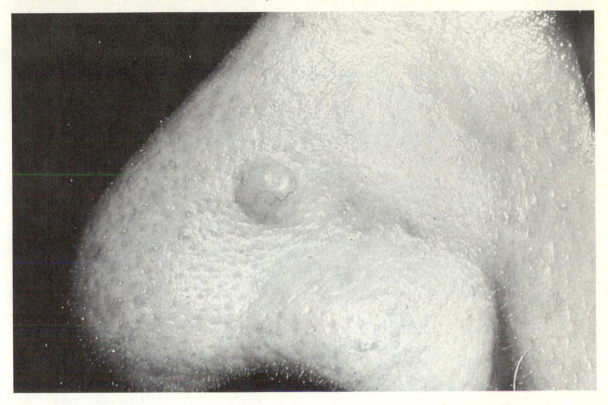

Basal cell carcinomas are very often curable. In fact, 95 percent of these cancers are cured. They rarely spread to the internal parts of the body, but can grow, and if they are not treated they can affect large areas of the skin. Basal cell carcinomas are sometimes removed surgically, sometimes frozen, and sometimes treated with an electric needle called a *hyfrecator*.

Squamous cell carcinomas are the second most frequently diagnosed form of skin cancer. They may look like red or pink solid bumps on the skin. They may appear as open sores or ulcers that do not seem to heal. They may look crusty, or the client may notice a crusty area that bleeds easily (Figure 16-4). Many clients notice this when washing or cleansing the face. Again, these lesions appear on chronically sun-exposed areas. Treatment is similar to treatment for basal cell carcinoma, but squamous cell carcinoma may sometimes spread to other areas of the body.

The least frequently seen form of the three major kinds of skin cancer is also the mostly deadly. **Melanoma** is characterized by moles or mole-like lesions that are dark in color. The Skin Cancer Foundation has coined an expression that is easy to remember when looking at suspicious lesions. They call this the

FIGURE 16-4 Squamous cell carcinoma. *Courtesy Michael J. Bond, M.D.*

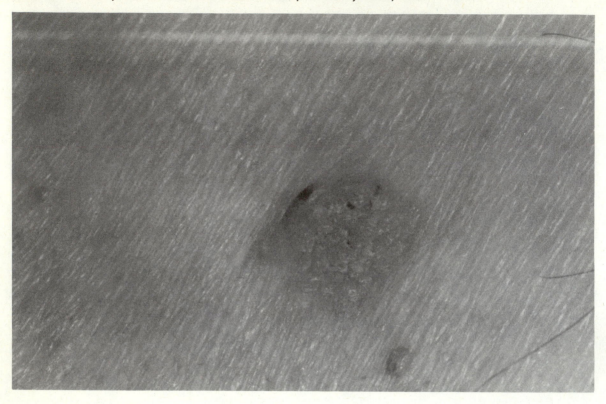

"ABCD's of Melanoma." "A" stands for asymmetric. The melanoma lesion is usually growing to one side of the lesion and is uneven. "B" stands for border. The borders of melanomas are uneven and not smooth. "C" is for color. Melanomas often have dark brown and black colors and are usually splotchy and not all one color. "D" stand for diameter. Melanomas are usually at least the size of a pencil eraser or bigger. Regular moles are usually smaller than this.

Melanomas can be found on any area of the body, but are most likely, again, to be found on areas that have had repeated sun exposure. They are most typically found on individuals with a history of sunburn and light-skinned individuals.

Other Sun-Related Growths

Actinic keratoses are rough areas of sun-damaged skin, indicated by dysplastic cell growth. **Dysplastic** means abnormal growth. Actinic keratoses are frequently found on the faces of individuals who have had chronic sun exposure. They are also prevalent in light-skinned individuals. They are rough patches of skin and can be crusty, scaly, and rough to the touch. Sometimes they feel like small needles or splinters sticking out of the skin when they are touched with the fingers. They frequently occur in small groups or patches. Because they are dysplastic cells, they can become cancerous, and are often referred to as **pre-cancers** (Figure 16-5).

Actinic keratoses may be treated surgically, with cryosurgery (freezing with liquid nitrogen), or with chemical therapy with a chemical called flourouracil (also commercially known as Effudex®).

Unusual looking moles or moles that are changing should be checked by a dermatologist. If you or your client notices changes in a wart or mole, refer the client to a dermatologist for diagnosis and treatment.

Sebaceous hyperplasias are small, donut-shaped lesions that look like large, open comedones surrounded by a ridge of skin. *Sebaceous hyperplasia* actually means "overgrown oil glands." They are frequently seen on oily skins that have had repeated sun exposure, but they can appear on any skin, usually in someone 25 years old and up. You will frequently find them on the forehead and temples, although they may appear anywhere on the face (Figure 16-6). Sebaceous hyperplasias are benign lesions that rarely cause any problems, except esthetically. They are rarely removed surgically, because the scar from excision is usually worse than the appearance of the lesion. Sebaceous hyperplasia can be treated with electrodessication or the electric needle. This helps to flatten the lesion, but may need to be retreated periodically, because the oil glands are deep within the skin and can still keep growing. Sebaceous hyperplasias are seen very frequently by estheticians, and clients are often concerned about them. Clients who have them also may have other symptoms of sun damage.

Seborrheic keratoses are large, flat, crusty-looking, brown, black, yellowish, or gray lesions that are often found on the faces of older, sun-damaged clients. They are frequently found on the temples or cheekbones, although they can appear anywhere on the skin. They look almost like a scab, and clients will sometimes pick at them, which they obviously should not do. They are usually harmless growths, but can occasionally turn into other more serious lesions, such as basal cell carcinomas. They are treated by the dermatologist, usually by curretage, in which a curette, a small, scoop-like instrument, is used to "scoop" the lesion off the face. Seborrheic keratoses are more of a cosmetic nuisance than anything, in most cases. Nevertheless, they should be referred to a dermatologist for treatment. Also, they may indicate other areas or other forms of sun damage that may require treatment.

After a dermatologist treats skin cancer, the doctor may suggest that the client not have skin-care treatments until the lesion is

FIGURE 16–5 Actinic kerotosis is frequently seen in sun-damaged clients. *Courtesy Michael J. Bond, M.D.*

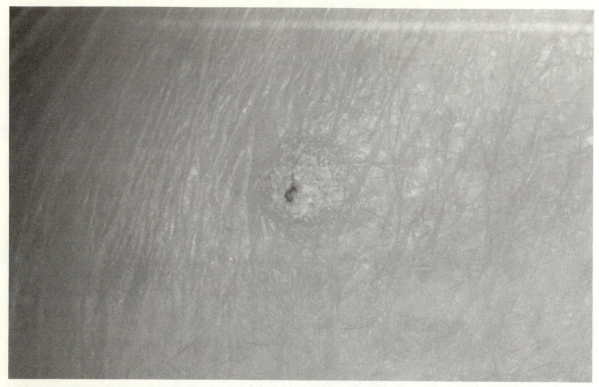

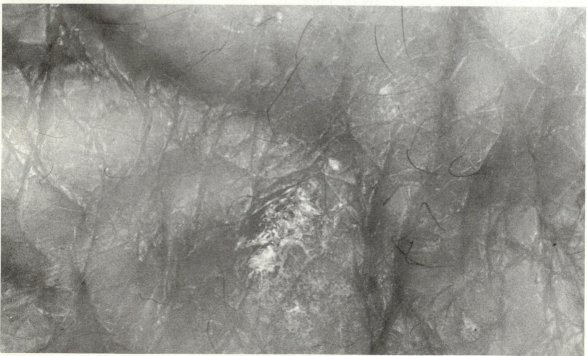

FIGURE 16–6 Multiple sebaceous hyperplasia in an adult male with oily skin and sun damage. Sebaceous hyperplasias are typically found on the forehead, temple, and upper cheeks, but can appear anywhere on the face. *Courtesy George Fisher, M.D.*

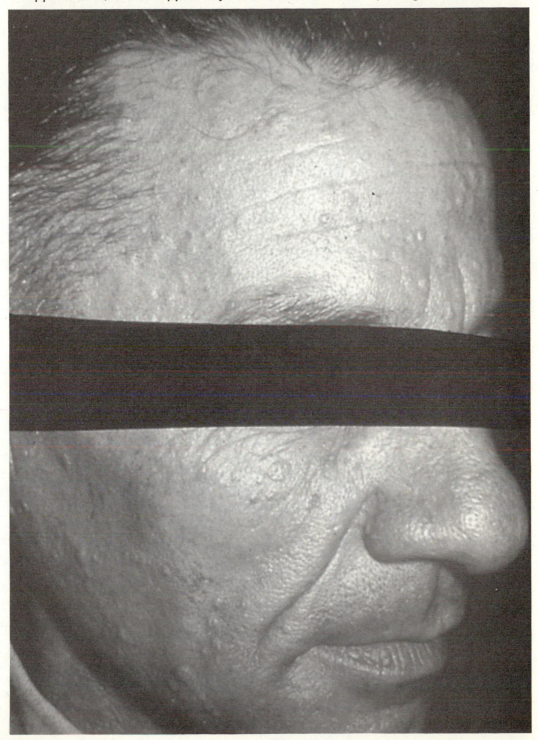

healed completely. As a general rule, clients should not have facial treatment if there are still **sutures**, or "stitches," present in a treated lesion. Clients treated with flourouracil should not have facial treatment until the therapy is completed, unless approved by the dermatologist, who may occasionally refer such a client for help with side effects. Make sure you have been properly trained by the doctor before treating these clients.

Other forms of growth treatment, such as electrosurgery or cryosurgery generally do not cause any problem for treatment, except that facial treatment should not be performed until the lesion is healed or unless the doctor advises otherwise. Avoid these areas completely, and simply treat the rest of the untreated areas of the face. If you have any questions, contact the dermatologist, and remember always—when in doubt, don't!

Solar freckles, also known as "liver spots," are clumps of hyperpigmentation caused by sun exposure. They can appear on any area, but frequently appear on the face and hands. These can be treated by the esthetician, and more severe cases can be treated by the dermatologist. More on treating hyperpigmentation will be covered in the chapter on therapy for photoaging.

Prevention of Sun Damage

Without question, the most effective treatment for sun damage is prevention. This involves routine use of sunscreen products. Sunscreen products are designed to filter, reflect, or absorb UVA and/or UVB rays emitted by the sun. Many different sunscreen chemicals work in different ways. Often chemists will mix two or more sunscreen chemicals together in a preparation. This type of product will filter more ultraviolet rays, and the combination will often also help to filter both UVA and UVB rays. Sunscreen chemicals may either absorb or reflect ultraviolet rays. Frequently used chemicals that absorb the rays are methoxycinnimate, para-amino-benzoic acid (PABA), padimate O, padimate A, oxybenzone, methyl salicylate, and benzophenone. Benzophenone and oxybenzone are primarily UVA absorbers, while the other chemicals listed are primarily UVB absorbers. This is why these chemicals are often combined to produce a sunscreen that blocks out a larger spectrum of ultraviolet rays. These screen products are sometimes referred to as broad-spectrum sunscreens.

Nonabsorbing, reflective sunscreen chemicals include titanium dioxide, a pigment that is also frequently used in foundation makeup to give opacity to foundations. Zinc oxide, a well-known sunscreen, is the chemical often used by surfers on their noses. Zinc oxide is also used in sunscreen products. Both of these chemicals reflect ultraviolet rays, rather than absorbing them. Their main advantages are that they reflect large amounts of ultraviolet rays and that they are less likely to cause allergic reactions than the absorbing chemicals. Their main disadvantage is that they are opaque and can be seen on the surface of the skin. Esthetically, many people will not use these products because, even in a refined form, they have some color and often appear pasty on the surface of the skin. A new form of micronized titanium dioxide has been developed and may in the future prove useful in sunscreen products, because it is less likely to be seen.

A new ingredient that is still in development at the time of this writing is a chemical called **parsol**, which is a new absorber that absorbs a large number of UVA rays. Also, scientists are now working on synthetic forms of melanin, growing melanin in plants. Because melanin is the body's own natural sunscreen, this may prove to be an excellent source of sunscreen chemical. Research continues in this area.

Sunscreen products may be either a cosmetic or a drug. Cosmetics that contain sunscreen usually do not make major claims concerning the products' sunscreening effects. This does not mean, necessarily, that the product is inferior. It simply means that the product contains sunscreen chemicals, but the company is not making any claims regarding how strong the sunscreen ingredient is. Cosmetic companies often do this to avoid the expensive testing of the strength of the sunscreen and to avoid listing the product as a drug with the FDA.

S.P.F. stands for "sun protection factor." This is a rating system that tells how long you can stay out in the sun while using the product without burning. It is not exactly a measurement of sunscreen strength, as the length of burn-exposure time varies greatly from individual to individual. If a person's skin normally burns in one hour without sunscreen, an SPF 2 sunscreen theoretically will allow the person to remain in the sun two times as long, or two hours, without burning. An SPF 4 sunscreen would allow the skin to be exposed four times as long, or four hours, without burning, etc.

As a general rule, most dermatologists, pharmacists, and estheticians consider an SPF 15 sunscreen product to be good protection against sun damage. It does not guarantee no sun damage. It simply means that an SPF 15 screen provides a fairly high amount of protection. Results will vary depending on the individual's heredity, method of application, frequency of application, his or her own skin, weather and climate conditions, and other factors. Sunscreens theoretically have no limit as to SPF ratings, although at the time of this writing many scientists con-

sider the value of an SPF rating above 30 to be hard to substanti-
ate. Sunscreen chemicals can be irritating to the skin, so the
more sunscreen chemical used in the product, the higher the
likelihood of allergic reaction or irritation.

Sun Skin Types

There is a universal system of classifying skin types when discussing sun exposure. This typing system is generally accepted
by the scientific community. The following is an excerpt from a
brochure provided by the Skin Cancer Foundation.

- Type 1: Always burns; never tans. Very fair, with red or
  blond hair and freckles.
- Type 2: Burns easily; tans minimally. Usually fair
  skinned.
- Type 3: Sometimes burns; gradually tans.
- Type 4: Minimum burning; always tans. Usually white
  with medium pigmentation.
- Type 5: Very seldom burns; always tans. Medium to
  heavy pigmentation.
- Type 6: Never burns, but tans darkly. Blacks as well as
  others with heavy pigmentation.

As you can see, the scale has a lot to do with heredity and
genetic skin characteristics. According to the Skin Cancer Foundation, your choice, or your client's choice, of a sunscreen
should be based on the sun skin type, the amount of time you
plan to spend in the sun, the intensity of the sun in your geographic region, and the preference of the formulation.

The geographic location does affect the intensity of the sun. As
a general rule, the closer to the equator that you live, the more
intense the sun's rays.

Types of Sunscreens

As we discussed before, a sunscreen can be a cosmetic or a drug.
Cosmetic sun preparations are usually "day creams," which
have also been discussed in the products chapter. Many companies now routinely use sunscreen ingredients in their day protection and moisturizing products.

Sunscreens that are marketed with an SPF rating and are registered as drugs with the FDA vary in strength and type. They provide an array of products for consumers to choose from.

Waterproof and water-resistant screens are designed for individuals who participate in water sports, or who are outdoors in hot environments, or who plan on staying out in the sun for long periods of time. These strong waterproof products are often used by fishermen, athletes, and people who work outdoors. They usually contain a fairly large amount of oil, petrolatum, or fat, which makes them highly water-resistant. These products sometimes cause problems for oily-skinned individuals, and often the waterproofing ingredients are also comedogenic or acnegenic.

Sunscreens that are made for oily skin are often in an alcohol gel. They are lighter weight and generally noncomedogenic. Unfortunately, they are also usually not very water-resistant, and therefore should be applied more frequently.

Sunscreens are also available in oils, creams, and lotions. These are choices that are really a matter of personal preference and individualized skin type. Many cosmetics companies make a variety of products that vary in SPF strength, vehicles, and usage directions.

Time of Day and the Sun

Because the earth revolves, during certain times of the day the sun is closer and more intense, and more ultraviolet rays reach the earth's surface. Most estheticians and dermatologists agree that the sun is at its most powerful between 10 A.M. and 3 P.M. Advise your clients not to go in the sun during these hours.

Frequent Misconceptions About Sun Damage and Sunbathing

Consumers have many misconceptions about sunbathing and the way the sun damages the skin. It is the duty of the esthetician to dispel these wrong ideas. Some of these misconceptions are:

1. *You cannot tan or burn if the weather is cloudy or rainy.* This, of course, is completely false. Clouds do filter a small amount of UV light, but not enough to affect damage to the skin. It is certainly possible to tan or burn even in cloudy, overcast weather, particularly without using sunscreen.

2. *You cannot burn if you are in the water.* This too is false. Water may feel cool to hot skin that has been basking in the sun, but it has no effect on the sun's burning and damage potential. The heat from the sun is caused by infrared rays, not ultraviolet rays. Swimming and going into the pool or ocean may indeed remove some or a large amount of the sunscreen applied earlier. If your client plans on swimming or participating in water sports, advise him or her to use a water-resistant sunscreen product. Sunscreens should be reapplied when swimming every time the client gets out of the water, or about once an hour.

3. *Umbrellas or large hats will prevent sun damage.* The real truth is that while these are a help, they do not prevent much sun from reaching the fragile skin and certainly do not replace a good sunscreen. They primarily cut down on glare so that the person does not squint as much, helping to prevent worsening of the expression lines. It's a good idea to wear lightweight, but sun resistant clothes, which also help filter light, but ultraviolet rays can burn the skin right through a lightweight shirt. Advise your clients to wear a hat, proper attire, and sit in the shade as much as possible, but to still wear a good sunscreen.

4. *Baby or mineral oil accelerates tanning.* This is simply not true. In fact, because these do not contain sunscreen, they may accelerate burning, and they provide no protection against sun damage.

5. *Applying moisturizer after sunbathing will prevent peeling.* This is completely false! If the skin has burned, it will peel no matter what is done to the skin. Applying moisturizer to well-protected skin may help replace some of the water in the dehydrated, exposed skin, or may lubricate peeling areas, making the skin look better, but it will not stop the sun-damaged skin from peeling.

6. *Applying lots of moisturizer will counter the damage the sun causes.* False again. Hydrating fluids do help replace some of the water that is also being robbed from the surface cells during sun exposure, but ultraviolet rays cut right through the skin. Remember, the UVA rays penetrate right through the dermis, destroying collagen and elastin fibrils, not to mention causing dysplastic cell growth and the other horrifying effects we have already discussed. Esthetically, you should administer good, soothing, hydrating facial treatments to your sun-worshipping clients, but this will not treat or prevent the damage the sun causes to these clients.

7. *Wearing sunglasses helps prevent sun damage.* True, only if the sun glasses contain UV filters, and only if they are worn constantly while out. When purchasing sunglasses, make sure to check to see if the glasses contain UV filters. The larger the glasses, the more area they will help protect.

The Quest for the Golden Tan

In medieval and Elizabethan times, a suntan was considered a sign of poverty. A suntan meant that the person worked outdoors on a farm or less prestigious job. White skin was considered fashionable and a mark of success and sophistication.

However, in the 20th century, as leisure time increased, many people considered a tan a mark of success, because the person was successful enough to afford leisure time spent in the sun. Some clients will always value this "beautiful tan." Unfortunately golden brown skin at age 20 translates to wrinkled, leathery, ugly, splotchy, old-looking skin at age 40 or 50. While some clients will never listen to reason about tanning, you should always make an effort to inform, educate, and save them from the ugly, long-term ravages of sun exposure!

Tell your clients that:

1. The best way to prevent sun damage is to stay out of the sun.

2. They should wear sunscreen every day, not just when sunbathing. We do not spend the majority of time at the beach. Hour for hour, most people receive more sun damage going to work, walking outside, and sitting by a window than we do basking in the sun. Sunbathing certainly makes the damage worse, but clients should use a good sunscreen moisturizer, for their skin type, daily.

3. As we discussed before, it is best not to go in the sun between 10 A.M. and 3 P.M.

4. Sunscreen should be applied 30 minutes before sun exposure. This provides better protection and allows the product to distribute itself more evenly.

5. Reapply sunscreen often if you are in direct light. While sunscreen applications are not cumulative (two applications of SPF 15 sunscreen do not make an SPF 30 sunscreen), they are at least reapplying protection to these areas where the screen may have rinsed off due to sweating or water exposure.

6. Consider using self-tanning milk instead of sunbathing. These new products cause surface tanning. Used on a regular basis, they can produce a beautiful golden color. Two

words of caution: Self-tanning products generally work better and more evenly on the body than on the face. A "tan" produced by a selftanning product provides no additional resistance to sunburning!

7. A tanning booth is not a safe alternative. These machines still use rays that promote long-term damage, which can cause premature aging!

The sun is the number one enemy of the skin. Educate, teach, and warn your clients about its effects!

TOPICS FOR DISCUSSION

1. Why is the sun the worst enemy of the skin?
2. Discuss what happens to the skin histologically after long-term sun exposure.
3. Discuss esthetic problems caused by long-term sun damage.
4. What are the ABCD's of melanoma?
5. Discuss some rules for sun exposure and some common misconceptions about sun exposure.

17

Therapy for Photoaging Skin

OBJECTIVES

Until recently there was relatively little that could be done to help the appearance of sun-damaged skin. In this chapter you will learn about some new developments in the treatment of photo-damaged skin and techniques the esthetician can use to help improve the appearance of sun-damaged, prematurely aging skin.

Photo Damage

We have already touched on the long-term damage that cumulative sun exposure does to the skin. We have also already defined the difference between intrinsic aging, or aging of the skin that appears normally over time, and extrinsic aging, aging of the skin that occurs from induced or environmental causes, such as sun damage from exposure. These signs of aging skin from extrinsic sources do not show up for years.

Sun-damaged skin is significantly more leathery, with deeper and more numerous wrinkles and severe loss of elasticity. Sun-damaged skin also has significant discolorations, splotching, and hyperpigmentation. Instrinsically aged skin does not have nearly as great a problem with hyperpigmentation and demarcation.

Histologically, sun-damaged skin shows very large differences from normally aging skin. The epidermis of photoaged skin is remarkably thicker. There is a large increase in elastic tissue in sun-damaged skin, but it takes on the form of a disorganized "blob," with little apparent organized structure. The fibroblasts in the thickened dermis of sun-damaged skin are considerably more numerous and are overactive, producing more collagen, but obviously in a disorganized fashion. There are also significant decreases in the vascular system of sun-damaged skin, which carries much needed blood to the various areas of the skin.

In short, the skin has obviously desperately tried to repair itself, producing an overabundance of tissue fibrils, but in a panicked and dysfunctional manner.

Treatment of Photoaging Skin

Esthetically, sun-damaged skin should be treated with a mild keratolytic, such as glycolic acid, to reduce the thickness of the epidermis. Exfoliation may also be helpful. This is why peeling treatments such as glycolic acid, enzymes, and salon cosmetic chemical peeling seem to have a positive esthetic effect on sun-damaged skin. Because this skin is also very dehydrated, use of good hydrating active agents such as sodium PCA, hyaluronic acid, sorbitol, and other good water-binders are helpful. These treatments, along with good general skin care, are helpful in controlling the bad appearance of sun-damaged skin.

It is not fully understood whether esthetic treatment has much long-term or significant effect on the dysfunction of the dermis as related to photo damage. To make such a claim would be a drug claim. We know that these treatments have esthetic benefits, and continual treatment seems to improve the appearance of the surface, which is the esthetician's utmost concern. But what, if anything, can be done to help truly restore or repair long-term dermal and epidermal damage caused by sun exposure?

Research on Retinoids

So far, no drug or treatment has been approved by the FDA for treatment or repair of photoaging. However, much research has been performed in the area of using retinoids, specifically tretinoin for photoaging. Tretinoin is also used for treatment of acne, under the trade name of Retin-A®, which is, at the time of this writing, approved only for the treatment of acne.

Treatment research has been performed by applying tretinoin to photoaged skin. Tretinoin was applied to the forearms and faces of patients in the study. As a control, just the vehicle of the cream was applied to the other arm. The vehicle cream contained the same ingredients, but without the tretinoin. This study took place over approximately four months. Each patient was checked carefully at regular intervals for appearance changes over the course of the study.

After 16 weeks, the appearance of the tretinoin-treated areas were visibly improved, showing less visible signs of sun damage. The areas of skin treated with only the vehicle did not show any significant improvement.

Improvement in the tretinoin-treated skin included improvement in both fine and coarse (deep) wrinkling, softness to the touch, as well as increased pinkness of the skin.

Upon closer examination, histologic changes were observed. The tretinoin-treated skin showed a thickening of the epidermis, with an even corneum. The vehicle-treated skin showed more of an uneven corneum. Cell division was increased in the tretinoin-treated skin.

In other related studies, researchers have reported a refinement of the cell structures and organelles, including changes in the melanocytes, showing a decrease in the activity of the melanosomes. The entire structure appeared to be more organized and defined, including refinement and increase in healthy-appearing fibroblasts; collagen and other fibrils appear more normal. There is also indication of increased vascularity, showing improvement of the blood vessels. There was no effect noted on telangectasias. The increase in blood flow may be responsible for the pinkness noted in the skin of the tretinoin-treated study patients.

In short, this research shows very positive effects of tretinoin on sun-damaged skin. Appearance is significantly improved. It appears that the use of tretinoin may be very helpful in producing changes within the skin structure of photoaged skin.

It should be emphasized that, at the time of this writing, tretinoin has still not received approval for treatment of photoaged skin by the FDA. Research using tretinoin for treatment of intrinsic aging has not been thoroughly investigated.

Analysis of Photoaging Skin

You will notice many symptoms of photoaging skin. Some of these symptoms may show up as early as the 20s. Severely sun damaged skin will appear thick leathery, rough to the touch, and will have many wrinkles, which may be both vertical and horizontal. Severe and multiple wrinkling in the non-intrinsic aging areas may be present. In other words, wrinkles around the eyes and nasolabial folds is normal, intrinsic skin aging. Severe wrinkling and surface roughness in the neck, cheek, chest, and other areas are usually not the result of intrinsic aging. These areas show cumulative effects of repeated sun exposure. Severe telangectasias (couperose) are also often present. The skin is muddy looking, with diverse dark coloration, lentigines, and general brown splotchiness.

Redness on the sides of the neck in a horseshoe pattern may be a definite sign of photoaging. These red areas may be accompanied by hyperpigmentation and telangectasias. This is known as **dermolichia of cevattes**.

In younger clients, you may notice all of the above symptoms in lesser amounts. The first sign may be hyperpigmentation, or dark blotchiness of the skin. Other signs might include rough, patchy skin, and the beginning of "chicken neck," in which the skin of the neck has constant "goose pimples," which is reflected by small, pinpoint, non-colored elevation of the follicles on the sides of the neck, like a plucked chicken. Wrinkles around the eyes and mouth may be especially severe for the client's age. However, brown splotchiness is the most evident sign of premature aging due to sun damage. The use of a Wood's lamp will indicate even more hyperpigmentaion beneath the skin's surface.

The Needs of Photoaging Skin

No Sun

The very first treatment should be a thorough discussion of the harmful effects of sun with the client. This author recommends a no-holds-barred lecture (in a friendly way!) about the ravages of cumulative sun damage. Emphasis should be placed on the cumulative nature of sun damage. Many clients will say, "I haven't had any sun in months!" The truth is that most of the sun damage you will see is from sunbathing that occurred twenty years ago, and years of daily exposure.

The client should be instructed in the proper use of sunscreens on a daily basis, including a moisturizer with sunscreen built in. They should use at least a 15 or 30 SPF sunscreen when out in direct sunlight.

Unless the client implements good sun habits, or better yet, stays out of the sun altogether, improvement will be minimal, if any improvement occurs. The first need of sun-damaged skin is to remove the source of damage.

Esthetic Techniques for Photoaging Skin

Exfoliation

The cell "turnover rate" slows down with aging anyway, but even more so in sun-damaged skin. Not only is the rate often slower, the cells are disorganized and are not in even layers. Use of exfoliants such as scrubs and mild enzyme treatments is helpful in the salon and at home. Glycolic acid is another good exfoliating agent. These treatments remove dead, crusty, dried-up cells on the surface of the skin, revealing younger cells and helping to smooth the surface appearance. These also help to increase the turnover rate, and the quality of the intercellular cement is improved, resulting in improved hydration of the skin's surface.

You must be careful, however not to over-exfoliate! This can severely irritate the skin. Be careful about combining exfoliating treatments, especially if the client is using glycolic acid or Retin-A.®

Hydration

Hydration is also very important in improving the appearance of photodamaged skin. The skin has lost its water-holding capability. While you cannot replace this ability, especially in the dermis, good hydrating agents, combined with the proper amount of emollients, will help improve the hydration of the surface, resulting in a smoother appearance. Be careful to use the proper amounts of emollients. Heavy emollients can still cause comedone development, especially if the skin is still oily or clog-prone. Always consider the skin type (oily, oil-dry, or combination) when selecting moisturizers and other products.

Stimulation

The circulation of sun-damaged skin is impaired by the malformation of blood vessels due to the sun damage. Therefore the skin is not nourished properly through normal blood flow. The use of good but gentle massage techniques is helpful in improving the circulation.

Be careful when massaging skin that is being treated with a keratolytic such as glycolic acid or Retin-A. This skin can be treated, but be careful not to over-stimulate.

Alphahydroxy Acids

One of the latest breakthroughs in the cosmetic treatment of aging skin are alphahydroxy acids. These are a family of acids that are extracted from natural sources. One of the first of the alphahydroxy acids used was lactic acid, which is derived from milk. Lactic acid is used in over-the-counter as well as prescription moisturizers. It has been used by dermatologists for some time. Lactic acid often works better on body skin than facial skin.

Alphahydroxy acids work by removing buildup of dead cells on the surface of dry and aging skin. The acids help to dissolve the "glue," or intercellular cement, that holds the clumped-up dead cells on the skin surface.

You must remember that sun damage causes abnormal cell growth and generally disorganizes normal cell patterns. This, of course, also affects the epidermis, piling dead cells on top of the skin in uneven patterns as they accumulate. Microscopic cross-section photographs of sun damaged skin show severe disfigurations of the normal patterns of the strata of the epidermis. This is both a medical and esthetic concern. The dysplastic cell growth can eventually cause skin cancer, but esthetically causes a rough, dry, scaly appearance on the skin's surface as well as contributing to the appearance of wrinkles.

By removing this conglomeration of dry, dead cells, the surface of the skin appears much smoother, and wrinkles appear much less deep. Hydrators applied over the acid treatments perform better because they are not having to moisturize the dead cell buildup. Instead they work to hydrate the skin more evenly, which results in a much smoother appearance of the skin.

Other forms of alphahydroxy acids include **glycolic acid**, which is the smallest, molecularly, of all the alphahydroxy acids. Because of this small molecular structure, glycolic acid appears to penetrate the skin better than the other alphahydroxy acids, making it the most useful for facial and cosmetic use.

Imagine a thick layer of dead cells lying on top of the skin. These cells are all dried up, like a thick layer of dust lying on top of a piece of furniture. This cell buildup makes the skin's surface look dull and flat, just as dust prevents light from reflecting from a piece of furniture. Surface mechanical peeling, which we have already discussed, helps to remove some of this "dust." Glycolic acid, however, works by loosening the bonds that hold the cells together, helping to continually shed off this sheath of dead cells (Figure 17-1).

This removal of dead cells is also beneficial to acne-prone skin, helping to loosen both surface cell buildup and impacted dead cells inside the follicle, which, as we have previously discussed, can lead to comedones and possibly acne.

Glycolic Home Treatments

Several types of glycolic acid treatment products are designed for use on a daily basis. These treatments can be used to treat a variety of skin problems including acne, clogged pores, hyperkeratinization, keratosis pilaris, hyperpigmentation, dry and dehydrated skin, dry body skin, foot and hand callouses, and the appearance of aging skin (Figure 17-2).

Different products are formulated differently with different vehicle ingredients, release systems, and different concentrations of glycolic acid, depending on the type of problem treated. Preparations for acne, oily, and problem skin are usually in a mild alcoholic liquid solution, so designed to combat oily skin. They are very helpful in conjunction with other acne treatments. As a word of caution, be careful when combining peeling agents. Combining glycolic acid with benzoyl peroxide, salicylic acid, resorcinol, sulfur, or retinoic acid must be done very carefully, if at all. Check the manufacturer's instructions well before combining home keratolytic treatments. The glycolic solution for oily and acne-prone skin should be applied to

FIGURE 17–1 Glycolic treatment is popular for lessening the appearance of facial wrinkles. Shown here are before and after photos of the eye area. *Courtesy Murad Skin Research Laboratories, Inc.*

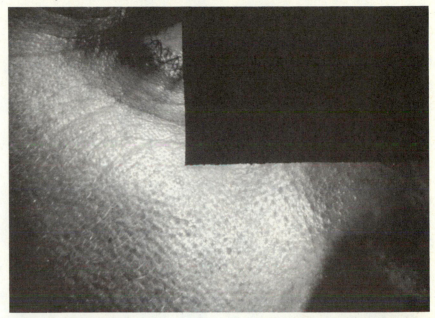

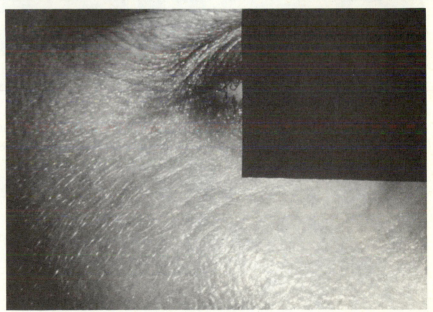

the face, usually twice daily, under a protective sunscreen moisturizer, or coupled with a light, noncomedogenic hydrating product at night. Some companies suggest treatments only once a day at home. Always check the manufacturer's instructions!

FIGURE 17–2   Glycolic acid used over a 25-month period shows dramatic improvement in the appearance of wrinkles. *Courtesy Murad Skin Research Laboratories, Inc.*

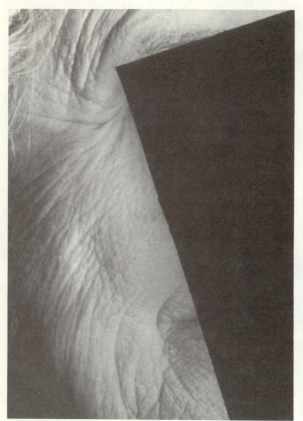 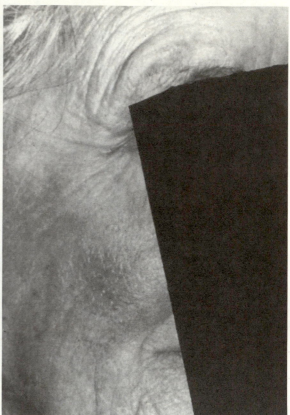

Glycolic products for the body are usually made in lotion form, to be applied like a body lotion. These are almost always oil-in-water emulsions and sometimes are not designed for facial use. Again, check the instructions.

Glycolic products for fading hyperpigmentation are in a gel or lotion form. The glycolic acid is mixed in the solution with a bleaching agent, hydroquinone. Glycolic acid helps to remove the buildup of dead cells, which helps the bleaching agent work better and faster. Age spots, sun freckles, pregnancy masks, and hyper-pigmented areas from acne all can be helped with such a solution. As with any bleaching solution, the client should be instructed to use a good sunscreen and avoid sun exposure, which, of course, can result in recurrence of the hyperpigmentation.

In the treatment of wrinkles and the appearance of sun damage, glycolic acid loosens the dead cell buildup, again helping to make the skin look smoother and softer. The appearance of wrinkles can be greatly improved with continued use. The creams available to help the appearance of aging skin are usually in a cream or lotion form. The cream form is for alipidic, dry, dehydrated, aging skin. Lotions are more appropriate for combination skin showing signs of aging including wrinkles, leathery texture, dull appearance, and uneven surfaces. The cream or lotion is applied under the moisturizer or sunscreen and under the night treatment. Most companies recommend twice daily application.

Recommending Glycolic Home Care

First, as always, carefully evaluate the appearance of the client's skin. You must also access the client's current home care. If he or she is currently using home care that is inappropriate, such as strong soap for aging skin, this must first be corrected. Glycolic treatment is most effective when used with a well-planned general home care program, designed for the skin type and conditions.

Explain how glycolic acid works on aging skin and the importance of the "program." Best results cannot be expected if the client is using a hodge podge of products along with the glycolic acid. Be careful to find out if the client is using other peeling-type products or drugs. Heavily scented products or products that are extremely stimulating should also be avoided when glycolic acid is being used. The client should also be instructed in the importance of regular use. No product will work if it is sitting in the medicine cabinet! Other problems such as hyperpigmented skin or problem oily areas should be addressed separately.

Glycolic acid often produces a mild to moderate tingling sensation when applied to the skin. Usually the tingling feeling lasts only 10 or 20 seconds. The client should wait for a short amount of time (a few minutes) before applying other hydrating or conditioning products. When a client first starts using glycolic acid, some slight cosmetic side effects might be experienced. In the case of dry or aging skin, the skin may show some flaking, which the client may misunderstand as dehydration. Explain that this is the dead cell layer coming off the surface, is a normal occurrence, and can be controlled by using the appropriate products along with the glycolic acid cream. This is another reason why the "surrounding" products are so important. If the client uses the wrong treatment cream or a cleanser that is too harsh, side effects will be more intense. The client's skin may feel "crunchy," as if it is peeling. Again, this feeling can be alleviated by using a good-hydrating fluid. In the case of clog-prone or combination skin, make sure that you recommend a moisturizer that is noncomedogenic.

If the client experiences severe peeling, tell the client to call you. Instruct the client to discontinue using the solution glycolic temporarily, until the peeling subsides. Then phase in the glycolic product, starting once a day, and eventually working back into twice daily application. Some clients with extremely thin skin may have problems with waxing. This is unusual, but it does occur sometimes. Waxing in these clients, or any other procedure that involves removing cells, should be discontinued. Allergic reactions to glycolic acid are rare, but like with any other cosmetic ingredient, allergic reaction is possible. Allergic symptoms are the same as for any other reaction. These may include redness, itching, and general irritation. The client should, of course, discontinue the treatment.

Treatments with glycolic acid are also performed in the salon. For more information, please see the chapter on chemical peeling.

Prevention Is Still the Best Treatment

Avoiding sun exposure and using sunscreens are still the best and most viable treatments for sun damage. Clients should always be instructed in the proper use of sunscreens to help prevent this terrible insult to the skin.

TOPICS FOR DISCUSSION

1. What are some signs of the beginning of sun damage?
2. Discuss the research on the use of retinoids for photoaging skin.
3. What would you say when discussing sun damage with a client?
4. What precautions would you take to avoid overstimulating photoaged skin?
5. Discuss alphahydroxy acids and their effect on the appearance of photoaged skin.
6. How does glycolic acid improve the surface of aging skin?

18

Chemical Peeling

Many different types of peeling treatments are available, ranging from brushing treatment and light enzyme peels to strong surgical peels that are administered by dermatologists and plastic surgeons. This chapter will discuss the various types of peeling treatments, both cosmetic and medical, and the various conditions that can benefit from different types of peeling treatments. This chapter is not a substitute for hands-on training in the use of superficial salon chemical peelings. The esthetician should always receive hands-on training before attempting any of the procedures discussed in this chapter.

The process of peeling the surface of the skin dates back to the 19th century in Europe. Chemical peeling was actually brought to America by a young esthetician, the daughter of a European doctor, who immigrated to America. The process of peeling the skin can take place in varying degrees, ranging from scrubs to salicylic creams to surgical level phenol peeling. Removing cell layers from the surface of the skin can be used to treat a variety of both cosmetic and medical problems.

Surface Peeling

There are basically two types of peeling treatments. Mechanical peeling uses some method of physical contact to literally scrape or bump cells off the skin. Granular scrubs, such as honey and almond scrubs, preparations with polyethylene granules, or the use of a brushing machine are all examples of mechanical peeling treatments. When the granules of these products or the bristles of a brushing machine come in contact with the surface corneum cells, the movement of the product or the brush literally "bumps off" cells from the surface of the corneum.

Many skin-care companies include brushing as a standard part of their salon treatments. The brushing machine is used over a layer of cleanser or moisturizer, which helps to buffer the contact with the skin. The skin should be thoroughly cleansed, toned, and steamed before the brushing machine is used. Applying a noncomedogenic hydrating fluid before steaming the face is helpful in hydrating the dry surface cells, also helping to loosen dead cell buildup on the surface. This makes removal of the dead cells much easier, and gentler pressure can be used.

Removing the surface cells help the skin in the following ways:

1. The procedure helps to remove uneven buildup of dead cells, so the skin appears much smoother.

2. It helps to clear away dead cells and debris from the pore openings, making extraction and other treatment of clogged pores much easier.

3. By removing the dead cell layer, the lower level cells are moved to the surface more quickly, improving the moisture content of the surface.

4. Mechanical treatment stimulates blood flow to the surface of the skin.

5. Removing the dry, dead cell buildup helps to deliver moisturizers and other treatment deeper into the epidermis.

All of these advantages generally help to smooth the skin's surface, which makes makeup apply more evenly. The dead cells will eventually build back up on the surface, making this procedure only a temporary appearance change. However, regular use of mechanical exfoliators such as granular scrubs helps to maintain this appearance. Granular scrubs for normal to dry skin are usually recommended two to three times per week.

Disadvantages of Mechanical Treatment

There are many circumstances when mechanical treatment is not appropriate. Do not use brushing machines or any harsh mechanical feeling techniques on the following skin types and conditions:

1. Couperose skin, or telangectatic skin, with many visible capillaries and blood vessels. The blood vessels in these skin types are very fragile and should not be subject to brushing treatment.

2. Fragile, thin skin that reddens easily. The epidermis of this skin is considerably thinner than other skin types. Brushing or abrasive treatment may redden and irritate this skin easily.

3. Older skin that is thin and bruises easily.

4. Severely sun-damaged skin. This skin also will often have many distended capillaries and redness.

5. Skin that is being treated with retinoic acid, glycolic acid, or flourouracil. (See the chapter on therapy for photoaging skin.)

6. Acne-prone skin types, particularly those with inflamed acne, papules, and pustules.

7. Accutane® patients.

8. Any skin that is red, irritated, thin, or extremely fair.

Other Mechanical Peeling Techniques

As an alternative to using a brushing machine, you may choose to use a granular scrub, such as honey and almond scrub, after steaming. Apply the scrub with your fingertips and gently massage in upward, outward circular movements. Do not scrub the face for more than 1 or 2 minutes. Be extremely gentle with the pressure you apply. For thinner skin types, you may dilute the scrub with cleanser or moisturizer before applying the preparation. This dilution helps to provide a buffer between the skin's surface and the scrub, which cuts down on irritation potential.

For oilier skins, you may apply a granular scrub made with fine polyethylene beads or granules. These preparations often contain a small amount of sulfur or salicylic acid as additional chemical exfoliators and antiseptics. These scrubs are generally excellent for oily, problem skin and will help to clear the surface of dead cells and other debris, making extraction easier.

Home Care Using Mechanical Exfoliation

For dry to normal skin, recommend a light scrub such as honey and almond scrub two or three times per week. The client should apply the scrub after cleansing with a milk-type cleanser. Instruct the client to be very gentle with the scrub. Home care scrubs should not be recommended for extremely thin skin or skin that is being treated with the therapies already listed in the precautions.

For oily and problem skin, granular scrubs are sometimes recommended on a daily or twice daily basis. This, of course, will depend on the skin type, contraindications previously discussed, and what other drug or esthetic therapies are being used to treat this skin type. Exfoliation and removal of dead cells is usually very helpful in treating problem oily and clog-prone skin.

Salon Peelings

These treatments are actually a type of chemical peeling, but they are extremely gentle. They are sometimes appropriate to use when mechanical peeling is not appropriate. These procedures involve the use of enzymes, specifically proteolytic enzymes. *Proteolytic* means "protein dissolving." The enzymes work to destroy the keratin in the dead cells on the surface of the skin. These are often referred to as enzyme peeling or enzyme treatments.

The enzyme often used in these treatments papain, which is derived from the papaya fruit. Papain is also used in meat tenderizer for its ability to soften tissue and dissolve protein. In Europe, this type of treatment is known as a lysing or lysis.

There are two basic types of proteolytic enzyme peeling. One is a cream that is applied to the skin after steaming and initial preparation. The cream dries in about 10 minutes, and then is massaged or "rolled" off the skin. Treatments of this type are often called "vegetal" or "vegetable" peelings. This treatment is actually a combination of enzyme and mechanical peeling. The "rolling" provides friction that physically removes dead cells. They can also be irritating for the skin types listed previously.

The second, and probably more popular, type of enzyme treatment uses a powdered form of enzyme. Mixed with warm water immediately before application this treatment stays soft during application, and does not dry. It is easily removed because it is soft and moist. This type of enzyme treatment generally produces a more even peeling of the cell buildup and helps to slightly dilate the follicle openings, helping make extraction much easier. Brushing the skin may miss some of the cells, while this type of enzyme treatment works evenly across the surface of the skin. Enzyme peelings are often available in varying strengths and suitable for the following conditions:

1. Oily, clogged skin with open and closed comedones and minor acne breakouts.

2. Dry or dehydrated skin with cell buildup, flaking, and tight dry surface.

3. Dull, lifeless looking skin. This skin condition actually has a tremendous buildup of dead cells that produces a slight gray color on the surface of the skin.

4. Skin with multiple milia.

5. Clients who desire a smoother appearance to their skin and a more even surface for makeup application.

Enzyme treatments are generally gentle enough to repeat even on an every two week schedule, although most clients have them with their regular monthly facial treatments. Most clients notice immediate softening of the skin after the very first application of the enzyme. Because enzyme treatment slightly dilates the pore openings, which helps with extraction, clients notice that extraction is more comfortable and that gentler pressure may be used to facilitate extraction of the clogged pores, comedones, and other impactions.

Procedure for Enzyme Treatment

Caution: Always follow manufacturer's directions for using particular peeling treatments! The following is an example of typical treatment with enzymes, but these directions may vary with the manufacturer.

1. Remove all makeup and cleanse the skin well, using a milk cleanser appropriate for the skin type.

2. Apply a pre-peel lotion, usually furnished by the manufacturer. This solution is applied in a similar method as a toner. This solution is normally slightly alkaline, which helps to remove excess oils on the surface of the skin, making the enzyme come in better contact with the dead surface cells.

3. Choose the appropriate strength of enzyme preparation for the particular skin type, thickness, and condition. Most companies make at least two strengths or furnish formulas to dilute the enzyme action of the product.

4. Mix the powder with warm water in a small mixing cup or beaker. Most enzyme treatments have the consistency and thickness of mayonnaise when mixed with warm water. Stir the preparation until the treatment is smooth and free of powder lumps.

5. Apply the enzyme to the face with a soft mask brush. Stay clear of the eye area and other sensitive areas unless otherwise directed by manufacturer's instructions.

6. Many companies recommend steaming during the application of the treatment and during treatment setting time. The steam helps to keep the treatment warm and also helps to keep the preparation from drying out on the surface. It is important to keep the preparation moist. If enzymes are allowed to dry on the face they can be irritating to the skin and are also hard to remove. Allow the treatment to set for about 8 minutes. Remove with tepid, damp sponges or a damp, soft, facial cloth. Be careful to remove the enzyme treatment thoroughly. It is easy to leave remnants of the peeling, particularly around the perimeter of the face, such as under the chin, on the jawline, and in front of the ears. This leftover enzyme can be irritating if not removed after the appropriate amount of time.

7. Brushing is not necessary when using an enzyme treatment. In fact, it can be irritating. Do not use the brush during an enzyme treatment.

8. Because of the follicle dilation caused by the enzyme, desincrustation using galvanic current is usually not necessary. It can also be irritating to thin, sensitive, or dry skins when combined with enzyme treatment. Excessively

oily skin, acne-prone skin, and thick, oily skin with multiple comedones may benefit from galvanic desincrustation after an enzyme treatment. Use your best judgment and remember, when in doubt, don't!

9. Proceed with extraction in a normal manner. You will probably find that you do not have to use nearly as much pressure during extraction. This will appeal to the client as well, as treatment is more comfortable.

10. Apply a toner to lower the pH of the skin immediately after extraction. It is important to lower the pH after the enzyme treatment.

11. Proceed with the rest of treatment as normal. You should not massage the skin before applying the enzyme. This may increase irritation potential. Any facial waxing should be done toward to end of the treatment session, not before the enzyme is applied. The waxing procedure will also physically remove dead cells. It is best to perform waxing after the enzyme is removed, or, on sensitive skin, suggest that the client make a separate appointment for a different day.

12. You may find that you do not need to use as aggressive a mask as usual after an enzyme treatment. Some masks also remove dead cell buildup. On dry or thin skins, apply a gel mask, a cream mask, or simply apply a thick layer of hydrating fluid as a mask. These types of masks are non-hardening and are easier to remove for sensitive or thin skins.

Most skin-care salons charge an additional fee for enzyme treatments. You may want to allow the client to try the enzyme treatment once at no charge so that the client can see the nice results.

Glycolic Peeling Treatments

Before reading this section, review the section on glycolic acid in the chapter on therapy for photoaging skin. Glycolic-acid is available in a variety of strengths for salon use. The typical concentration of glycolic acid used in salon treatment is between 15 and 30 percent. Higher strengths are usually used only by dermatologists. It is strongly suggested that you not experiment with higher percentages of glycolic acid!

There are two methods of treatment with glycolic acid. The most commonly used method uses a lower strength of glycolic acid. The client should already have used glycolic acid at home for at least two to four weeks before using the higher concentration in the salon. A 15 to 20 percent solution of glycolic acid is applied for 10 minutes only, usually twice a week for three weeks. This technique exposes the skin to lower concentrations of glycolic acid, which is less irritating. The procedure, however, can be repeated more often than if using higher percentages.

Glycolic acid peeling has a similar action as enzyme peeling, but goes slightly deeper. It can be used to treat the same basic conditions listed as indications for enzyme treatment. Again, take the same precautions as for enzyme treatment, and always follow manufacturer's instructions to the letter!

Mild glycolic treatment may be influenced by the cleansing procedure that takes place before extraction. The cleansing procedure determines how much surface oil is removed prior to applying the glycolic peeling treatment. The following is a typical procedure for glycolic treatment, but read the instructions of the particular product you are using and follow them.

Procedure for Glycolic Peeling

1. Cleanse the skin with a mild cleansing milk, removing makeup.
2. Apply a compress to the eyes to avoid accidentally spilling the solution into the eyes.
3. Set a timer for 10 minutes, or the length of time suggested by the manufacturer. Apply the glycolic acid gel with two cotton swabs held together. Begin with the forehead, and apply the gel using small, circular motions with the cotton swabs. Proceed to other areas in a precise clockwise pattern. It is important to follow a precise pattern to ensure even application of the gel.

The glycolic treatment is allowed to stay on the skin for the prescribed amount of time, as recommended by the manufacturer. A typical time for a low-strength solution is 10 minutes. After 10 minutes remove the gel from the face with cool, wet, gauze pads. Rinse the face well with the wet gauze. You may follow this with a cool spray of plain water in an atomizer and another clean-up with wet gauze. Finish by applying a sunscreen moisturizer.

This treatment is normally performed twice a week for the first three weeks. The pretreatment prior to application of the glycolic acid gel can influence the strength of the treatment. The strength of the cleansing products used will determine the amount of surface oils and corneum cells removed prior to application of the gel.

You should, during the first treatment, cleanse with a very mild cleansing milk. If the first treatment does not produce any redness or irritation, the second treatment may be preceded by a slightly stronger milk cleanser. For the third visit, again assuming there is no irritation, you may add a mild toner to complete the cleansing. The fourth treatment may be strengthened by using a slightly stronger milk cleanser with a slightly stronger toner. The cleansers and toners used should never be extremely strong or alcoholic.

It is strongly recommended that a minimum of six treatments be given before assessing the results. When using a low-strength glycolic acid, results will not be particularly dramatic after one treatment. It takes several applications of low-strength glycolic acid, over several weeks, to see appreciable results in many cases (Figure 18-1).

FIGURE 18–1 Glycolic acid is applied to the skin of a client who has been using a lower strength glycolic treatment product for at least two weeks at home. This treatment is applied with cotton swabs and carefully monitored according to manufacturer's directions. *Courtesy Murad Skin Research Laboratories, Inc.*

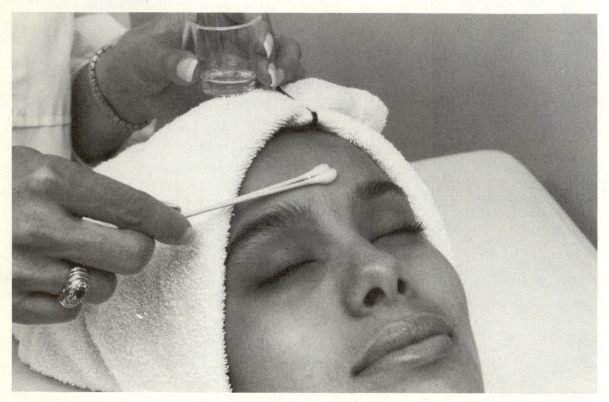

After the initial treatment, you may decide to repeat the treatment weekly, biweekly, or monthly, depending on the results. You should reassess the condition of the skin after the first few applications to determine a further treatment course.

Precautions to Take when Administering Glycolic Peelings

1. Always make sure the skin has been pretreated with lower strength glycolic acid at home for several weeks before administering salon-strength treatment. Failure to do this may cause irritation. For instructions on home care glycolic treatment, see the chapter on therapy for photoaged skin.

2. Do not use the glycolic treatment if the client is currently using retinoic acid. Treatment with retinoic acid should be discontinued for several weeks before using salon glycolic peelings.

3. Do not use glycolic acid on Accutane® patients.

4. Do not administer glycolic peelings if the client is under a dermatologist's care for any skin disorders, without first obtaining approval from the dermatologist.

5. Be careful to use eyepads, and avoid getting the glycolic acid close to the eyes.

6. Do not use the peeling gel on a male client immediately after he has shaved. It is best to wait several hours after shaving to apply glycolic salon treatment.

7. Check with the client before each successive treatment to make sure the client has not experienced any irritation from the previous treatment. If irritation developed after the previous treatment, do not add pre-cleansing steps as discussed earlier. Avoid any area that is peeling, red, or irritated, or wait a few days before resuming treatment.

You should not combine professional glycolic acid application with other salon facial treatments when first beginning glycolic treatment. After the initial series of glycolic salon applications, you may administer glycolic treatment during facial treatments, depending on the client. As always, check manufacturer's instructions for instruction regarding combining glycolic treatment with other types of salon skin-care treatments.

The skin should never be exfoliated prior to glycolic application. Avoid pretreatment with any technique or product that is stimulating, heating, or irritating.

Glycolic treatment with low-strength gel can be administered indefinitely on a weekly, biweekly, or monthly basis, depending on the client and the skin type.

Using Glycolic Treatment for Acne

The procedure is essentially the same as we have just discussed. You may notice an apparent increase in comedones and blackheads during the first few treatments. Because glycolic acid is a peeling treatment, it uncovers closed comedones and loosens open comedones while exfoliating the dead-cell layer on the surface of the skin, which can be fairly heavy on oily, problem skin. You should explain the possibility to the client that the skin may seem to get worse before it gets better. Continued treatment, along with alternating extraction treatments on different days, will help to loosen the acne impactions (Figure 18-2).

FIGURE 18–2 Glycolic treatment can significantly improve the appearance of problem and acne-prone skin. (Before and after.) *Courtesy Murad Skin Research Laboratories, Inc.*

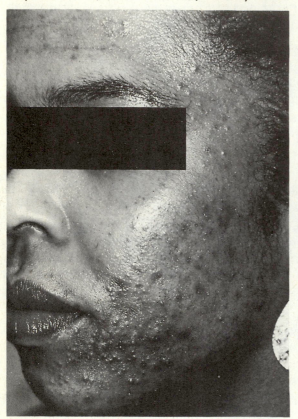 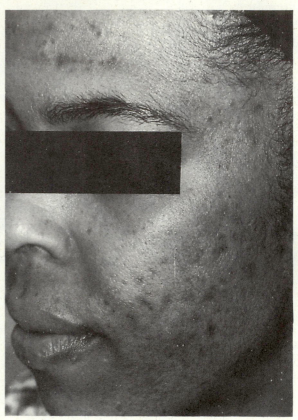

Treatment for Hyperpigmented Skin

Again, the treatment method is essentially the same. The client should, as always, be pretreated at home for several weeks before starting salon treatment. The client should use a glycolic product with hydroquinone (a bleaching agent) at home. There are such premixed solutions available. The hyperpigmented client should always wear a good sunscreen and completely avoid the sun for best results (Figure 18-3).

Stronger Glycolic Peeling

Stronger solutions are available for salon use, but with added strength comes added risk. Thirty percent solutions are available for salon use, but they should be used conservatively and should never be left on the skin for more than 2 minutes. The amount of time glycolic acid is allowed to contact the skin is

FIGURE 18–3 Glycolic treatment can help the appearance of hyperpigmented skin conditions. *Courtesy Murad Skin Research Laboratories, Inc.*

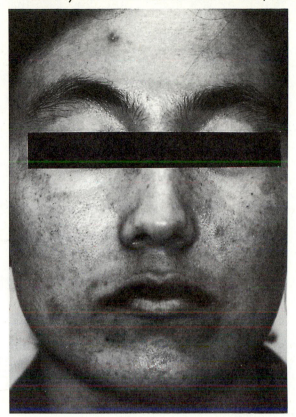 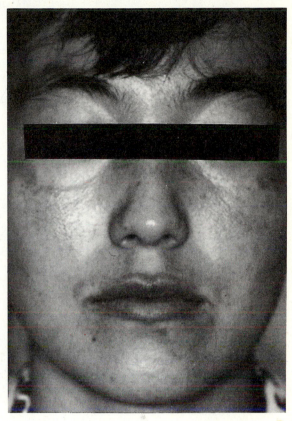

directly related to the strength and depth of the treatment. Do not experiment! Stick to manufacturer's directions at all times!

Medical Glycolic Treatment

Dermatologists and plastic surgeons may use glycolic acid solutions in concentrations of 50 to 70 percent. These are medical grade strengths and should never be used by estheticians. High strengths are used to treat deeper wrinkles, solar lentigines, and actinic keratoses.

Stronger Peeling Treatments

The treatments we have been discussing using 20 percent glycolic acid are generally very safe and helpful for cosmetic effects. This level of glycolic acid is acceptable for almost all skin types and produces a good cosmetic effect with a very low amount of potential irritation. One company calls their treatment "rapid exfoliation," indicating that it is actually a "high-tech exfoliator," rather than a "chemical peel."

The stronger peels are of three types and three levels.

Surgical phenol peeling is a deep peeling procedure that should only be administered by a dermatologist or a plastic surgeon. This procedure involves applying a very strong solution of a very strong chemical called phenol. Phenol peeling must be administered in a doctor's office or surgical unit. Phenol, in large amounts, can be absorbed into the bloodstream and rarely can cause heart fluctuations. The heart is monitored during this procedure to ensure safety. The phenol peel penetrates to the reticular layer of the dermis. It is used for severely sun-damaged, severely wrinkled skin, and can also be used to treat skin growths such as repeated instances of skin cancers and actinic keratoses (Figure 18-4). It may produce hypopigmentation of

FIGURE 18–4 (a) Phenol solution is used on the wrinkled lip of this patient. Shown here is the "frosting" effect after application of the phenol solution. (b) Several months after the peel, the lip is much smoother. *Courtesy Kirk Smith, M.D.*

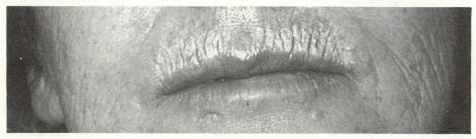

a

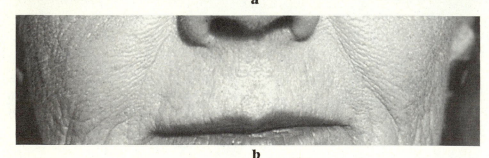

b

the skin and a ruddy surface to the face (Figure 18-5). For further information on phenol peeling, please read the chapter on treating the plastic surgery patient.

Medium depth peels include 50 to 70 percent glycolic acid applications and 40 to 50 percent trichloroacetic acid, better known to the medical community as TCA. TCA at this strength penetrates to the layer of the dermis, and again is a procedure that should only be administered by a dermatologist or a plastic

FIGURE 18–5 In-depth phenol peel—before and after. *Courtesy Melvin L. Elson, M.D.*

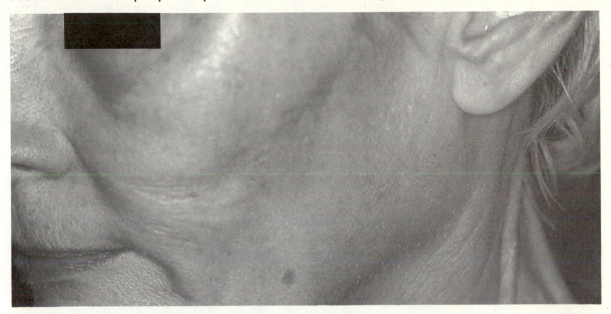

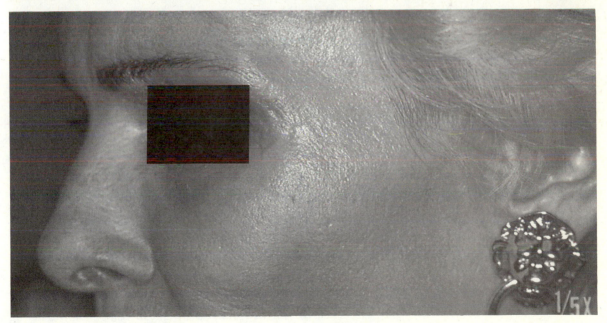

surgeon. Combinations of TCA and glycolic acid are sometimes used by doctors to treat deeper wrinkles.

TCA does not have the potential for absorption into the bloodstream like high concentrations of phenol. Lighter peelings can be given with TCA at concentrations of 15 to 35 percent, but they do not have the dramatic results of the deeper phenol peels. Some doctors will use repeated treatments with these smaller concentrations of TCA. TCA in general also does not have as great a potential for scarring as phenol peeling.

Superficial peeling is the deepest type of chemical peeling performed by estheticians. Superficial peelings, unlike deep and medium medical peelings, only remove cells from the stratum corneum. The most frequently used type of chemical is known as Jessner's Solution, which is a mixture of salicylic acid, resorcinol, lactic acid, and ethanol. Some superficial peeling formulas also contain a small amount of phenol, usually 2 percent, and sometimes sulfur. While Jessner's Solution is a liquid, some cream forms of peels are similar and produce similar effects on the skin.

These superficial chemical peels are helpful for treating small, superficial wrinkles, dark spots, and other forms of hyperpigmentation, melasma, and acne-prone skin.

The superficial peel evens the surface skin pigment, smoothes the appearance of the skin, and dries the surface of acne and problem skin. Like glycolic acid, superficial peeling may also increase the amount of surface acne lesions, because it loosens impactions and causes them to move toward the surface. In other words, it may cause acne to get worse before it gets better.

Candidates for Salon Superficial Peelings

Clients who have sun damage, hyperpigmented skin, or other forms of melasma are the best candidates for superficial peeling. Technically, most adult clients can benefit from peelings, because most adults do have some form of fine wrinkling or hyperpigmentation.

There are, of course, many other alternatives for treating these cosmetic problems. Glycolic acid, hydroquinone solutions, or a combination can be very effective for many forms of hyperpigmentation. Low-strength glycolic peelings are also another alternative. Most estheticians will attempt to treat these cosmetic conditions with more conservative treatments, such as the ones listed above before resorting to superficial chemical peeling.

It is best to have a client started on home care before administering superficial chemical peeling. This pretreatment will ensure that the client's skin is in better shape before using chemical peelings. Many estheticians insist that a client have facial treatments for a period of time prior to administering a chemical peel. This is not a bad idea, because it allows you to learn about the client, the client's skin, and the client's needs before using peelings.

Many clients will call the salon specifically asking about chemical peels. Information given out over the phone should be minimal, because you have not seen the client's skin. Ask the client to make an appointment for a consultation before you issue an opinion about her skin. Many clients have cosmetic problems that can be treated by other simpler methods than chemical peels. Some clients are not using proper home care. Good home care and salon care may make the difference they need and establish a good, healthy program for their skin for a lifetime. Chemical peeling should not be looked at as a "band-aid" for skin problems. The client needs to continually take care of the skin at home on a regular basis.

Other forms of lighter peelings such as enzyme or glycolic acid may be sufficient for treating the client's problem.

Chemical peeling is probably the most drastic and dramatic treatment administered by an esthetician. There are some disadvantages to superficial peeling. These include discomfort, temporary discolorations, a small risk of allergic reaction, a bad appearance to the skin during the actual procedure, and a possibility of hyperpigmentation. All of these disadvantages should be explained to the client long before the procedure is administered. When the client agrees to have the superficial chemical peel, the client should be required to sign a release saying that the client has been informed of all the possible side effects and discomfort that may be associated with chemical peeling. Clients should also be shown pictures of what clients look like during the peel so that they know how they might look.

These few paragraphs are not meant to discourage the use of chemical peelings. They are meant to clarify that clients do not always fully understand chemical peeling or for what conditions it is intended. Clients who are not familiar with good skin care and do not use a regular skin-care program will generally not have as good or as long-lasting results as clients who have regular salon treatments and are good about home care.

You should also get to know a client's personality. Chemical peeling is uncomfortable, and during the procedure the skin looks terrible. A client who is nervous or who becomes hysterical easily should not have chemical peelings. You will save yourself a world of trouble by getting to know your client well before performing chemical peeling.

Other clients who should not have chemical peeling are:

1. Clients who are pregnant or lactating.
2. Clients who have a history of heart problems.
3. Clients who have a history of medical problems. These clients should have written permission from their physician. Examples of these conditions include, but are not limited

to, eczema, sebhorrea, psoriasis, bacterial skin infections, mental disorders, extremely sensitive or hyperallergic skin, and other systemic problems. Take a thorough health history, and refer the client to a medical doctor if you have any questions.

4. Clients who have a history of fever blisters or herpes simplex, which can be stimulated by chemical peeling. Clients should discuss this with a physician.

5. Clients using Accutane® or other dermatological drugs.

6. Clients using retinoic acid (Retin-A), which should be discontinued about three months before superficial peeling is administered.

7. Clients who have extremely thin telangectatic or couperose skin.

The Pre-Peel Consultation

At least a week before the peeling is scheduled, you should have a consultation appointment with the client. Explain to the client what normally happens, step-by-step. Make sure the client understands the discomfort and how the client will look during the procedure. Explain that the client should not have any sun for eight weeks after peeling and must use a sunscreen at all times. Clients who are being treated for hyperpigmentation should always be very careful about sun exposure.

Show the client pictures of what a normal peel looks like during the process. Take pictures of the client's skin before and after the procedure. This will allow you to show the client the improvement in the skin's appearance.

Have the client sign a release saying that the client has been fully informed about the possible disadvantages of peeling and the actual procedure that takes place. It is very important to be honest with the client.

Superficial peeling will not:

- Remove deep wrinkles.
- Remove scarring or acne pocks.
- Repair severe sun damage to any appreciable degree.
- Cause a lifting effect on the skin.

Superficial peelings will:

- Improve the skin's texture.
- Even the coloring.

- Help to lighten hyperpigmentation.
- Improve fine lines and rough textures.

The Superficial Peeling Procedure

Several different procedures are used for superficial salon chemical peeling, which will vary according to the manufacturer. The following are two examples of typical procedures for liquid and cream peelings. These are meant to serve only as examples. Always follow the manufacturer's direction for the preparation that you are using.

Liquid Peeling

The liquid type of peeling solution is normally Jessner's Solution. It is applied with cotton swabs to the face. The following procedure is typical:

1. Complete all the pre-peel consultation procedures discussed.
2. Remove the client's makeup thoroughly with a cleansing milk.
3. Apply a "prep" lotion furnished by the manufacturer. This solution is usually acetone, which removes excess oils and surface dead cells.
4. Turn on a small fan and place it so it blows gently on the client's face. Do not turn the fan to high speed, as this may blow the liquid. Some fans are small enough for clients to hold them in their hands.
5. Put on a pair of latex gloves. Paint the liquid solution onto the face using two cotton swabs held closely together. Begin with the forehead and apply the solution in small, gentle, circular motions. Do not apply pressure with the swabs. Proceed from the forehead down the cheek and around the face. It is very important that the application be as even as possible. Do not apply the solution to the lips, ears, or upper lids. Lower lids may be treated, but it is strongly suggested to stay within 1/8-inch of the lower lid edge. The client should keep the eyes shut during the procedure.
6. Allow this coat to "dry" for two minutes. If you notice any white areas forming on the face, this is known as frosting. Frosting occurs when the peel is complete. Some clients will frost after one coat, and some after two or three coats of solution. If frosting does not occur after the first coat, repeat the application procedure, and wait for

another four minutes. Occasionally areas of the face will frost when other areas will not. If this happens, reapply the solution to the unfrosted areas only.

7. Apply the solution at 4-minute intervals until frosting occurs. Most clients will only require one to three coats.

The solution remains on the face, and the client should stay in the salon for about an hour.

A strong burning sensation will be felt when application starts. The intensity of the burning sensation will vary with the client. This is the reason for the fan, which helps to cool the sensation. After about 15 minutes, this burning sensation will stop, and the skin feels numb and slightly tingly.

The Cream Peel

The preparation procedure is the same as for the liquid peel. No prep solution is used with the cream peel.

1. With gloved hands apply the cream peel to the forehead, cheeks, nose, chin, neck, and finishing with a very light application to the lower lids using a cotton swab. Apply evenly. The face will begin to burn and sting. Again this sensation can be lessened by the use of a fan, and usually subsides after 15 to 20 minutes.

2. You do not have to watch for frosting with this treatment. It will happen automatically. There is no need for a second application until the next day. This thick treatment stays on the face for 1 1/2 hours. After this time the cream is gently removed with a tongue depressor and then cleansed well with cool, wet, cotton compresses.

3. After removing the treatment, apply the thick moisturizing cream furnished in the peeling kit. The client will continue to apply this emollient cream to the face at home. The skin should be well lubricated with the emollient at all times.

4. The second day, with this cream peel, the same procedure is repeated in the salon. The client continues to keep the skin moist with the emollient cream.

While these procedures sound fairly simple, you must be thoroughly trained and experienced to perform them correctly. You must have hands-on training to perform chemical peeling. Do not think you are qualified simply from reading this chapter or a manufacturer's handbook. You should observe several peeling procedures before attempting to perform peeling!

After the Treatment

Immediately after treatment the skin often looks slightly red and flushed. There is often little change the first day. The second day of either peel, the skin will become tan-looking, sometimes splotchy.

The third day the skin becomes very dark, and often splotchy, and will feel very tight and dry. Peeling will begin around the mouth and chin first, then the cheeks, then the eyes. The neck and forehead are the last to peel. The skin will peel for usually the third through the sixth or seventh day. Occasionally the peeling will continue for several more days. The client should be warned not to pull on the loose skin. This can cause infection and possible hyperpigmentation. It is best for the client to visit the salon daily for a quick check, and the esthetician can gently peel off areas that are ready.

Clients should not wash the face at all during the peeling procedure. They may use moisturizer, depending on the manufacturer's instructions. Cool water may be applied, but no cleanser.

Granular scrubs and other keratolytic preparations should be discontinued for at least the first two weeks after peeling. These include glycolic acid, benzoyl peroxide, sulfur, resorcinol, Retin-A, salicylic acid, lactic acid, or any other peeling or exfoliating agent.

The skin should be completely protected with a daily sunscreen for at least eight weeks after peeling. Direct sun exposure must be avoided.

Reactions to Peeling

Rarely, a client will have an allergic reaction to a chemical peeling. The symptoms may include severe itching, swelling, severe redness, and stinging. Refer this client to a dermatologist who is familiar with your services, particularly your peeling procedures. Normally, a steroid cream is prescribed, which quickly alleviates the problem.

Dark skin types will sometimes have a tendency to hyperpigment after a peel. Many estheticians will not administer chemical peeling to darker or black skins. If the client pulls off skin that is not ready, splotchy hyperpigmentation can occur. Normally this fades within a few weeks, as long as the skin is protected with a sunscreen. Sometimes you may need to treat the skin with a mild bleaching cream, if the hyperpigmentation does not decrease within two or three weeks after peeling.

Your proficiency in chemical peeling will increase as you perform more and more peelings. This is why it so important that you thoroughly train with someone accomplished in the practice of superficial peeling and observe the actual peeling that takes place during the six or seven days after the procedure is performed. With this training you can become proficient at superficial chemical peeling.

TOPICS FOR DISCUSSION

1. Discuss the difference between mechanical and chemical peeling.
2. What are some skin conditions that can benefit from enzyme peeling?
3. What are the differences between deep, medium, and superficial peels?
4. Discuss the consultation procedures for superficial chemical peeling.
5. What conditions will not be improved with salon superficial peeling?
6. Discuss the procedures and possible problems associated with salon chemical peeling. Why is it so important to receive hands-on training?

19

Treating the Plastic Surgery Patient

More and more frequently, clients are having plastic surgery performed. In this chapter we will discuss the many types of plastic surgery procedures used, and common problems of the plastic surgery patient. We will also discuss treatments for preparing the patient for plastic surgery, counseling the plastic surgery patient for referral, and how to treat cosmetic side effects of plastic surgery.

Again, it is very important that the esthetician have hands-on experience with the plastic surgery patient. Do not attempt any of the treatments listed in this chapter without the instruction of a licensed qualified instructor or a plastic surgeon.

Years ago plastic surgery was considered by many to be a sign of vanity and to be reserved only for the rich and famous. Now plastic surgery is performed daily in every major American city. It is no longer considered unacceptable for people to want to look better. There are two basic types of plastic surgery—*cosmetic* surgery and *reconstructive* surgery.

Cosmetic surgery generally refers to surgical procedures used for cosmetic purposes only. These procedures include eyelid, face, and forehead lifts, dermabrasion, chemical peelings, liposuction, collagen injections, and other procedures. Body cosmetic surgery includes body sculpting contour surgery, body liposuction, tummy tucks, and breast augmentation or reduction.

Reconstructive surgery generally refers to surgical techniques used to correct noncosmetic abnormalities such as skin cancer removal, surgery needed due to accidental injury, and other physical deformities. These surgical procedures are often medically necessary, and in some cases, such as melanoma, can be treatment for serious, life-threatening diseases.

For the purposes of this discussion, we will primarily discuss facial cosmetic surgery, although we will briefly discuss reconstructive surgery.

Types of Surgeons

Several different types of physicians perform plastic, reconstructive, and cosmetic surgery. All of these doctors receive four years of medical school training, followed by an internship and residency that takes four or more years to complete. These various specialists are then board-certified by their particular specialty associations.

General plastic surgeons perform all types of plastic, reconstructive and cosmetic surgery. They often also perform hand surgery. They perform surgery on all areas of the face and body. They are board certified by the American Board of Plastic Surgery, which is in association with the American Society of Plastic and Reconstructive Surgeons (ASPRS). These doctors generally limit their practices to plastic surgery.

Facial plastic surgeons specialize in plastic surgery of the face, head, and neck. They generally do not perform body surgery. They are usually trained in otolaryngology, the specialty area of medicine that treats diseases of the ears, nose, and throat, and head and neck surgery. Their professional association is called the American Academy of Facial Plastic and Reconstructive Surgeons. They may perform facial cosmetic, or reconstructive surgery, but may also perform surgery on the sinuses, ears, nose, and throat.

Opthalmic surgeons are medical doctors who treat eye diseases and perform eye surgery. They perform eyelid surgery, or reconstructive surgery involving the eyes.

Dermatological surgeons are dermatologists who also perform plastic or cosmetic surgery.

You should always work with surgeons who are board certified in their specialty areas.

Common Types of Cosmetic Surgery

We will first discuss the various types of facial cosmetic surgery procedures. We will break these procedures down into several subjects: symptoms of need for plastic surgery, discussion of the actual surgical procedure, suggestions for pre- and post-care treatment (salon treatment and home-care recommendations for before and after surgery), makeup needs of the postoperative patient, and long-term needs of the patient.

Rhytidectomy

Rhytidectomy is the medical term for a face lift.

Presurgical Facial Characteristics

These characteristics include sagging skin with marked lack of elasticity, folds of skin in the jawline and neck area, jowls in the cheek and jawline area, and general lack of skin tone.

Surgical Procedure

Incisions are made in front of, or inside, the ears, following around the back of the ears, and into the hairline in the back of the head. After the incision is made, the face is literally "pulled up," and excess skin is clipped away. In some cases, the underlying muscle structure may also be surgically altered, or excess fat may be removed. In some cases a small incision may have to be made under the chin. After the excess skin is removed the skin is reconnected in the areas of the incisions and sewn together with materials called **sutures** (often called "stitches" by lay people). In some cases surgical staples are used instead of suture material (Figure 19-1).

After surgery the face is very swollen and bruised. The head is wrapped in gauze dressing to provide support for the surgical area. The patient is instructed to keep the head elevated for several days, even when sleeping, to provide gravity for draining fluids. Skin discolorations, mainly due to bruising, are typical after surgery and may last for weeks. Some patients notice numbness in certain areas, particularly in front of the ears.

The sutures and dressings are removed a few days after surgery by the plastic surgeon. Most patients are pleasantly surprised how little pain is associated with rhytidectomy, but any pain can be managed with medication. The skin may feel very tight at first, but generally feels better after a few weeks when the facial swelling has subsided.

Pretreatment for the Lift Patient

The same pretreatment procedures are followed for blepharoplasty, rhytidectomy, and forehead lift. Ideally, treatment should begin at least three months before surgery. Treatments should be administered weekly or biweekly for a minimum of six treatments. The purposes of these treatments is to thoroughly cleanse the skin, to improve circulation through massage and electrical treatment, and to have the skin in the best condition before surgery. Skin that is in prime condition prior to surgery will most often look better after surgery, and the good condition will aid healing.

Before starting the treatment program, you should talk to the client extensively about plans for the surgery, including the

FIGURE 19–1 Rhytidectomy, or face lifting, can dramatically improve the appearance of sagging facial skin and elastosis. A forehead lift has also been performed on this patient. *Courtesy Samuel J. LaMonte, M.D.*

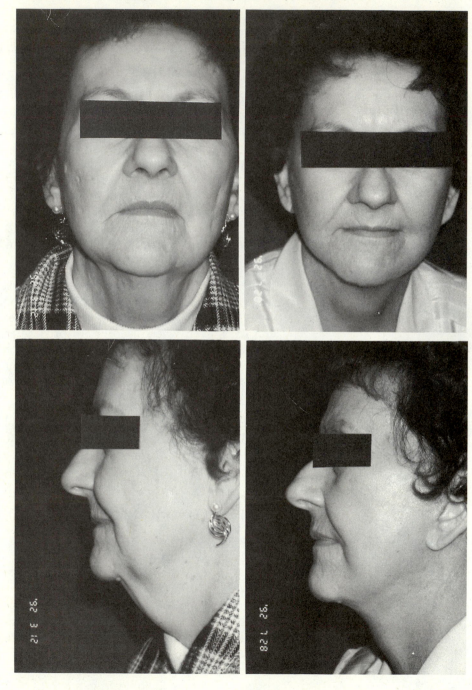

dates of the surgery. Plan your treatment schedule around the date of the actual surgery. You should explain all the benefits of skin treatment in general, as well as how important it is for the patient to take perfect care of the skin before and after the surgery, as well as emphasizing the need for ongoing care after the surgery is completed. You should give the client realistic expectations of what you will accomplish, and the differences between what the surgeon and the esthetician will do to improve the appearance of the skin and face.

1. To begin treatment, thoroughly cleanse the face.

2. Thoroughly examine the face under a magnifying lamp, making notes of all problems, especially conditions that will not be improved by plastic surgery, such as comedones, milia, fine wrinkles, hyperpigmentation, rough, dehydrated areas, etc. Type the skin and write up a detailed analysis as you would for any new client.

   Regardless of the surgery, you should treat the skin as you always would for the analyzed condition. Design treatment based on the examination. Client home care will also be directly related to the analysis, as always.

3. Begin the procedure by using the steamer on the skin for 8 to 10 minutes. During the steam you may apply an exfoliating treatment if necessary. Scrub creams are frequently helpful, provided the skin is suitable for scrubs. Brushing may be used over a layer of hydrating fluid. Using hydrating fluid during steam can greatly help to soften a rough-textured surface. If the skin is oily, apply a desincrustant pre-mask to the skin to help soften comedones and sebaceous filaments. Enzymes or scrubs may also be helpful to this skin.

4. After steaming, proceed with galvanic desincrustation (assuming there are no contraindications) to all areas with comedones, sebaceous filaments, or other impactions. Oil-dry (alipidic), poreless areas of the skin should not be treated with galvanic desincrustation.

5. Begin extraction of any impacted areas. Be thorough, but do not perform more than 10 minutes of extraction in one visit.

6. After extraction, apply a toner with an antiseptic.

7. Apply a lightweight, noncomedogenlc hydrating fluid to the face and begin a thorough massage appropriate for the skin type. Oily skin should not be excessively massaged, nor should areas that are still clogged. A good facial massage will be excellent for improving the circulation before surgery.

8. Apply more hydrating fluid and apply high frequency to the skin with the mushroom electrode for 2 to 3 minutes.

9. Apply a mask appropriate for the skin type. You may need to use more than one mask, such as a cleansing clay mask for the oily areas and a soft-setting gel or cream mask for dry areas. After the setting time has passed, remove the mask and apply a moisturizer with sunscreen.

Home Pre-Care

The main difference between this home-care procedure and that of a regular client is that the client must be very diligent about performing home care daily. Not enough emphasis can be placed on good routine home care. You should mention that home care may need to be altered after surgery depending on the case and the surgeon's wishes.

Postsurgical Skin Care

Immediate post-care for the patient will be handled by the surgeon. The client should check with the surgeon to see when regular home care can resume.

After the client has been given the approval by the surgeon to continue home care, the client should be instructed to be extremely gentle with the skin, being careful not pull on the skin or apply significant pressure to the suture areas. Light massage at home, always using a hydrating fluid, will help to dissipate bruising. Instruct your client how to perform light effleurage and tapotement (piano massage) to the face nightly.

Post-Care Salon Treatment

Never begin treatment of a postsurgical client without the approval of a plastic surgeon. After you have established a good working relationship with a plastic surgeon, you should sit down and discuss both of your expectations for post-care of the patients he or she sends you. The plastic surgeon may establish a general set of rules for administering postsurgical treatment to patients. You will both be fully informed of each others' procedures and precautions. The patient should not have treatment while sutures are still in the skin, unless otherwise directed by the surgeon. Be extremely gentle with all facial procedures. The client may still be sensitive from the surgery, and you do not want to pull on the suture areas or apply firm pressure, especially immediately after surgery. Generally salon treatment can resume about two to three weeks after surgery.

The main objectives of post-care are to help improve the circulation, reduce swelling, and help dissipate any discolorations from bruising. Long-term goals of postsurgical treatment are to improve the texture and appearance of the surface of the skin, putting the "icing on the cake" by routinely providing care to improve the surface appearance.

Assuming the patient has approval from the surgeon, the following is a typical postsurgical treatment:

1. Apply liquid cleanser to the face with gloved hands, using very gentle application movements. Use very soft facial cloths or sponges, or cotton pads to remove the cleanser, being careful not to pull on the skin too much.

2. Apply a light hydrating fluid to the skin and allow it to be steamed for about 8 minutes.

3. Remove the hydrating fluid and examine the skin under a magnifying lamp. Check for bruised areas and look carefully at the suture areas. In general, suture areas should be avoided during treatment.

4. If there is a lot of surface flaking, apply a diluted nondrying exfoliator, such as honey and almond scrub, and gently massage, removing the scrub with the same careful technique. Avoid using brushing or suction immediately after surgery. Wait about three months before using these techniques after rhytidectomy.

5. Any extraction should be very minimal. In general, unless there are large open comedones, extraction should be avoided at this particular time.

6. Apply a lightweight hydrating fluid and begin a thorough but gentle massage, using light effleurage and tapotement. Avoid petrissage, rolling, friction or any rough type of massage. Plenty of hydrating fluid should be used to keep the skin slippery during the massage, which helps to avoid excessive pulling. Concentrate on the eyes and neck, using gentle, circular effleurage movements.

7. Apply more hydrating fluid and apply high frequency with the mushroom electrode set at a very low intensity. Move around the face in small, gentle, circular movements for about 3 to 4 minutes.

8. Apply a non-setting, nonstimulating mask, or apply a thick coat of hydrating fluid. It is very important that whatever you put on the face be easy to remove. Setting masks and thicker creams may be more difficult to remove, causing you to pull on the face more than normal.

9. After the mask has processed for 10 minutes, wet the mask well using a spray of cool toner to help loosen it for removal. Remove the mask gently using soft facial cloths, sponges, or cotton pads. Apply a moisturizer-protectant appropriate for the skin type with sunscreen.

10. While it is best to avoid makeup immediately after treatment, this may be impossible for the plastic surgery patient. Be understanding, and help her with makeup after treatment. Do not start any "new" treatments on the client immediately after surgery. There is a rare possibility of allergic reaction, particularly with new products that the client has not tried. Do not recommend new products for home use at this point. Wait until the healing process is further along to start any new procedures.

Makeup Needs

The postsurgical rhytidectomy patient will likely experience extensive bruising. There is no conclusive evidence, but many patients who undergo extensive presurgical skin care at home and in the salon seem to have less bruising, and any bruising seems to dissipate faster.

Bruises are the main problem immediately after surgery. As soon as the surgeon approves, the esthetician may help the client with camouflage makeup for the bruising. You should make available to the client a heavy coverage camouflage makeup to help conceal the bruises. The bruising usually occurs under the eyes, on the lids, in a half-moon pattern on the upper cheeks, in front of the ears, and sometimes along the jawline and neck.

Prepare the skin in the normal manner. Yellow toner may help to conceal purple bruises. You may wish to apply a layer of amber or yellow toner prior to applying the coverage.

Apply the coverage makeup with dabbing movements using a latex makeup sponge. Blend in the edges with the client's normal foundation. As the patient heals, bruises will start to change color as the blood is absorbed by the body. Bruising also tends to shift with gravity; i.e., bruises that start on the jawline may slowly seem to move down the neck and decollete, and occasionally onto the chest. During this time there may be variation in color, ranging from normal black-purple bruising to yellow or green. Apply the proper color toner to help neutralize the colors.

After the bruising has totally subsided and the suture lines have healed completely, have a second makeup lesson with the client and teach her to cover the incision scars. Work with her hairstylist to establish a good hairstyle that will help conceal the scars from the incisions. This is particularly necessary in front of the ears. Occasionally a plastic surgery patient will experience a small amount of hair loss in the surgical area, and sometimes hair areas from above the ears end up in back of the ears. Again, the skills of a good hairstylist are very important.

Within a few months of surgery, after all swelling has subsided, the client should have a new makeup lesson, teaching her how to best complement her new look, emphasizing the new contours that the surgeon has created.

Long-Term Needs

The main long-term need is great skin care! Clients will often be interested in new products and treatments to improve the look created by the surgery. Most patients are very interested in protecting their "investment" by taking good care of their skin.

Blepharoplasty

Blepharoplasty is the surgical procedure for "lifting" the eyes and removing excess skin from the eye area.

Presurgical Facial Characteristics

These characteristics include puffiness, bags under the eyes, drooping or flapping upper lids. Sometimes the drooping of the upper lids is so dramatic that it actually interferes with the patient's vision.

Surgical Procedure

The patient is anesthetized or sedated. Incisions are made in the normal fold of the upper lid, and excess skin is trimmed away. The suture line is made in the actual fold of the lid, rendering it practically invisible when it heals.

Lower lids are corrected by making an incision in the lower lash line. The fat pocket in a "bag" is removed, and, again, the excess skin is trimmed away and sutured along the lowerlash line.

The brows are lifted by making an incision in the lower part of the browline. Excess skin and fat is removed from this area as well. More and more patients are having a forehead lift at the same time as their eyes are corrected. Much of the sagging of the upper lid may be attributed to elastosis in the forehead. In a forehead lift, an incision is made about an inch back into the hairline. The excess skin is removed from the hairline incision, simultaneously lifting the brow area. This procedure is becoming more and more popular. Forehead lifts may be a problem in persons with extremely high foreheads or in men who have receding hairlines or male pattern baldness, because the scars will not be concealable (Figure 19-2).

Pretreatment

The same basic procedure is followed as is already outlined in the pretreatment section for rhytidectomy.

Home Pre-Care

Use the same procedures as for rhytidectomy patients.

FIGURE 19–2 Blepharoplasty, or eyelid surgery, along with a face lift, can help tc significantly restructure the eye contours, achieving a more alert, youthful look. *Courtesy Samuel J. LaMonte, M.D.*

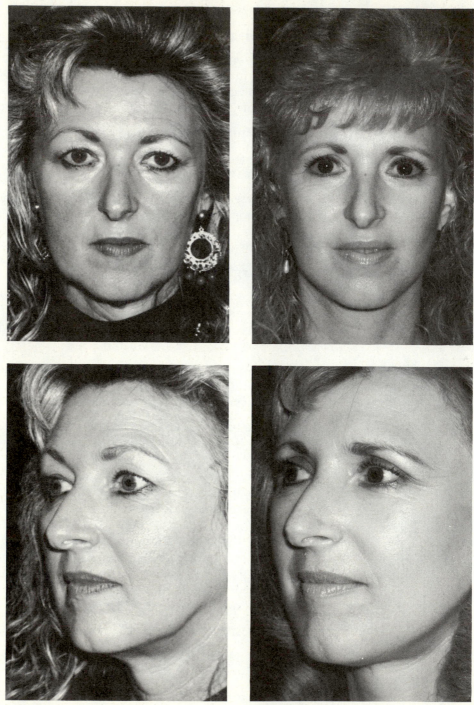

Postsurgical Skin Care

Follow the same post-treatment recommendations for post-rhytidectomy patients. Mild massage of the lids, after they have healed and with the surgeon's approval, may help to dissipate discoloration from bruising and swelling. Makeup needs will be the same.

A patient may occasionally choose to have only a forehead and eye lift, without a general face lift. While this is sometimes appropriate, particularly in young individuals who only have eyelid drooping and puffiness, in most cases, general face lifting is also necessary. Most plastic surgeons will encourage these clients to proceed with face lifting at the same time as the corrective procedure for the eyes.

Rhinoplasty

Rhinoplasty is the term for surgically altering the nose. Commonly called a "nose job," many clients of many different ages request this procedure. In an older individual, a rhinoplasty may make the entire face looks younger, particularly if the nose is "drooping."

Presurgical Facial Characteristics

This will vary in the rhinoplasty procedure. The nose may be crooked, too long, too short, upturned, or drooping. In many cases rhinoplasty is medically necessary to correct internal blockages of the breathing passages caused by chronic sinus problems or a deviated septum (Figure 19-3).

Surgical Procedure

An incision is made inside the nostrils. The bones of the nose are reshaped using special surgical tools. The nose is then "redraped" over the new bone structure. Occasionally excess skin and cartilage is removed, and any internal problem affecting breathing is corrected. After surgery a splint is placed on the nose, which is removed after a few days. The nose will be quite swollen immediately after the surgery. Swelling may last for weeks after surgery, and results cannot be assessed until the swelling has completely subsided.

Pretreatment

In the salon, the follicles of the nose should be cleaned routinely before surgery. It is advisable for the client to have about six weekly or biweekly treatments, concentrating on deep-cleansing as well as general skin care. The same procedure should be followed as for rhytidectomy, outlined earlier in this chapter. If the general skin of the face is in excellent shape, the skin in general will be in better condition for healing.

FIGURE 19–3 These views feature the patient before and after a rhinoplasty. Note the reduction of the nasal bone protrusion, the straightening of the nostrils, and the softer look of the face in general after surgery. *Courtesy Samuel J. LaMonte, M.D.*

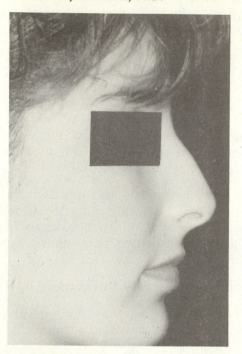
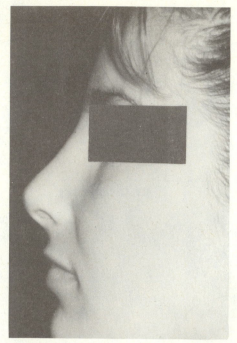
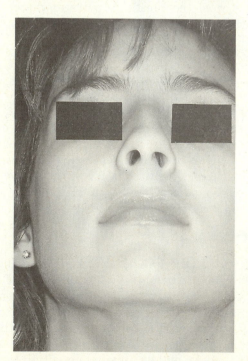
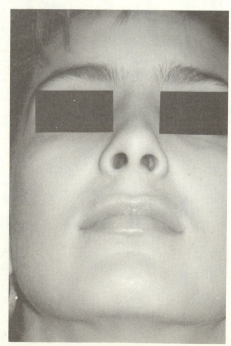

Home Pre-Care

Again, the procedure is the same used for rhytidectomy patients. You may recommend that the client apply a deep cleansing mask to the nose, especially clients with extremely oily skin, with many clogged follicles on the nose.

Postsurgical Skin Care

You must be extremely careful with treatment of the nose for several months after surgery. Remember, the bones have been re-shaped, and no pressure should be applied. This is particularly important regarding extraction. Essentially, no extraction on the nose or on surrounding tissue should take place for several months after surgery.

In lieu of extraction, you may use enzyme treatment on the nose to help remove excess cell buildup. Comedones on the nose may be increased after surgery due to trauma, surgical dressings, and because cleaning the nose may be uncomfortable for the client. Use of enzyme peelings or desincrustant pre-masks on the nose will help to soften pore accumulations.

If this is followed by clay-based deep cleansing masks, improvement may be obtained without extraction on the nose area. The tissue around the nose and upper cheeks should be treated in the same manner. Use "wet" treatments—do not apply treatments that need to be rubbed or lifted off. Stick to fluid type treatments that can be easily removed. Clay-based masks should be thoroughly moistened before removal. After the clay mask dries, spray it with a cold spray of diluted toner to loosen and wet it before removal.

You may notice that the client is uncomfortable, even during massage and basic cleansing. Be very gentle when cleansing the nose area, and avoid any movements that pull upward on the nose.

Avoid the use of brushing or suction on the nose area. Galvanic desincrustation can be beneficial, but be careful with the amount of pressure used.

Makeup Needs

Because of swelling, clients may need help with contouring makeup for minimizing the appearance of swelling, particularly during the first few weeks after surgery. Bruising of the eyes and cheeks may occur. Use the same procedures outlined earlier in this chapter to help the client cover these areas.

Long-Term Needs

After several months have passed, you may proceed with extraction, being very careful and gentle. The client may need frequent treatments to help with clogged pores, especially while extraction is being avoided.

Dermabrasion

Dermabrasion is the technique of reducing acne scarring, scar tissue, and in some cases wrinkles.

Presurgical Facial Characteristics

These characteristics are acne scarring, "icepick" scarring, "pock" marks from acne, hypertrophic (raised) scarring, and wrinkles in limited areas, such as around the mouth.

Surgical Procedure

The patient is anesthetized or sedated. The surgeon uses a rotating attachment, similar to an esthetician's electric brush, except the attachment is an abrasive steel instrument. The skin is literally "sanded," and the tissue is "planed" to a low level, helping to smooth out imperfections.

Generally only areas that are affected by the scarring are treated. While the treatment sounds painful, most patients are surprised at how little pain is involved (Figure 19-4).

Pretreatment

This procedure probably requires the most intensive pre- and postoperative salon treatment. Many dermabrasion patients are present or former acne sufferers, and often still have very oily, problem skin. If the acne has been or is cystic, the client should be seen by a dermatologist for treatment. It is vitally important to be sure that acne is not recurring before performing surgery. If the surgery is performed while cysts are still developing, the patient may risk more scarring after surgery.

Assuming the client has finished any dermatological treatment, treat the client as you would any acne or oily skinned client, using deep cleansing treatments routinely in the salon prior to the surgery. Frequent treatment, weekly or biweekly, prior to surgery is usually necessary. Follow the treatment program outlined in the acne chapter. The ultimate goal is to have the skin completely clear, oiliness under control, and as clean as possible before surgery.

Home Pre-Care

Again, follow the procedures outlined in the chapters on acne and comedogenicity. The client should use completely non-comedogenic products at home. Use of keratolytics such as salicylic acid, resorcinol, sulfur, glycolic acid, and benzoyl peroxide are useful before surgery. Because of the nature of the dermabrasion procedure, keratolytics must be discontinued after the

FIGURE 19–4 (a) Acne scarring in the cheek of this former acne patient. (b) After dermabrasion, the cheek area is much smoother. (c) This patient needed both a dermabrasion and revision of this large surgical scar. (d) Revision of the scar and dermabrasion result in a much smoother appearance. *Courtesy Kirk Smith, M.D.*

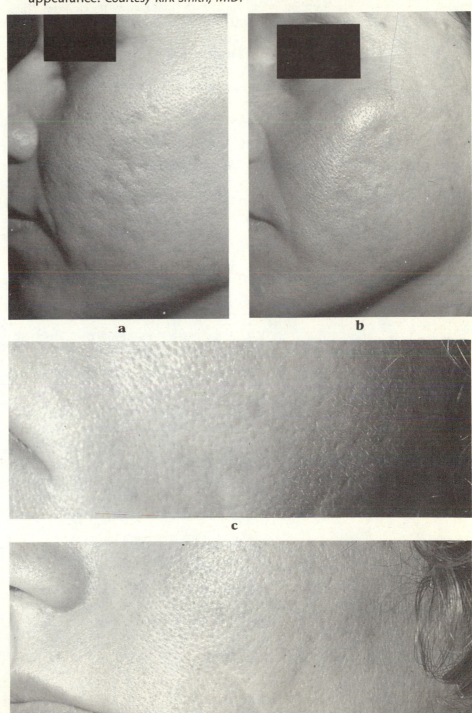

surgery, unless otherwise prescribed by the plastic surgeon or dermatologist.

Postsurgical Skin Care

During the dermabrasion procedure, the skin is traumatized, and this often results in multiple milia development. Sometimes dozens and dozens of milia appear after a dermabrasion. After the surgeon has approved your treatment of the skin, you may begin treatment of the milia. There is also a lot of redness usually present. Normally treatment in the salon may resume three to four weeks after surgery. The following is a suggested treatment for post-dermabrasion clients with multiple milia:

1. Cleanse the face thoroughly with cleansing milk.

2. Steam the face with lukewarm steam over a layer of desin-crustant pre-mask or solution. Do not use brushing, enzymes, or suction on the skin at this time.

3. Using a sterile lancet, begin extraction of the milia, which are usually very soft and easily removed. Do not perform this procedure unless you have been thoroughly trained in extraction of milia! Only extract for a few minutes, and discontinue immediately if redness seems to worsen. The skin is still erythemic from the surgery. You must be very careful not to traumatize the skin.

4. After extraction, spray the skin with an antiseptic toner solution.

5. Apply cold aloe compresses to the extracted area. Allow to sit for 15 to 20 minutes.

6. Do not apply tightening or abrasive masks to freshly dermabraded skin. The skin has already been exfoliated through the surgical procedure.

7. After the aloe compresses have set on the face for 15 to 20 minutes, remove them and apply a noncomedogenic moisturizer-protectant with sunscreen.

Treatment for the milia may take several weeks. The client should visit for treatment either weekly or biweekly.

Postsurgical Home Care

Advise the client to use a rinseable cleanser, a mild toner, a protectant with sunscreen, and a night hydrating fluid. Remember, you are still dealing with oily skin, but this oily skin has been severely exfoliated! Avoid the use of any keratolytic or peeling agents for at least the first eight or ten weeks, depending on the surgeon's recommendations. All home care should still be completely noncomedogenic, as it should be for any oily skin. You should explain the differences in home care to the client before the surgical procedure so that the client can anticipate and understand the need for the change of products.

Makeup Needs

The client will need help in concealing the redness caused by surgery. Using a green-colored toner and beige-based makeup is helpful in concealing the redness in the areas treated. The client's normal makeup can be blended into the outer nontreated areas. Remember to keep all makeup products noncomedogenic!

Long-Term Needs

After the initial post-treatment is completed, the milia have subsided, and the redness has diminished, the client generally has much smoother skin. The client should have a makeup lesson to learn to best complement the change in skin texture. The skin normally still has oily tendencies, and treatment for the skin should be adapted to treat the current conditions of the skin four to six months after surgery. At this time it may be appropriate to return to the keratolytic treatments previously used.

Chemical Peeling

We have already discussed surgical chemical peeling in the chapter on chemical peeling. Here we will discuss only phenol-type peeling treatments administered by plastic surgeons or dermatologists.

Presurgical Facial Characteristics

These characteristics include multiple deep wrinkles and superficial lines in the areas to be treated. Treatment may be isolated to one or two areas, such as around the mouth. Many clients will often seek information about chemical peeling for acne scarring, but dermabrasion is the most commonly used procedure for acne scarring. Chemical peeling can also be used for medicinal purposes to treat recurring skin cancers and pre-cancers.

Surgical Procedure

After sedating the patient, the plastic surgeon paints the affected areas of the face with a phenol solution. The patient is closely monitored. The face may or may not be taped with adhesive-like tape strips. The tape, if used, is removed within a few days of the procedure. The skin looks very red and scabbed at this point. Patient discomfort is common and is controlled by prescribed medication. The doctor will often recommend a special ointment to keep the skin lubricated at this point.

Pretreatment

Salon pretreatment should begin about twelve weeks before the treatment. Treatment every two weeks is typical. Several layers of skin are actually "burned off" during phenol peeling. The main reason for treatment is to have the skin in the best shape possible before surgery. Postoperative care, and particularly makeup, is often more important in the phenol peeling patient.

Home Pre-Care

Designed for the sun-damaged, but sensitive skin.

Postsurgical Skin Care

Extensive redness is typical for several weeks after chemical phenol peeling. Treatment should not begin in the salon until approved by the surgeon, usually about three weeks after surgery. All keratolytic and exfoliating treatments should be completely avoided, unless otherwise recommended by the surgeon.

Use an extremely gentle, soothing treatment. Avoid the use of any scrubs, peels, or stimulating treatment. Cool aloe compresses are often used as a mask. The primary purpose of esthetic treatment for postoperative peel patients is to help with redness. Effleurage and very light tapotement are the only massage movements that should be used. Masks should be gels or liquid hydrating treatments that do not tighten and can be easily removed. Milia may form during healing, similarly to dermabrasion, but usually not as severe. Patients who have received chemical peeling often need more emotional support than other plastic surgery patients. The skin may be red for weeks after surgery, and hypopigmentation is sometimes a side effect. The skin may appear grainy, and pores may appear larger than before surgery. The client will need esthetic help to minimize these problems with proper skin care or makeup.

Post-Home Care

The client, with the surgeon's approval, should use very mild cleansers, usually milks or liquid rinseable cleansers followed by a mild, nonalcoholic toner. Sunscreen must be used. Skin often no longer tans after a chemical peel, making routine use of sunscreen a must. Hydrating products that are fragrance-free are the best bet. Azulene or bisabolol based creams may help to minimize redness. The client, again, should avoid scrubs or keratolytic products.

Makeup Needs

Plastic surgeons frequently refer chemical peel patients for makeup lessons to help conceal the redness after a chemical peel and to help the patient conceal any lines of demarcation that may be present as a result of the peel treatment. Application of a green-colored toner after proper skin preparation will help neutralize redness. Then apply a liquid foundation, carefully matching the patient's neck color. In some cases cream makeup may provide better coverage, but liquid generally looks more natural, if it is feasible to cover with a liquid. Teach the client to carefully blend in any lines of demarcation, such as darker areas that have not been treated by the chemical peel. Makeup designs that focus attention on the eyes may help to draw attention away from other treated areas of the face.

Long-Term Needs

Besides good general skin care, the chemical peel patient will need help with the aforementioned possible side effects of the peel.

Phenol peeling is most often recommended for seriously sun-damaged, wrinkled, and leathery skin. Although the peel procedure does seem to tighten the face, it is not a substitute for face lift. The phenol peel is often reserved for patients who need serious help because of severe wrinkling and rough textures from sun damage. The possible side effects of phenol peelings must be considered acceptable risks for this sun damaged skin.

Other Surgical Procedures

Liposuction is the term for surgical removal of fat deposits. The procedure uses a vacuum-like instrument, which suctions away fat from areas such as the chin or the cheeks. Liposuction is often also used on the body, such as the hips and thighs. A small incision is made in the skin, and the instrument is inserted into the subcutaneous fat layer, where treatment is administered. Bruising is the main side effect of this procedure. Chin or cheek liposuction is often performed at the same time as a face lift.

There are no specific additional pre- or postoperative salon procedures for facial liposuction, except as already outlined for facelift surgery. Treatment of the incision areas should be avoided, and harsh massage should be avoided. Treatment, as always, should not begin until the surgeon approves.

Collagen injections are almost always an in-office procedure. Bovine (cow) collagen is injected into the dermis through an **intradermal** injection. The wrinkle depression in the dermis is "inflated" with the collagen, immediately reducing the appearance of the wrinkle. Collagen injections are frequently used for treatment of nasolabial wrinkling, eyelines, and small depressions, pocks, and hypotrophic scars (Figure 19-5).

Treatment should be avoided in the freshly treated area. The area may appear "lumpy" for up to several weeks after the injection. The body will slowly absorb the collagen, so collagen injections need to be repeated for best results, usually every few months.

FIGURE 19–5 (a) Note the deep nasolabial folds on this patient. (b) By injecting collagen, the surgeon achieves a remarkable reduction of the wrinkle. *Courtesy Kirk Smith, M.D.*

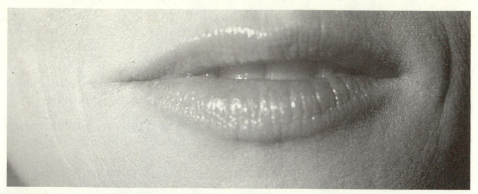

a

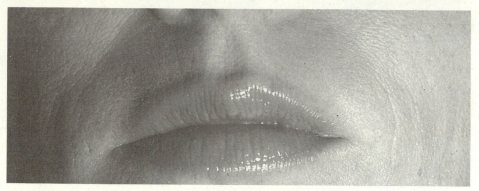

b

Collagen injections are often the first procedure sought by clients for minor wrinkles and other small imperfections. They are a good treatment for spot wrinkles, but are not a substitute for a face lift. Collagen injections appeal to clients because they are nonsurgical, but often the client needs other surgery in addition to collagen to "polish" the results of surgery.

Implants are used to improve the cheeks and chin. These are small "sacks" of silicone or saline (saltwater solution) that are implanted in the chin and cheek areas to improve low cheekbone appearance or receding chins. Avoid treating the area immediately after surgery, following the surgeon's recommendations. Implants are often performed at the same time as a face lift.

Permanent eyeliner or **makeup** is often performed by plastic surgeons, but in some states it is legal for estheticians to perform. The procedure involves a "tattooing" type process that implants small amounts of pigment in the skin. The procedure is often used to create a permanent eyeline or lipline, but can also be used in the cheek area, and occasionally to help correct dark, flat lesions, such as small, red macules. Courses available through many schools teach permanent makeup. Check with your instructor regarding the laws in your state affecting permanent makeup.

Reconstructive surgery as previously discussed, is used to help correct skin scars and abnormalities that are caused by accidents, disease, or congenital (birth) defects.

These procedures vary greatly, due to the many differences in the problems being treated. Plastic surgeons often remove facial skin cancers, using their skills to best conceal the demarcations from these treatments.

Often there is no time for pretreatment of these areas. The patient normally sees the esthetician after the surgery has occurred. Often seeking makeup help the patient is frequently referred by the surgeon for help with concealing scars from the surgery. Sometimes several operations may have to take place to help revise scars from accidents or skin cancer. Makeup help may be required for coverage during and between these operations.

We will not discuss the correction of these types of scars here. The esthetician should take specialty courses in paramedical camouflage makeup in order to help these patients.

Referrals

The plastic surgery candidate will often first seek counseling from the esthetician. Carefully evaluate the client's concerns, and then refer the client to a plastic surgeon. Because plastic cosmetic surgery is an elective procedure, the client will often want to think about the possibility of surgery for some time before proceeding.

You should have brochures available from your referring surgeon that briefly describe the various types of surgery. Plastic surgeons will gladly furnish these at no charge to you once you have established a working relationship.

You should have a working understanding with the plastic surgeon of each other's procedures and needs. Prepare a pre- and postsurgical brochure discussing esthetic procedures and how they help plastic surgery patients. Work with your plastic surgeon on this brochure, so that both of you are involved and are knowledgeable about typical procedures. When in doubt about treating a cosmetic or plastic surgery patient, always consult the doctor!

Many workshops and classes are available on paramedical makeup and working with plastic surgeons. You should take these courses to best prepare yourself for working with a plastic surgeon.

1. What is the difference between cosmetic and reconstructive surgery?

2. What are the various types of physicians who perform plastic surgery?

3. What are some general postoperative skin-care procedures that should be avoided?

4. Why is it important for the plastic surgery patient to have presurgical skin-care treatments?

5. What should the esthetician do when there is a question about a treatment procedure for a plastic surgery patient?

6. Discuss preparing a brochure about esthetic treatment for a plastic surgery patient. Why is it important for both the esthetician and the plastic surgeon to be involved in preparing such a brochure?

20

Recognize and Refer Medical Conditions

The esthetician should be trained to recognize common medical conditions and diseases of the skin and refer them to the proper medical authority—in most cases the dermatologist.

This chapter is designed to illustrate and briefly discuss some of the medical conditions that the esthetician may observe in routine practice. While not all of these conditions are life-threatening, many skin conditions need to be referred to the dermatologist for proper medical treatment.

The esthetician will often have clients who come to the salon for treatment of what they may think is a cosmetic disorder, but is actually a dermatological condition. The esthetician should never diagnose a medical condition, but should be able to recognize conditions that require medical treatment. The esthetician should be well educated about the different types of common skin diseases and conditions and should be able to discuss conditions with the dermatologist. The esthetician should also be familiar with the cosmetic effects of certain skin disorders and know how they can help with cosmetic symptoms that the client may need to conceal.

This chapter will teach you about medical conditions that need medical referral. You should always refer any condition that you do not understand or that is obviously not just a minor cosmetic problem.

Before discussing the medical conditions in this chapter, it is important to discuss common medical terminology—specifically dermatological terminology. The medical community has very precise descriptions for symptoms of the skin. Using these specific terms, dermatologists can very accurately describe lesions and therefore diagnose illnesses more efficiently. (The author wishes to thank Rube Pardo, M.D., Ph.D., of the Department of Dermatology at the University of Miami, for his assistance in preparing this section on dermatological terminology.)

Primary and Secondary Lesions

Primary lesions of the skin are lesions that are in the early stages of development. A **lesion** is any mark on the skin that is not a normal part of the skin. It does not necessarily mean that the skin is diseased. A freckle is a lesion; so is a wrinkle. However, lesions can also be symptoms of disease, such as melanoma, shingles, or measles.

Secondary lesions are lesions that primary lesions eventually become.

Macules are flat (nonelevated) marks on the skin in which there is only a change in the normal color of the skin. Again, a freckle can be an example of a macule, and the flat red mark left after a pimple has healed is also a macule. It is simply a descriptive term meaning that this is a flat area with a change in the normal color of the skin. The adjective used to describe a lesion is macular. Large macules, larger than 1 centimeter, are called **patches**. **Papules** are raised areas on the skin that are generally smaller than one centimeter. **Plaques** are papules that are larger than 1 centimeter.

Nodules are raised lesions that are larger and deep in the skin. A nodule looks like a lump, but the skin can be moved over the lesion. Very large nodules are called **tumors**.

A **pustule** is a lesion that is filled with pus, which we have previously discussed in the chapter on acne. Extremely deep infections with pockets of pus are called **abcesses**.

Vesicle is the medical term for blisters. They contain body fluids. A **bulla** is a large vesicle. A vesicle or bulla, that has ruptured so that the fluid is exposed to the surface of the skin is said to be weeping or oozing.

A **wheal** is a hive. Wheals are caused by a concentration of fluid in the tissue. Wheals are reabsorbed into the bloodstream via the lymphatic system.

Erosion refers to a shallow depression in the skin. Scratches on the skin are called **excoriations**, which we have already discussed in the acne chapter. Deep erosions are called **ulcers**, in which part of the dermis has been lost.

Diseased skin often has remnants of body fluids, pus, or blood caked to a lesion. This is described as **crust**.

Scales are patches of dry, dehydrated skin, without crust.

Erythema refers to any area of redness associated with a lesion. Bruises are known as **hematomas**. **Purpura** are hemorrhages of the blood vessels.

Atrophy means wasting away. Skin that has thinned from age or chronic sun exposure is said to have atrophied. **Hypertrophy** is thickening of a tissue. Hypertrophic scars are raised scars, due to thickening of the tissue. **Atrophic** scars are depressed scars, such as acne pocks, caused by loss of tissue.

A number of terms are used to describe the shapes of certain lesions. A **linear** lesion is a line-like lesion. A ring-shaped lesion is called **annular**. Lesions that have a snake-like pattern are called **sepiginous**. **Geographic** lesions look like a map. **Target** or **iris** lesions have a center with a round surrounding area, such as a pustule.

Keratosis is a general term meaning a thickening of the stratum corneum, such as seborrheic keratosis, described in the chapter on sun damage.

Eczematization refers to a combination of symptoms including erythema, weeping, crusting, and present vesicles.

A **nevus** is a mole. More than one mole are described as nevi. **Lentigines** are freckles. **Hyperpigmentation** refers to any condition that has more than the normal amount of melanin. **Hypopigmentation** refers to any area with less than the normal amount of pigment.

Acne

We have already thoroughly discussed acne in Chapter 13. Severe acne requires medical attention. Grade 4 acne is severe inflammatory acne with cystic lesions. Cysts should always be referred to the dermatologist. The medical treatments for cysts include injections with steroids, which help to shrink the lesion. Some cysts may be lanced by the dermatologist and drained. Both topical and oral antibiotics may be used to help control inflammatory acne conditions. Common topical preparations may include the antibiotics erythromycin (tradename ATS®) or clindamycin (tradename CleocinT®). These preparations are available only by prescription and are liquid roll-ons that are applied to the skin either daily or twice daily. The doctor may suggest that the client not use certain cosmetic products that will increase irritation. Frequently dermatologists will prescribe prescription keratolytic products such as prescription-strength benzoyl peroxide treatments or retinoic acid (Retin-A). These products are discussed in detail in Chapter 13.

Other acne-related medical conditions include *acne rosacea, perioral dermatitis*, and *seborrheic dermatitis*, which are all also discussed in Chapter 13.

Common Infections of the Skin

Infections of the skin may be grouped into three types: bacterial, fungal, and viral.

Common Bacterial Infections

Impetigo is a skin infection that is commonly seen on the face, particularly in the lower part of the face, but it can occur anywhere. This disease is characterized by large, open, weeping lesions. They look like large sores, similar to acne, except that impetigo lesions weep and appear damp. The lesions can range in size. Impetigo is frequently seen in children and is extremely contagious. Impetigo is caused by a staphylococcus bacteria. The disease is treated by the use of antibiotics (Figure 20-1).

FIGURE 20–1 Impetigo is commonly seen on the face. *Courtesy Timothy G. Berger, M.D.*

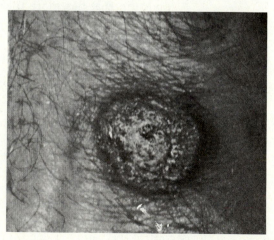

Folliculitis is a bacterial infection of the hair follicle. The infection results in irritation and is characterized by multiple pinpoint irritations around the pore openings (Figure 20-2). **Pseudofolliculitis** is caused by irritation from shaving. It also appears as irritated follicles, but is not usually infected. Ingrown hairs are the main cause of pseudofolliculitis, seen frequently in the beard area of male clients, especially the neck.

FIGURE 20–2 Folliculitis on the back. *Courtesy Rube J. Pardo, M.D., Ph.D.*

A more severe infection of the hair follicle is called a **furuncle**, also known as a boil. Large boils often result in abcesses and are referred to as *carbuncles*. Folliculitis, furuncles, and carbuncles are treated with antibiotics. If a furuncle or carbuncle bursts on the inside of the lesion, the bacteria may enter the bloodstream, causing *septicemia*, also known as blood poisoning. Septicemia is characterized by a red erythemic line running from the source of primary infection. Septicemia is extremely serious, and should be treated immediately by a physician. **Cellulitis** is a deep infection of the dermis, caused by streptococcus (Figure 20-3). A severe form of cellulitis is called *erysipelas*, also known as St. Anthony's Fire. Again, this is extremely serious and should be seen immediately by a physician.

Fungal Skin Infections

There are a large number of fungal infections of the skin. Fungal infections are called **mycoses**.

Tinea versicolor is sometimes called *sun fungus*. It is often seen on the backs and chests of persons who are tan. Tinea versicolor inhibits the production of melanin in the skin, which results in its appearance as white patches. It is not actually directly related to sun exposure, but is often seen on tanned persons, because the skin will not tan in the areas where tinea versicolor is active. The disease is easily treated with the use of antifungal prescription medications.

Tinea pedis is commonly known as *athlete's foot*, which is a fungal infection of the skin on the foot. The disease is character-

FIGURE 20–3 Facial cellulitis. Note the severe swelling and inflammation. *Courtesy Rube J. Pardo, M.D., Ph.D.*

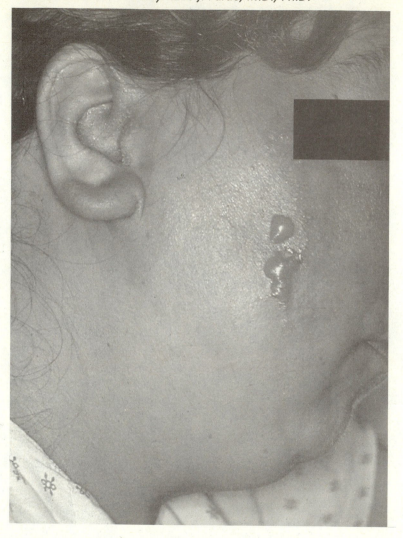

ized by severe itching and scaling, particularly on the sole of the foot. Again, tinea pedis is easily treated by the use of antifungal prescription medications (Figure 20-4).

Tinea corporis is better known by the public as ringworm. It can occur on any area of the body and presents itself as a ring-like lesion.

Tinea infections are extremely contagious and should be treated promptly.

Candidas are yeast infections. They can cause a variety of skin infections. Oral thrush, seen often in infants and persons with

FIGURE 20—4 Tinea corporis infection on the leg. *Courtesy Rube J. Pardo, M.D., Ph.D.*

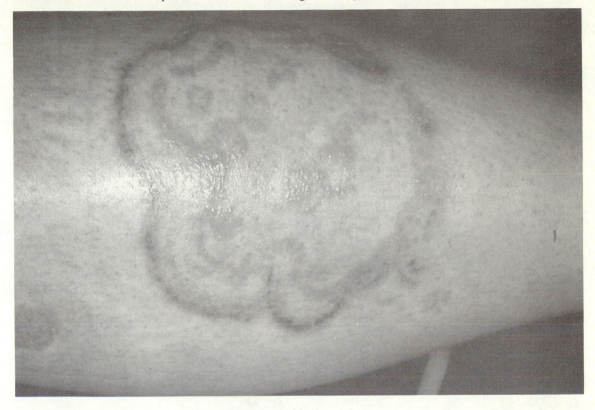

suppressed immune systems, such as AIDS patients, is a yeast infection of the mouth characterized by white patches inside the mouth.

Viral Skin Infections

Herpes refers to a group of viruses. Herpes simplex is the cause of common cold sores, which generally appear on or around the mouth and often appear as oozing red ulcers (Figure 20-5). They are very contagious, and should be treated by a physician. Facial treatments should be avoided for clients with active lesions. Certain facial treatments, such as chemical peels have been know to cause a flareup of the herpes virus.

Herpes zoster, better known as *shingles*, is caused by the same virus that causes chicken pox. Herpes zoster is harboured by the nervous system and generally follows a pattern along the nerves in the skin. The lesions of herpes zoster look like multiple red blisters (Figure 20-6). Subjective symptoms may include burning, tingling, or numbness, and severe cases can result in extreme pain. Minor infections can be only a nuisance, and the disease subsides by itself. However, the infection can reoccur and in some cases causes scarring and pain due to nerve inflam-

FIGURE 20–5 Herpes simplex causes common cold sores. *Courtesy Timothy G. Berger, M.D.*

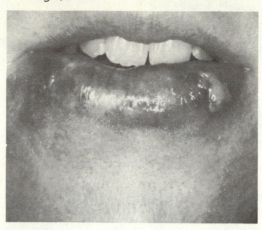

FIGURE 20–6 Typical case of herpes zoster (shingles). Note the lesions follow a typical nerve-route pattern. *Courtesy Rube J. Pardo, M.D., Ph.D.*

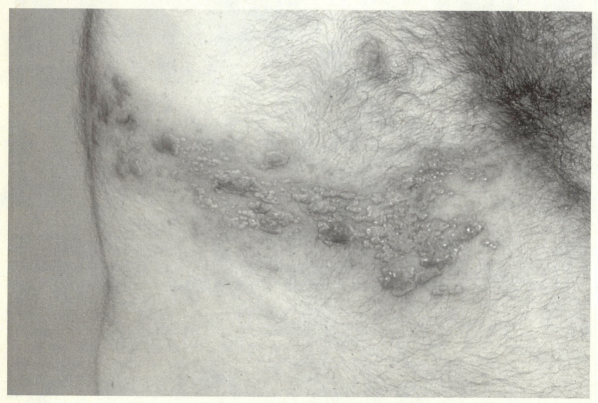

mation. There is no cure for herpes zoster, although there are some prescriptions helpful in controlling it. Herpes zoster is another infection that may be especially a problem in immuno-suppressed individuals, such as AIDS patients.

Molloscum contagiosum is a viral infection frequently seen on the faces of children, which appears as groups of small, flesh-colored papules. They often resemble milia, but are in groups or clusters and are hard to the touch (Figure 20-7). They must be treated by a physician.

FIGURE 20–7 Molloscum contagiosum. *Courtesy Melvin L. Elson, M.D.*

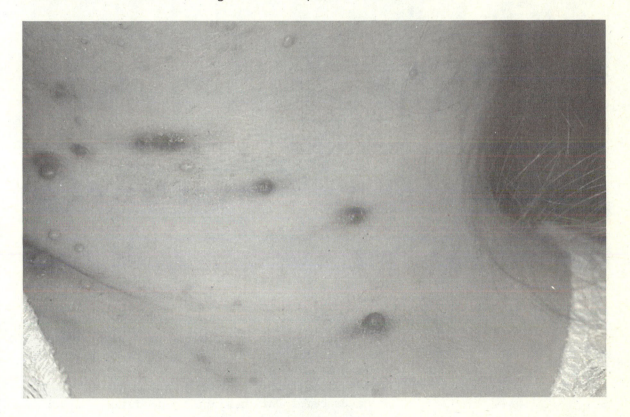

One of the most frequent viral lesions seen are warts. **Warts** are caused by a variety of viruses known as *papovaviruses* or *veruccae*. Wart treatment varies with the lesion, including topical acid therapy using salicylic acid or trichloroacetic acid. Other dermatologic treatments include freezing the lesions with liquid nitrogen or cautery with an electric needle. Warts are contagious, especially to the same individual, and can be spread to another area of the body easily. Warts may be seen by the esthetician on the face, feet, and hands, especially the nails, and should be referred to a dermatologist for treatment (Figure 20-8).

FIGURE 20–8 Warts. *Courtesy Rube J. Pardo, M.D., Ph.D.*

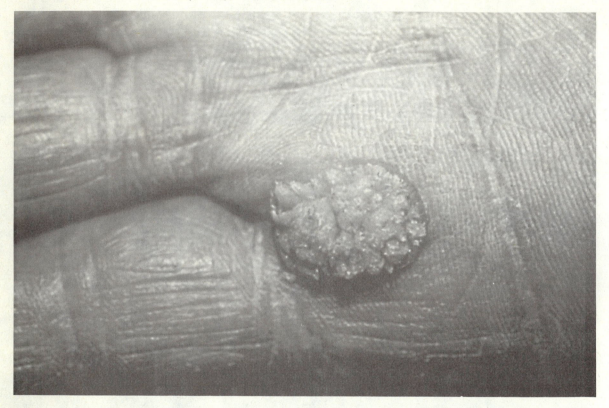

Pityriasis rosea is a patchy, red, rashlike disorder. It can occur anywhere on the body, but is frequently seen on the trunk. Groups of patches may develop. Many outbreaks resemble the pattern of a Christmas tree on the trunk. There is no real cure for pityriasis rosea, but it usually subsides after a few weeks. Itching associated with infection can be treated with topical prescription steroid creams (Figure 20-9).

Common Reactions, Rashes, and Irritations

In the chapter on allergies we have already discussed common allergies that the esthetician sees routinely. **Dermatitis** means inflammation of the skin. It is a descriptive term used to

FIGURE 20–9 Pityriasis rosea. *Courtesy Melvin L. Elson, M.D.*

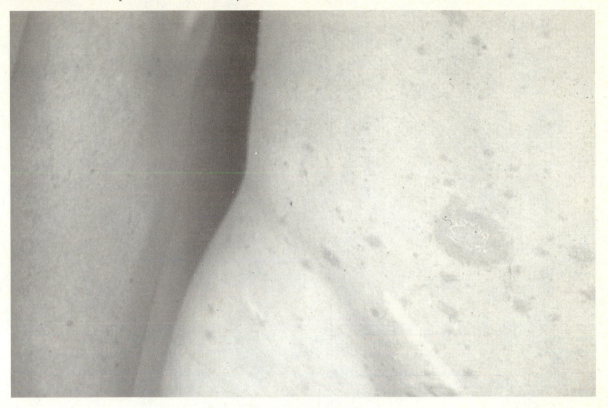

describe many different types of skin inflammation and irritation. Dermatitis is an irritation, rather than a disease. It is generally not caused by pathological organisms, such as infections caused by viruses, bacteria, and fungi. Many of the other terms already discussed in this chapter are used as adjectives to describe different types and patterns of dermatitis.

Contact Dermatitis

Contact dermatitis is probably the most common form of dermatitis observed by the esthetician. Contact dermatitis is an irritation caused by either an allergic reaction or irritation to something or some substance touching the skin or coming in contact with the skin's surface. Cosmetics are a frequent cause of contact dermatitis. Other frequent causes of contact dermatitis include jewelry, laundry products, clothing fabrics and dyes, plants (such as poison ivy), and other substances (Figure 20-10).

There are two basic treatments for contact dermatitis. The first, of course, is to avoid contact with the offending substance. This is sometimes hard to pinpoint, because we touch so many substances on a daily basis. Often the dermatologist can tell much about the source of irritation by the location of the dermatitis. Irri-

FIGURE 20–10 (a) Contact dermatitis in a hairdresser due to parapheneline-diamine. (b) Contact dermatitis due to nickel allergy. *Courtesy Rube J. Pardo, M.D., Ph.D.*

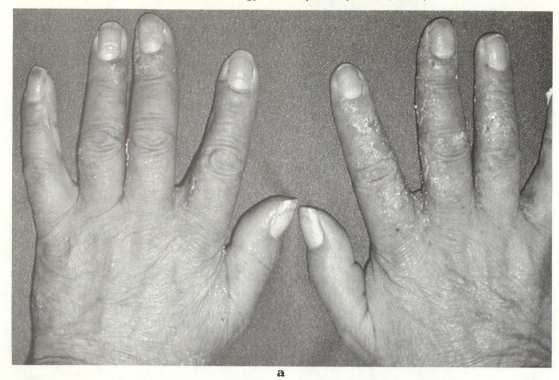

a

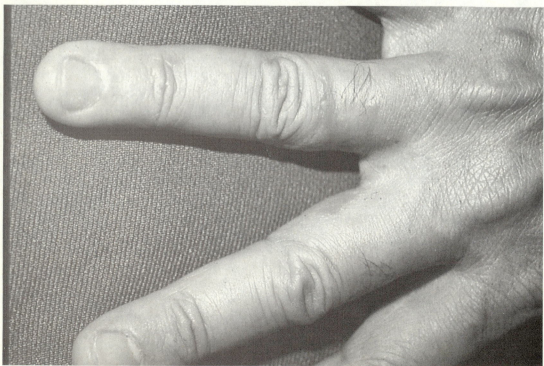

b

tation of the hands is often caused by household products. Health and personal care professionals, including estheticians, often suffer from dermatitis related to substances they touch at work.

Irritation from hand washes, disinfectants and antiseptics, and even allergies to latex gloves are frequently seen in these professionals. Estheticians also come in contact with a large number of cosmetic products, which can also be a source of irritation.

The process of eliminating the offending substance is often a matter of trial and error, eliminating one or all substances and testing by slowly adding steps of substance contact. Allergies are sometimes easier to detect. The dermatologist can often run allergy patch tests, and allergies have a tendency to be more acute, or sudden, than irritation dermatitis.

Topical steroid creams are often prescribed by the dermatologist to ease the symptoms of allergic or irritant dermatitis. These prescription creams usually work fairly quickly, assuming that the source of irritation has also been eliminated.

Dermatitis can have many characteristics visually, but is usually red (erythemic), and often itchy or burning. The term *eczema* refers to the same condition as *dermatitis.*

Atopic Dermatitis

Atopic eczema or dermatitis is a more complicated form of dermatitis. It is a more severe and chronic condition, and is associated, in most cases, with heredity. It may be affected by illness, stress, and other changes. Some patients suffer with atopic dermatitis all their lives.

Atopic eczema can be controlled with the use of prescription steroid creams and oral antihistamines. Cosmetologically, the atopic eczema patient will be more likely to have irritant reactions to cosmetics. If you have a client with atopic eczema, discuss any cosmetics with the client's doctor. In general, stick to fragrance-free, simple products—the simpler the better, and the fewer ingredients, the better. Use the same care as discussed in the chapter on allergies and sensitive skin.

Occasionally you may notice a rash following a pattern on the face that does not clear up. Rashes in a butterfly pattern across the cheeks can be a symptom of lupus erythematosus. We have already discussed lupus in the chapter on the immune system. If you notice a recurrent rash on a client's face, you should refer the client to a physician, as you should all rashes and chronic redness (Figure 20-11).

Psoriasis

Psoriasis is an inflammatory disorder of the skin that is caused by the skin and epidermis "turning over" faster than it does in a normal individual. Largely hereditary, it can be chronic and last over a

FIGURE 20–11 Discoid lesion in systemic lupus. *Courtesy Rube J. Pardo, M.D., Ph.D.*

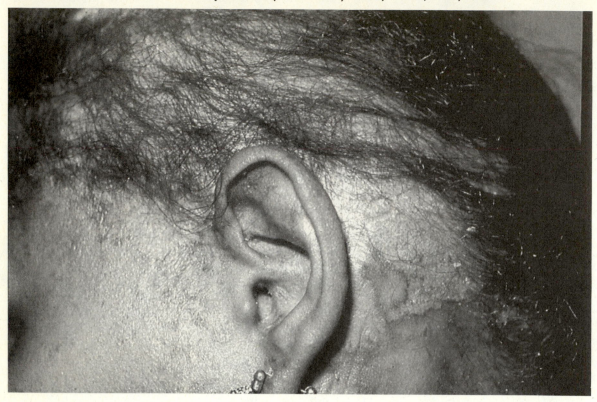

lifetime. The disorder is not contagious and is not related to any pathological organism. It is a disorder, not a disease (Figure 20-12).

Psoriasis primarily affects the skin on the body and is often symmetrical, which means it occurs simultaneously on both sides of the body in the same place. It often affects the elbows, the knees, and other extremities.

Treatments used to control psoriasis include steroid creams, antihistamines, and light therapy using controlled exposures of UVA. Some new oral drugs are also being used to treat chronic cases

Urticaria

An outbreak of **urticaria**, or hives, is due to allergies. Urticaria often quickly fades without treatment, but the source of the allergy should be identified. Dermatologists use topical steroids, oral steroids, antihistamines, and allergy testing to treat and identify causes of urticaria.

Keratosis Pilaris

Keratosis pilaris is a condition in which the skin exhibits redness and irritation in patches, accompanied by a rough texture, and small pinpoint white papules that look like very small milia. Keratosis pilaris is often found on the cheeks and upper

FIGURE 20–12 Psoriasis. *Courtesy Rube J. Pardo, M.D., Ph.D.*

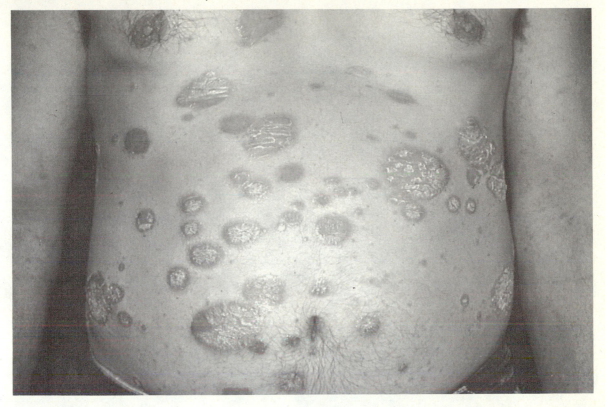

arms. It is often seen in children and teenagers, but can affect any age group. In most cases, it is a nuisance disorder. Doctors have been successful in treating keratosis pilaris with glycolic or lactic acid solutions, but it often goes away by itself.

Telangectasias are enlarged or broken capillaries, often referred to as *couperose* by European estheticians. Telangectasias are permanent and are caused by a variety of factors including chronic sun exposure, exposure to extreme temperatures, friction, or injury to the skin. They can also be caused or worsened by use of vasodilators, which are drugs or substances that cause dilation of the blood vessels. Included in the category of vasodilators are tobacco and alcohol. Alcoholics often have many telangectatic vessels. Treatment ranges from freezing and electrocautery to laser and injection of saline (salt) solution. Most telangectasias are only a beauty nuisance, but clients with multiple telangectasias should be referred to a dermatologist for treatment or evaluation.

Growths

We have already discussed solar-induced growths of the skin. These include sebaceous hyperplasias, seborrheic keratoses, basal and squamous cell carcinomas, solar lentigenes, and melanoma. Solar-induced skin growths are seen frequently by estheticians.

You should review the chapter on sun damage and be very familiar with identifying these growths, especially cancers and pre-cancers.

Skin tags are very small, threadlike growths. They are frequently seen on the eyelids, neck, and decollete. They are benign lesions, but frequently are irritated by jewelry or clothing, rubbing against them. Most people find them unattractive, and they should be removed. They are easily removed by the dermatologist using freezing, electric needle, or scissors (Figure 20-13).

FIGURE 20–13 Skin tags are often seen on the neck and in the chest area. *Courtesy Michael J. Bond, M.D.*

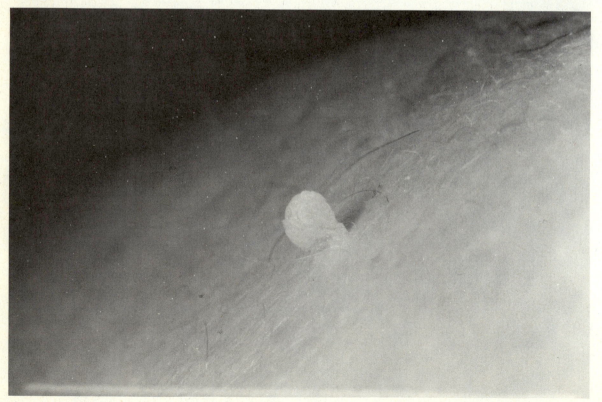

Skin tags are largely hereditary, and have been associated with pregnancy, post-menopause, diabetes, and intestinal disorders. These medical associations are another reason that skin tags should be seen by a physician.

Xanthomas or **xanthalasmas** are fatty pockets found on the eyelids. They look like large closed comedones, and are frequently found on the upper and lower lids. They are somewhat flat and are usually oval or egg-shaped.

Xanthalasmas should be referred to a dermatologist for removal by extraction or excision. They are often associated with high cholesterol, and often the dermatologist will order tests to determine cholesterol levels.

We have only touched on the many disorders and diseases that can affect the skin. We have however, discussed many conditions frequently observed by the practicing esthetician.

Again, this chapter should educate you, to recognize symptoms that could indicate conditions that should be referred to a dermatologist or other appropriate physician. Estheticians treat cosmetic disorders of the skin. They should never attempt to diagnose or treat a disease or medical disorder.

Always refer any suspicious rash, growth, or other abnormality to a dermatologist.

TOPICS FOR DISCUSSION

1. What is the difference between a primary and a secondary lesion?
2. What are some common infections of the skin? What are their causes?
3. What are some common fungal infections?
4. Use your knowledge of dermatological terminology to describe a grade 3 acne condition.
5. Why should estheticians be familiar with common forms of skin disease?

21

Medical Relations

The esthetician and the medical doctor can beautifully complement each other's work. It is important to learn to work with doctors, especially dermatologists and plastic surgeons.

In this chapter you will learn about medical relations, and you will learn important factors in having good relationships with the medical community. We will also discuss common problems between the two professions and what you can do to make these relationships successful.

More and more estheticians routinely work with physicians, usually dermatologists and plastic surgeons. In many instances estheticians work in the offices of doctors.

This chapter will address how esthetics and medicine relate. Specifically, we will discuss how physician-esthetician relationsships work and how to establish working relationships with members of the medical community.

How Estheticians Work with Physicians

Estheticians can provide many services that complement a medical practice. For example, estheticians can provide deep cleansing facial treatments for acne patients and problem skin clients who also receive medical treatment from a dermatologist. Estheticians can help educate the patient about home care and can help recommend proper home care. They can also teach clients how to cope with the cosmetic side effects of many dermatological drugs.

The dermatologist may refer a client to an esthetician for help choosing noncomedogenic cosmetics or they may ask the esthetician to find a cosmetic that will work for a specific client without certain ingredients to which the patient may be allergic.

Paramedical camouflage makeup cases are often referred by dermatologists.

There are literally hundreds of reasons that estheticians and dermatologists should work together!

Patient Referrals from the Esthetician

You are in a position, seeing dozens of clients a week, to send many referrals to the dermatologist for problems such as cysts, rashes, allergies, possible skin cancers, sun damage, and other skin afflictions that we have discussed in the previous chapter. So many skin diseases and abnormalities require medical care. Always refer any cases that you are not sure about!

Medical Training

Let us discuss the kinds of doctors you may work with and what kind of training they have.

Dermatologists are specialists in the diseases of the skin, hair, and nails. They treat diseases, while estheticians treat cosmetic disorders. They study for four years of college and then four years of medical school, at which time they are awarded the Medical Doctor degree (M.D.). After medical school, they generally have a year of internship and then two to four years of specialty residency in dermatology. They train under dermatologists at major hospitals or universities. After all these years of training, they take their board exam in dermatology, administered by the American Academy of Dermatology, the professional association for dermatologists. This special certification is what dermatologists refer to when they say they are board-certified.

Dermatologists may also sub-specialize in several fields. MOHS surgeons have further specialty training in micrographic surgery, a specialized form of surgery for hard-to-treat skin cancers. Other dermatologists may be dermatological surgeons, specializing in skin surgery, or may practice plastic surgery.

Another up-and-coming field in dermatology is cosmetic dermatology. This field certainly relates well to the field of esthetics. These dermatologists have specialty training in cosmetic disorders and diseases of the skin and have a good understanding of human appearance and beauty. Cosmetic dermatologists generally have a really good understanding of esthetics and the needs of the esthetic client.

Plastic surgeons have four years of college and four years of medical school, internship, and then several years of residency in plastic surgery.

Qualifications for board exams and the different types of physicians who practice plastic surgery have already been discussed in Chapter 19.

Other Doctors

Besides dermatologists and plastic surgeons, there are other types of doctors that estheticians should be acquainted with and be able to refer cases to. Generally these physicians are M.D.'s who are board certified in their various fields of specialty.

Endocrinologists specialize in treatment of diseases of the endocrine system. The glandular system, if it is diseased, can seriously affect the skin. Thyroid or adrenal disorders, for example, can affect the skin, hair, and nails. **Rheumatologists** are specialists in rheumatoid diseases, including lupus.

Internists specialize in the treatment of internal diseases, including heart problems, diabetes, and other internal afflictions. Clients who have body massage may need referral to orthopedic surgeons, neurologists, or chiropractors. Cosmetic dentists, who specialize in the treatment of cosmetic disorders of the mouth and teeth, can also help make the client look better.

Your First Contact with a Physician

You must establish contact with a physician in order to have a working relationship. Many doctors are not familiar with estheticians or their training. This is why it is so important to have a complete resume listing all your credentials. You should also list any specialty you have and any additional degrees you may hold. List only academic training. In other words, do not list particular product training that you may have had, unless it includes training in a specialized area, such as acne, paramedical camouflage, comedogenicity, etc.

Make sure you list all the positions you have held, any professional affiliations, such as membership in esthetic organizations, and special awards. Make sure your resume looks very professional. It may be beneficial to contact a resume service organization, to help you write it.

What Doctors Like...and Don't

Doctors have very serious, scientific training. They generally do not have much training in artistic fields and are not well-acquainted with special techniques in the esthetics field. Be specific about what kind of special training you have had. Doctors are trained in the scientific method—make sure you read the chapter on the scientific approach. This will help you better understand why doctors are sometimes skeptical about estheticians.

Sometimes it may seem that doctors do not care much about esthetics. Often a doctor is more concerned about a patient's medical condition than about a cosmetic problem. Medical concerns outweigh cosmetic concerns. In other words, a physical reaction is more important than how something looks. If a patient has skin cancer, for example, getting rid of the cancer outweighs how the skin will look after medical treatment. Ideally, of course, both factors will be taken into consideration, but the patient's life and medical condition is always first!

Doctors in general are impressed with estheticians who have a good working knowledge of dermatology and how the human body functions in general. It helps to have additional training in other medically related fields. Estheticians who are also nurses, for example, often do very well working with dermatologists. If you have a good background in a science-related field, it will help you greatly when communicating with physicians. Doctors also appreciate it when an esthetician is scientific in an approach to cosmetic treatment. Examples of this are practicing clinically, using sterile techniques, using time-tested methods, and respecting when a client needs dermatological care, rather than esthetic care.

The biggest dislike of dermatologists, and doctors in general, is unscientific, "miraculous" approaches to beauty. If you make exaggerated claims or always tout the latest "miracle" treatment, you will not get much respect from the medical community. "Natural" treatments also raise medical eyebrows. There are advantages and disadvantages to using "natural" products. As one prominent dermatologist said, "Tuberculosis is natural, and so are scorpions!" For more information on why "natural" is not always best, read the chapter on allergies.

The bottom line is that doctors are honest with patients and expect the same from you. They know that neither of you can perform miracles. Be honest with your medical colleagues. Admit when you don't understand something. And don't act as if you are the dermatologist's equal. You are in entirely different, related fields.

The Interview

Call and make an appointment with the dermatologist to talk. Explain to the receptionist who you are and briefly why you would like to talk to the dermatologist. If the receptionist is hesitant about making the appointment, leave a message for the doctor to call you. If the doctor returns your call, ask for an appointment to come by and talk.

Remember, not all doctors understand what estheticians do. Briefly explain what services you perform and your particular specialties. Bring your resume. You may want to bring a good book with you to show what kind of education you have had.

Ask if the doctor has any particular specialties, and suggest working with you. Relax and get to know the doctor as a person. You will often find you have more in common than you think.

Ask the dermatologist for any patient brochures distributed in the office. Familiarize yourself with these brochures and any other patient education materials the doctor uses routinely. This will acquaint you with the doctor's techniques and may also give you an idea of how you could fit into the practice.

Invite the doctor to visit your salon. Offer a free treatment, and after the treatment offer some samples of free products. Do everything just as you normally would. Tell the doctor that you will act as if he or she was any other client. This way the doctor will see how you really work. Most dermatologists are actually very impressed with a good facial treatment. You might also offer a free treatment to the doctor's nurse or assistant. They often are involved with patient education in the office!

After you get to know the doctor you may ask if you may observe some procedures. Spending a day with a dermatologist is a truly enlightening experience! You will see cases you never see in the salon, and you will leave with a better understanding of medicine in general.

Doctor's Concerns

Allergies

Have a good understanding of how allergies develop and how irritation occurs. Dermatologists see a lot of allergic reactions and a lot of contact dermatitis. Be knowledgeable about common cosmetic ingredient allergies and patch testing. Ask the doctor to help you understand the method of allergy testing.

Comedogenic Cosmetics

This is an area where you can really win a dermatologist over. If you have a good understanding of comedogenicity and acne, you can provide an excellent service to the dermatologist, helping patients find noncomedogenic, nonacnegenic cosmetics and skin-care products.

Sun Damage

Dermatologists are impressed if you have a good knowledge of skin cancer and sun damage. They will be equally unimpressed if you offer tanning sessions in your salon!

Electrolysis

Here is another excellent service for esthetic referral. Dermatologists see a lot of cases of unwanted hair that may be a result of another medical condition. Electrolysis is generally very well accepted by dermatologists, and doctors in general.

Paramedical Makeup

In general, you will receive more referrals for paramedical makeup from doctors than for any other service you perform. You must be trained to do paramedical camouflage makeup. Doctors will frequently refer patients with scars, birthmarks, accident victims, post-skin-cancer treatment patients, and patients with disfigurements for help with makeup. Do not be discouraged if this is all they refer at first. Eventually one of those patients will have skin-care treatments and will return to the doctor with glowing results and comments!

Extraction

Dermatologists often refer patients for treatment of comedones. They are often already treating the patients with other prescription drugs. Knowing how to treat these patients will help you prove yourself to the doctor. Discuss your extraction techniques with the doctor and set up a list of rules for various types of patients.

Retinoic Acid

Retinoic acid (Retin-A) is frequently prescribed by dermatologists. You must know how to work with these patients. See the chapter on acne and on retinoids for further information.

Seborrhea and Other Inflammations

The doctor will be interested in how you deal with the patient who has a history of seborrheic dermatitis or other dermatitis.

Perhaps you are lucky enough to have attended a school that has a lecturing dermatologist on staff. This type of learning experience is extremely valuable preparation for working with a dermatologist. Try to take continuing education classes with dermatologists or take classes that address some of the pertinent topics we have discussed as being important issues to them. Read all that you can, obtaining brochures and purchasing dermatology textbooks to study on your own. There are several condensed versions of these types of texts, and a variety of good books are available, written in easy-to-understand language, that discuss common dermatological problems.

Some pharmaceutical companies are progressive enough to offer training to allied health professionals, including estheticians. Many of these programs are new, and more will, no doubt, be offered in the future. Many of the esthetician's journals offer regular interviews with medical experts and frequently contain articles about the subjects we have discussed. Taking a course in medical terminology is also a good idea so you will better understand medical language.

How to Refer a Client

When you notice that a client has a problem that needs referral, tell the client to call your referring dermatologist for an appointment. Send the dermatologist a referral slip telling about your client, why you are referring the client, and what services you have been performing to help the client. Many doctors will return a referral letter letting you know what their diagnosis was and what treatment they have prescribed. In this letter they will tell you what should be done in the salon as a followup. Occasionally a dermatologist will tell a client not to have esthetic services for a period of time. This should be explained in the doctor's letter, as well as the reason for this recommendation. Sometimes, particularly if the patient has minor skin surgery, or has recurrent dermatitis, or has a communicable disease, it is necessary to discontinue esthetic treatment.

Some Common Problems

Many estheticians have discussed problems they often have in their relationships with dermatologists. Many of these are caused by miscommunication between the doctor and the esthetician. This is why it is so important to have an open line of communication with the dermatologist. We will discuss some of the most common complaints estheticians have about dermatologists and the common problems dermatologists have with estheticians.

Why Do Dermatologists Only Recommend Certain Product Lines?

Just as you are educated about certain product lines, dermatologists receive training about certain products. Drug companies sponsor product knowledge classes and workshops, just as cosmetic companies do. So it is only natural that the doctor recommend familiar products. An esthetician would not recommend unfamiliar products either.

Doctors recommend what is widely available to their patients. They also recommend products they know their patients can afford. Dermatologists are particular about many allergy-causing, comedogenic, or irritancy-inducing chemicals used in cosmetics. Therefore it is important that you have products available that meet these standards. You should try to have available moderately priced, noncomedogenic, hypoallergenic cosmetics that are as fragrance-free as possible. Dermatologists are concerned about allergies, and fragrances frequently cause allergies. This does not mean that this type of product is all you should carry, but you certainly should have a specialty line available for this type of client. Furnish information to dermatologists about your products, and furnish them with some sample products to try themselves.

Why Do Dermatologists Always Recommend Soap and Water?

Soap and water is readily available to most patients in all income groups. Soaps that dermatologists recommend rarely cause allergy problems. Soaps are more rinseable than many cleansing milks, an important factor in treating skin problems. Talk to the dermatologist about recommending rinseable "soapless" soaps, which have the same rinseability as soap, but without the residues and possible higher pH. Again, you should have this type of product available, and it should be fragrance-free.

When I Send a Client to a Dermatologist, the Client Doesn't Come Back to the Salon!

This could result from different situations. First, get the doctor to agree to send you a referral letter letting you know about the client's progress, if esthetic treatment should be discontinued, and, most importantly, why.

Occasionally a client will find that the visit to the dermatologist solves the problem and simply elects not to return to the salon at that time.

Occasionally you will discover that you are working with an "esthetician-basher!" The best way to deal with this kind of doctor is to find another doctor who you can work with!

Dermatologists' Problems with Estheticians

Here are some common complaints dermatologists have about estheticians.

The Esthetician Is Not Scientific

To fully understand this, please read the chapter on the scientific approach. Many products on the market were developed based on anecdotal evidence, which is not scientifically sound. If you use and recommend products with exaggerated claims, or that have no scientific basis, this is a problem for many dermatologists. The solution to this problem is to carry products that are as scientific as possible and that do not make unbelievable claims.

The Esthetician Uses Products that Are Too Heavy or Comedogenic

Both of these are "no-no"'s with dermatologists. As previously discussed, carry a good line of lightweight, fragrance-free, non-comedogenic cosmetics.

Patients Complain that
the Esthetician Is "Hard-Sell"

An esthetician should never take a "hard-sell" approach, no matter what kind of client you are dealing with. Carefully evaluate each client's individual needs, as well as lifestyle, budget, and skin-care needs. You should let the doctor know the range of what your products cost so they can brief their patients.

Some patients simply cannot afford esthetic services. Medical doctors see patients with serious medical problems, many of whom may not be able to afford esthetic services. Try your best to help these patients find an affordable product that they can use at home, even if they don't visit regularly for services.

Working with
the Plastic Surgeon

Plastic surgeons are generally easier to work with than dermatologists. Cosmetic surgeons have clients who can afford elective cosmetic surgery. These clients can usually also afford esthetic services and more upscale products.

Because plastic surgery is often elective, plastic surgeons are more interested in esthetics, due to the artistic aspects of their specialty. They are interested in having their patients look as good as possible. Esthetic services "put the icing on the cake" by accentuating their work. Good skin care and proper makeup really enhances a good cosmetic surgery procedure. As previously discussed in the chapter on treating the plastic surgery patient, you should establish a relationship with a plastic surgeon and have an understanding with the surgeon about treatment procedures so that you both know what to expect from one another.

The bottom line is that good communication and a healthy respect for each others' professions is the key to a successful working medical relationship.

TOPICS FOR DISCUSSION

1. What are some services that you can provide to the dermatology patient?

2. What type of conditions might you refer to the dermatologist?

3. Discuss a physician's training.

4. Discuss scheduling a first-time meeting with a dermatologist.

5. What are common communication problems between estheticians and dermatologists?

6. Discuss some ways to improve relations between the esthetics and medical communities.

22

The Scientific Approach

Improving your education is a vital part of professional growth. Setting standards and learning to evaluate new developments is an essential part of any profession.

In this chapter we will discuss the need to be scientific in your approach to the practice of esthetics and the many educational opportunities that are available for advancement in the profession of esthetics.

Esthetics, like other health-related fields, is not an exact science. Too many factors are involved to determine the exact cause of a skin problem or to suggest an exact solution to a skin problem. So many factors are involved in any treatment involving the human body, whether the treatment is esthetic or medical. Therefore estheticians can only give a "best guess" opinion about skin conditions and what they recommend to help.

We can, however, make an educated guess, taking the time to learn as much as we can about the human body in general and the skin in particular.

The Scientific Method

The scientific method refers to the experimental technique of developing a hypothesis, or idea, based on available information. After the hypothesis is established, the method involves testing the idea and interpreting and publishing the results of the experiment. Let's look at an example. Years ago, doctors observed that certain keratolytic agents helped to peel the skin. They knew that many forms of acne were essentially caused by dead cells building up and clogging the follicles. It made sense that a keratolytic agent applied to the skin of acne patients would help loosen and remove dead cell buildup, opening the follicle and therefore increasing the oxygen content of the follicle canal. They also knew that acne bacteria could not survive in the presence of oxygen. They assembled a group of acne sufferers and experimentally applied keratolytic agents routinely to the skin of these patients. They tried to control the patients' other habits. In other words, if some of these patients were using special soaps, or vigorously scrubbing the skin, this could affect the results of the study. Factors that can affect an experiment are called *variables*. If there are too many variables in a study, it is hard to determine what causes changes that occur in an experiment.

In order to see if other factors caused changes besides the keratolytic agents, these scientists assembled a **control group**, a group of acne patients who did everything the same as the experimental group but did not apply the keratolytic. Instead they were given a product that looked the same as the keratolytic product but that did not actually contain the keratolytic. Such a product is call a *placebo*. Scientists observed that the group of acne patients that used the product with the keratolytic experienced marked improvement in their acne, whereas the group who applied the product without keratolytic had no improvement.

This method of research showed the keratolytics can help acne patients. The scientists carefully observed the number of acne lesions present on all of the patients' faces before and after the experiment. They carefully calculated the percentage of decrease in acne lesions of the group using the keratolytic and compared it to the control group. They then applied specially designed mathematical formulas to measure the differences they observed. Using this type of mathematical calculation is called **statistics**. If there is a measurable difference in factors before and after the experiment, as there was in the group using the keratolytic, the results are said to be statistically significant. The scientists then published the results of their study, and the theory of using keratolytics to help acne eventually became standard practice.

This is a very simplified example, but it illustrates the scientific method. Other factors can influence a study. The number of subjects (patients) studied is an important factor. If too few people are studied, the study will not be significant. If the study does not take place over a long enough period of time, the study will not be significant. Research like this takes a lot of time and money. Drugs may be tested for years and years before being released. Side effects and possible dangers of using the drug must also be studied. If a drug helps a certain condition, but at the same time hurts another area of the body, it often cannot be practically used. Cosmetics generally have less research performed on them than drugs. The main reason for this is money. It is very expensive to perform complicated research studies. Also, as we learned in the chapter on claims, if a cosmetic manufacturer makes a claim that it affects anything but appearance, it is considered a drug and is subject to governmental regulations that require much more research. This is why doctors often consider the need for cosmetic treatment to be questionable. Cosmetics are generally not tested nearly as extensively as drugs and therefore are not as scientifically sound as pharmaceuticals, according to many scientists.

Research on cosmetics is often performed on the ingredients rather than the product itself. The active agent is tested in the laboratory to determine its benefits, and then it is mixed with a usable vehicle, such as a cream or lotion. More and more cosmetic companies are testing their products and measuring improvement in the subjects' appearance.

If a product contains ingredients that are thought to be beneficial for the skin, this theory is called *anecdotal*. Anecdotal evidence is based on observation and theory, but the theory has not been thoroughly scientifically tested, as we discussed earlier. This doesn't mean that the product has no beneficial cosmetic effects; it simply means that the results and use are based on anecdotal, rather than scientific, findings.

An example of anecdotal information is the use of plant extracts and essential oils. There has been some scientific research in the use of these extracts, but not enough to establish scientifically significant findings for all of the many extracts that are used in cosmetics. Pharmaceutical companies frequently use chemicals that are actually extracted from plants, but the chemicals are isolated and pure, rather than using the entire extract, as many cosmetic companies do.

This brings up the subject of "natural" versus "synthetic." Natural cosmetics are regarded by some estheticians as superior to "chemicals." But plant extracts are nothing more than a group of different chemicals, because all materials on earth are made of chemicals! This is the main, and justified, argument against "natural" products. As we discussed in the allergy chapter, if a person experiences an allergic reaction to salicylic acid, it is easy to determine that the person is allergic because salicylic acid is used as an isolated chemical. But if a client has an allergic reaction to a product containing sweet birch extract, a plant source for salicylic acid, it is hard to determine if the client had a reaction to salicylic acid or to one of the many other chemicals that comprise sweet birch extract.

This example is why dermatologists are often skeptical about the use of plant extracts and essential oils in cosmetic products. In general it is accepted that the fewer and more isolated ingredients that are used in cosmetics, the less potential there is for allergic reaction.

Evaluating Products

When you talk to a manufacturer about a new product or line of products, you should try to establish how scientific the research has been on the products. Ask many questions. Has the product been evaluated as thoroughly as possible? Do their claims sound believable? Or are they using "puffing" descriptions. **Puffing** refers to using complicated descriptions of the products to describe their effects on the skin. Some companies have excellent products and still use "puffing" because they are attempting to avoid making drug claims. If a company claims that a product has an effect on the functioning of the body, it is making drug claims.

What is the company's approach to skin care? Are formulations based on current research and do they use techniques that have been time-tested? What are their developer's credentials? If they make claims for hypoallergenicity or noncomedogenicity, how are the products tested?

You must have a sound background to be able to ask good questions and evaluate a product. How do you prepare so you know what questions to ask? There are many things you can do to improve your scientific approach to skin care.

Go Back to School

Take some courses in chemistry, biology, and other sciences at your local community college or university. Start with beginning level classes. Many estheticians go back to school for additional classes and even degrees! A college degree in a related field such as health, chemistry, nutrition, or biological sciences is very helpful in the practice of esthetics. Many very successful estheticians have degrees in other related fields. You don't have to give up your practice to expand your education. More and more colleges offer night or weekend classes for working people. Some major universities now offer special two to five day classes in cosmetic sciences. One of these is the University of California at Los Angeles. For further information on this program, contact UCLA Extension.

Read Your Journals

You should subscribe to every journal in the beauty business. Contacts for magazines are listed in the bibliography section of this book.

These journals contain a wealth of information including information about the many products available to estheticians. Many excellent estheticians write for these journals, describing their good and bad experiences. There is so much you can learn each month from reading these magazines.

Buy Any Book You Can About Skin

Visit your bookstore every month and purchase any new books about skin or health. Visit your college bookstore and purchase beginning level textbooks in anatomy, chemistry, biology, and other subjects related to esthetics.

Go to Trade Shows

An extremely important learning source is trade shows! You will meet and learn from some of the top estheticians, dermatologists, chemists, and researchers in the industry!

Stay for the whole show, and attend all the classes you can. You will learn a lot from your fellow attendees. The fellowship and learning experience has no price and is an extremely valuable learning tool. But you won't meet them if you don't go to the shows!

While at the shows, talk to the exhibitors and speakers and see from whom you feel you can learn the most. Ask if they offer additional training or classes. Make arrangements to attend classes offered by these specialists. Get on their mailing lists so you can receive a calendar of upcoming events or speaking engagements.

Three types of classes are generally offered at trade shows.

General education is taught at a "main stage" routinely throughout the convention. This is included in your admission fee. Usually held in a large ballroom, speakers discuss their specialties, or there are panel discussions. These lectures are usually less than an hour each.

Manufacturer education is offered in private classrooms. This is where the manufacturers teach you about their products. Obviously manufacturers want you to buy their products after the classes. This is an excellent opportunity to evaluate new products. Remember, these lectures are usually commercial, but they are still a great way to learn more about your profession.

Workshops and seminars are often offered after the main convention. These are usually referred to as post-classes. Post-classes usually carry a separate fee and allow you to spend two or more hours with an accomplished speaker. If you read journal articles that you like or find helpful, the authors of these articles may be featured at trade-show post-classes. The education in these classes is often call generic, meaning that it is not commercially product-oriented. Spending this kind of time with a top esthetician is by far the best learning experience you can have.

Regional Seminars

Most skin-care companies have educational programs available, both product classes and general advanced esthetics classes. These classes often last a day or more and are offered frequently. Of course, this involves traveling to the city where the seminar is held, but you will usually find it very worthwhile.

Join Your Professional Associations

At the time of this writing, there are two major trade associations. The National Cosmetology Association (NCA) is the United States affiliate of CIDESCO International, the oldest and best-established esthetics organization in the world. CIDESCO helps to set standards for the industry and administers the CIDESCO International Examination, a board-certification exam for estheticians. In many European countries, estheticians attend schools that have been accredited by CIDESCO and are eligible to take the exam upon graduation. At the time of this writing, there are no CIDESCO-accredited schools in the United States. For graduates of schools that are not accredited, CIDESCO offers the "Three Year Exam." This means that if you have graduated from a licensed esthetics school, have practiced as a licensed esthetician for three years, and have been a member of the National Cosmetology Association for at least one year, you may take the exam. The exam is difficult, and you should plan on several months of preparation for the test. If you pass the test, which is both written and practical, you are awarded the CIDESCO International Diploma. Estheticians who pass the exam are called CIDESCO Diplomats. The CIDESCO diploma is accepted as the highest earned title in the world for estheticians.

The NCA also offers other examinations. The NCA offers programs on the national and state level. The Esthetics America committee is a group of accomplished estheticians who have passed the Esthetics America exam, a national level test that is administered by the NCA. There are also state-level examinations that must be passed to qualify for the national exam. For further information on NCA programs, contact NCA, 3510 Olive St., St. Louis, Missouri 63103, or call 314–534–7980.

Aestheticians International Association, 4447 McKinnney Ave., Dallas, Texas 75205, 1–800–950–8707, is another professional association. AIA also offers certification exams, the AIACA examination. They also offer special certification programs in different advanced areas.

Most professional organizations also offer special seminars, conventions and congresses, magazine subscriptions and journals, special insurance programs, and many other benefits.

Strive to obtain the highest credentials you can. There are three special secrets to being a great esthetician. You must receive the best education possible. You have to communicate well with people, and you have to, most of all, love your profession!

TOPICS FOR DISCUSSION

1. Describe the scientific method.
2. What does *statistically significant* mean?
3. What kind of factors can affect a study?

4. What is the difference between scientific and anecdotal evidence?

5. Discuss how to evaluate products.

6. Why is it important to read and subscribe to esthetic journals?

Bibliography and Recommended Readings

Bark, J. (1989). Retin-A and other youth miracles. Rocklin, Calif.: Prima Publishing.

Bevan, J. (1979). The Simon and Schuster handbook of anatomy and physiology. New York: Simon and Schuster.

Chase, D. (1989). The new medically based no-nonsense beauty book. New York: Henry Holt & Co.

Desowitz, R. (1987). The thorn in the starfish. New York: W.W. Norton & Co.

Dwyer, J. (1990). The body at war. New York: Mentor Books.

Flandermeyer, K. (1979). Clear skin. Boston: Little, Brown and Co.

Fulton, J. (1984). Dr. Fulton's step-by-step program for clearing acne. New York: Barnes & Noble books.

Gerson, J. (1992). Standard textbook for professional estheticians. Albany: Milady Publishing Company.

Goodman, T., & S. Young (1988). Smart face. New York: Prentice-Hall.

Gray, H. (1974). Gray's anatomy. Philadelphia: Running Press.

Haberman, F., & D. Fortino, (1983). Your skin. New York: Berkley.

Jovanovic, L., & G. Subak-Sharpe (1987). Hormones – The woman's answerbook. New York: Fawcett Columbine.

Otto, J., & A. Towle (1985). Modern biology. New York: Holt, Rinehart & Winston.

Pugliese, P. (1991). Advanced professional skin care. Bernville, Pa.: APSC Publishing.

Winter, R. (1984). A consumer's dictionary of cosmetic ingredients. New York: Crown Publishers, Inc.

Wolfe, D. (1988). Introduction to college chemistry. New York: McGraw-Hill.

Periodicals:

Dermascope Magazine
4447 McKinney Ave.
Dallas, TX 75205
1–214–526–0752

Les Nouvelles Esthetiques
12880 Hillcrest Suite 235
Dallas, TX 75230
1–214–934–3072

Skin Inc.
362 Schmale Rd.
Carol Stream, IL 60188
1–708–653–2155